M.P. Fink P.M. Suter W.J. Sibbald (Eds.)

Intensive Care Medicine in 10 Years

With 70 Figures and 43 Tables

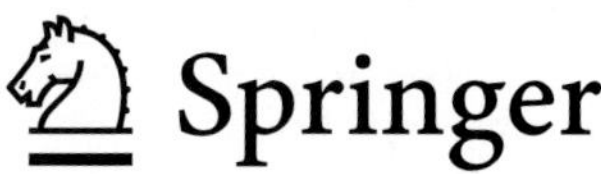

Series Editor

Prof. Jean-Louis Vincent
Head, Department of Intensive Care
Erasme University Hospital
Route de Lennik 808, 1070 Brussels
Belgium
jlvincen@ulb.ac.be

Volume Editors

Professor Michell P. Fink
Chair, Department of Critical Care Medicine
University of Pittsburgh
School of Medicine
Suite 616A, Scaife Hall
3550 Terrace St.
Pittsburgh, PA 15261, USA

Professor Peter M. Suter
Head, Department of Anesthesiology, Pharmacology,
and Surgical Intensive Care
University Hospital
Rue Michel-du-Crest 24
1211 Geneva 14
Switzerland

Professor William J. Sibbald
Physician-in-Chief
Department of Medicine
Sunnybrook & Women's College
Health Sciences Centre
University of Toronto
2075 Bayview Avenue, Suite D4, 74
Toronto, M4N 3M5
Canada

ISSN 0933-6788
ISBN-10 3-540-26092-7 Springer-Verlag Berlin Heidelberg NewYork
ISBN-13 987-3-540-26092-9 Springer-Verlag Berlin Heidelberg NewYork

Library of Congress Control Number: 2005932381

Springer is a part of Springer Science+Business Media

springeronline.com

Editor: Dr. Ute Heilmann, Heidelberg, Germany
Desk Editor: Hiltrud Wilbertz, Heidelberg, Germany
Typsetting: Satz-Druck-Service, Leimen, Germany
Production: Pro Edit GmbH, Heidelberg, Germany
Cover design: design & production GmbH, 69126 Heidelberg, Germany
Printed on acid-free paper 21/3152/Re – 543210

Contents

Setting the Stage

Setting the Scene 3
J. L. Vincent

Managing and Leading in Critical Care 23
W. J. Sibbald

Critical Care from 50,000 Feet................................ 41
D. C. Angus

Expectations around Intensive Care – 10 Years on 55
K. Hillman

The Safety and Quality Agenda in Critical Care Medicine....... 61
T. Dorman

The Challenge of Emerging Infections
and Progressive Antibiotic Resistance......................... 69
S. M. Opal

Technology Assessment 87
J. Bakker and P. Verboom

Trends in Pediatric and Neonatal Critical Care
in the next 10 Years 99
R.C. Tasker

Diagnostic, Therapeutic and Information Technologies 10 Years from Now

The Patient Process as the Basis for the Design of an ICU 115
B. Regli and J. Takala

Information Technology. 133
G.D. Martich, D.C. Van Pelt, and D. Lovasik

Diagnostic Technologies to Assess Tissue Perfusion and Cardiorespiratory Performance 153
M.R. Pinsky

Microcirculatory Distress in Critically Ill Patients: Meaning and Future 165
C. Ince

Managing Infection: From Agar Plate to Genome Scan 177
J. Cohen

Immunological Monitoring, Functional Genomics and Proteomics 189
E. Abraham

Improving Organ Function 201
M. Singer

The Profile and Management of Acute Respiratory Distress Syndrome. 213
L. Gattinoni, P. Caironi, and E. Carlesso

The Ventilator of Tomorrow 227
L. Brochard, M. Dojat, and F. Lellouche

My NeuroICU 10 Years from Now. 239
D.K. Menon

Disaster Medicine 257
P.E. Pepe, K.J. Rinnert, and J.G. Wigginton

How Might Critical Care Medicine be Organized and Regulated?

Hospital and Medical School Organization of Critical Care Services 273
M.P. Fink

Physician Staffing in the ICU 10 Years from Now 279
J.A. Russell and A. Sutherland

ICU Research – One Decade from Now 291
J.J. Marini and D.J. Dries

Organizing Clinical Critical Care Research
and Implementing the Results. 311
D. Cook and S. Finfer

Funding and Accounting Systems 325
P.M. Suter

Measuring Performance 335
G.D. Rubenfeld

Ethics and End-of-Life Care. 345
J.R. Curtis

Rationing in the ICU: Fear, Fiction and Fact 363
M.M. Levy

Training

Training Pathways – Physician and Non-Physician 377
J. Bion, H. Barrett, and T. Clutton-Brock

Simulation Training in Critical Care Medicine 389
P.B. Angood

The Critical Care 'Agenda'

The Agenda for the Intensivist 401
V.M. Ranieri and G.L. Rosboch

Transforming Adult Critical Care Service Delivery in Ontario. . . 413
H. MacLeod

Subject Index 431

Contributors

Abraham E
Division of Pulmonary Sciences
and Critical Care Medicine
University of Colorado Health
Sciences Center
4200 E. Ninth Avenue
Denver, CO 80200
USA

Angood PB
Office of Patient Safety
Joint Commission for Accreditation
of Healthcare Organizations
One Renaissance Blvd
Chicago, IL 60181
USA

Angus DC
Dept of Critical Care Medicine
University of Pittsburgh
604 Scaife Hall
3550 Terrace Street
Pittsburgh, PA 15261
USA

Bakker J
Dept of Intensive Care Medicine
Erasmus Hospital
PO Box 2040
Room V-212
3000 CA Rotterdam
Netherlands

Barrett H
Dept of Intensive Care Medicine
The University of Birmingham
Edgbaston N5
Birmingham, EH4 2XU
United Kingdom

Bion J
Dept of Intensive Care Medicine
The University of Birmingham
Edgbaston N5
Birmingham, EH4 2XU
United Kingdom

Brochard L
Dept of Intensive Care Medicine
Henri Mondor Hospital
51, avenue du Maréchal de Lattre de
Tassigny
94010 Créteil
France

Caironi P
Institute of Anesthesiology and
Intensive Care Medicine
Ospedale Maggiore Policlinico-
IRCCS
Via Francesco Sforza 35
20122 Milan
Italy

Carlesso E
Institute of Anesthesiology and
Intensive Care Medicine
Ospedale Maggiore Policlinico-
IRCCS
Via Francesco Sforza 35
20122 Milan
Italy

Clutton-Brock T
Dept of Intensive Care Medicine
The University of Birmingham
Edgbaston N5
Birmingham, EH4 2XU
United Kingdom

Cohen J
Dept of Medicine
Brighton & Sussex Medical School
Falmer, BN1 9PX
United Kingdom

Cook D
Dept of Medicine and Epidemiology and Biostatistics
McMaster University Health Sciences Center
Room 2C11
1200 Main Street West
Hamilton, ON L8N 3Z5
Canada

Curtis JR
Dept of Pulmonary and Critical Care Medicine
Harborview Medical Center
Box 359762
325 9th Avenue
Seattle, WA 98104-2499
USA

Dojat M
UM 594 INSERM-UJF
University Hospital Center
Pavillion B
BP 217
38043 Grenoble
France

Dorman T
Dept of Anesthesiology and Critical Care Medicine
Johns Hopkins Hospital
Meyer 291
600 N. Wolfe Street
Baltimore, MD 21287-7294
USA

Dries DJ
Dept of Pulmonary and Critical Care Medicine
Regions Hospital
640 Jackson Street
St. Paul, MN 55101
USA

Finfer S
Dept of Intensive Care Medicine
Royal North Shore Hospital
2065 Sydney
Australia

Fink MP
Dept of Critical Care Medicine
University Hospital
606 Scaife Hall
3550 Terrace Street
Pittsburgh, PA 15261
USA

Gattinoni L
Institute of Anesthesiology and Intensive Care Medicine
Ospedale Maggiore Policlinico-IRCCS
Via Francesco Sforza 35
20122 Milan
Italy

Hillman K
Dept of Intensive Care Medicine
University of New South Wales
The Liverpool Health Service
Locked Bag 7103
Liverpool BC, NSW 1871
Australia

Ince C
Dept of Physiology
Academic Medical Center
Meibergdreef 9
1105 AZ Amsterdam
Netherlands

Lellouche F
Dept of Intensive Care Medicine
Henri Mondor Hospital
51, avenue du Maréchal de Lattre de Tassigny
94010 Créteil
France

Levy MM
Dept of Pulmonary and Critical Care Medicine
Brown University Rhode Island Hospital
593 Eddy Street
Providence, RI 02906
USA

Lovasik D
Critical Care Information Systems Dept
University Hospital
3550 Terrace Street
Pittsburgh, PA 15261
USA

MacLeod H
Ministry of Health and Long-Term Care
8th floor, Hepburn Block
80 Grosvenor Street
Toronto, ON M7A 1R3
Canada

Marini JJ
Dept of Pulmonary and Critical Care Medicine
Regions Hospital
640 Jackson Street
St. Paul, MN 55101
USA

Martich GD
Dept of Critical Care Medicine
University Hospital
3550 Terrace Street
Room 602B
Pittsburgh, PA 15261
USA

Menon DK
Dept of Anesthesia
Addenbrooke's Hospital
Box 93
Cambridge, CB2 2QQ
United Kingdom

Opal SM
Infectious Disease Division
Memorial Hospital of RI
111 Brewster Street
Pawtucket, RI 02860
USA

Pepe PE
Dept of Emergency Medicine
University of Texas Southwestern Medical Center
5323 Harry Hines Boulevard, Mail Code 8579
Dallas, TX 75390-8579
USA

Pinsky MR
Dept of Critical Care Medicine
University Hospital
606 Scaife Hall
3550 Terrace Street
Pittsburgh, PA 15261
USA

Ranieri VM
Dept of Anesthesiology and Intensive Care Medicine
San Giovanni Battista Hospital
Corso Dogliotti 14
1026 Torino
Italy

Regli B
Dept of Intensive Care Medicine
University Hospital
3010 Bern
Switzerland

Rinnert KJ
Dept of Surgery
University of Texas Southwestern Medical Center
5323 Harry Hines Boulevard, Mail Code 8579
Dallas, TX 75390-8579
USA

Rosboch GL
Dept of Anesthesiology and Intensive Care Medicine
San Giovanni Battista Hospital
Corso Dogliotti 14
1026 Torino
Italy

Rubenfeld GD
Dept of Pulmonary and Critical Care Medicine
Harborview Medical Center
Box 359762
325 9th Avenue
Seattle, WA 98104-2499
USA

Russell JA
Dept of Medicine
St. Paul's Hospital
1081 Burrard Street
Vancouver, BC
Canada

Sibbald WJ
Dept of Medicine
Sunnybrook and Women's College
Health Science Center
2075 Bayview Avenue, Suite D474
Toronto, Ontario M4N 3M5
Canada

Singer M
Bloomsbury Institute of Intensive
Care Medicine
University College
Gower Street
London, WC1E 6BT
United Kingdom

Suter PM
Department APSIC
University Hospitals
24, rue Micheli-du-Crest
1211 Geneva
Switzerland

Sutherland A
Dept of Experimental Medicine
St. Paul's Hospital
1081 Burrard Street
Vancouver, BC
Canada

Takala J
Dept of Intensive Care Medicine
University Hospital
3010 Bern
Switzerland

Tasker RC
Dept of Pediatrics
Addenbrooke's Hospital
Hills Road
Cambridge, CB2 2QQ
United Kingdom

Van Pelt DC
Dept of Critical Care Medicine
University Hospital
3550 Terrace Street
Room 602B
Pittsburgh, PA 15261
USA

Verboom P
Institute for Medical Technology
Assessment
Erasmus Hospital
PO Box 2040
3000 CA Rotterdam
Netherlands

Vincent JL
Dept of Intensive Care Medicine
Erasme University Hospital
Route de Lennik 808
1070 Brussels
Belgium

Wigginton JG
Dept of Surgery
University of Texas Southwestern
Medical Center
5323 Harry Hines Boulevard, Mail
Code 8579
Dallas, TX 75390-8579
USA

Common Abbreviations

ALI	Acute lung injury
ARDS	Acute respiratory distress syndrome
CIS	Clinical information system
CT	Computed tomography
DNR	Do-not-resuscitate
EBM	Evidence-based medicine
EKG	Electrocardiogram
EMR	Electronic medical record
ICU	Intensive care unit
LAN	Local area network
MET	Medical emergency team
MRI	Magnetic resonance imaging
MRSA	Methicillin-resistant Staphylococcus aureus
PEEP	Positive end-expiratory pressure
RCT	Randomized controlled trial
SARS	Severe acute respiratory syndrome

Setting the Stage

Setting The Scene

J. L. Vincent

Introduction

Intensive care medicine of today is almost unrecognizable when compared to its humble beginnings following the polio epidemics of the 1950s. This relatively young field of medicine is growing at such a pace that it is interesting, and indeed important, to speculate on how we will be practicing intensive care medicine 10 years from now.

In this chapter, I will focus on what has altered in the last 50 years in various aspects of intensive care medicine. Playing Devil's advocate somewhat, I will consider changes in each field from a positive and negative viewpoint. Looking into the recent past (and the present) raises many questions and many uncertainties, but sets the stage for the future, and I believe that we must use the past to define future priorities.

Intensive Care in General

The Optimist's View

The quality of intensive care has improved over time; changes have not necessarily been made in great strides, but multiple small improvements have led to a progressive reduction in morbidity and mortality. Despite the altered population of intensive care patients with more elderly, more debilitated, and more immunosuppressed patients being treated, there is some evidence that mortality has decreased among patients with sepsis [1] or the acute respiratory distress syndrome (ARDS) [2-4]. The recent rush of guidelines and protocols for everything from administration of sedation to management of septic shock to end-of-life patient management has caused a reduction in the wide variability in medical practice, thus improving its overall quality.

The Pessimist's View

What actual progress has been made over the last few decades? After all, there has been no outstanding breakthrough, like insulin for diabetes or thrombolysis for acute myocardial infarction, in our field. Indeed, much of the apparent progress in intensive care medicine has been borrowed from other specialties, e.g., surgery, immunology, cardiology. We are not even sure that mortality from sepsis and ARDS has decreased substantially [5]. The major development could be said to be a decrease in iatrogenic events as we have realized the negative impacts of some common interventions (Table 1). However, with newer therapies, invasive monitoring, and more complex interventions, we have also increased the potential for iatrogenicity.

Mechanical Ventilation

The Optimist's View

Early respirators were large, unwieldy pieces of equipment that delivered established minute ventilation at a given, fixed rate. Modern machines are increasingly streamlined and portable and provide the physician with an almost unlimited range of ventilatory modes and options that enable mechanical ventilation to be targeted at individual patients and adjusted according to their needs and response. Improved understanding of the use and potential of non-invasive mechanical ventilation has enabled the rates of endotracheal intubation, and consequently the risks of ventilator-associated pneumonia (VAP), to be reduced [6]. This technique can even decrease mortality rates in patients with hypercapnic respiratory failure [7, 8].

The Pessimist's View

Modern respirators have so many options and knobs that they can be difficult to use and it takes some time to become familiar with each new machine. Indeed, many of the options are never used at all! The development of newer ventilatory modes, such as pressure support ventilation, has not been shown to improve outcomes. The success of non-invasive mechanical ventilation just demonstrates the risk of iatrogenic complications due to our interventions. However, we still do not know how best to apply non-invasive mechanical ventilation or which patients will benefit most from it. While it does seem to be beneficial in hypercapnic respiratory failure, what about in non-hypercapnic respiratory failure? More questions remain unanswered than have been answered.

Acute Respiratory Failure

The Optimist's View

Major advances have been made in our understanding of respiratory mechanics, and application of this knowledge has improved outcomes. For example, large tidal volumes, long considered as useful to improve tolerance and prevent the development of atelectasis, have been shown to promote inflammation and worsen outcomes in ARDS [9]. Patients both with and without ARDS are now being managed with lower tidal volumes than in the past [10].

The Pessimist's View

The optimal respiratory conditions for the patient with ARDS remain undefined. What is the optimal tidal volume, level of positive end-expiratory pressure (PEEP), or alveolar recruitment strategy? Respiratory monitoring systems at the bedside are unimpressive, and pharmacological interventions including surfactant [11], inhaled nitric oxide [12], and anti-inflammatory agents [13] have not been shown to reduce mortality. Even prone positioning, although shown to improve gas exchange, has not been shown to definitely improve outcome [14].

Sepsis Therapies

The Optimist's View

Better understanding of the complex network of mediators involved in the immune response to infection has led to the development of new strategies specifically targeted against sepsis. The development of new drugs in sepsis has certainly not been a smooth ride. Still, one new agent, activated protein C, has been licensed for use in patients with severe sepsis and septic shock and has been shown to decrease mortality [15]. Now, other new agents will certainly follow. Many others are already in the pipeline and several are currently undergoing clinical trials. Combinations of these agents in the future will further improve outcomes.

The Pessimist's View

The list of negative studies of sepsis therapies is actually far more impressive than the list of positive studies. Particularly notable have been the negative results from clinical trials of agents that had been clearly shown to improve outcomes in pre-clinical and sometimes even in phase I and II clinical trials, for example, endotoxin antibodies [16, 17], anti-tumor necrosis factor (TNF) strategies [18], and interleukin-1 receptor antagonist [19]. For all the time and money that has been expended in this field, only one agent has been licensed, activated protein C, and even with this drug, the survival advantage remains limited, and high costs restrict its use.

Steroids in Septic Shock

The Optimist's View

The use of massive doses of methylprednisolone to limit the inflammatory response, which failed to improve outcomes [20], has been replaced by the concept of relative adrenal insufficiency, leading to the administration of low doses of hydrocortisone in septic shock, which has been shown to reduce mortality rates [21].

The Pessimist's View

The evidence for relative adrenal insufficiency is actually not so strong. The study by Annane et al. [21] was not entirely positive (significant differences were obtained only after adjustment for several factors), so that the potential benefits of corticosteroid administration in septic shock is not yet convincingly proven [22]. Moreover, the need for an ACTH test is unsettled. In the study by Annane et al. [21], many patients had received etomidate to facilitate endotracheal intubation, and this product is known to alter adrenal function. Hence, there is a need for further study to finally answer some of these questions (the Corticus prospective, double-blind, multicenter study of hydrocortisone in patients with septic shock is ongoing).

Vasopressin Administration In Septic Shock

The Optimist's View

Vasopressin is one of the most important endogenous stress hormones during shock, and increased interest in metabolic alterations during sepsis has led to the realization that vasopressin levels are inappropriately low in patients with severe sepsis and this phenomenon may contribute to the hemodynamic perturbations that are characteristic of septic shock [23]. Addition of vasopressin to standard vasopressors, such as norepinephrine, can improve hemodynamic status [24] and recent guidelines for the management of patients with septic shock support its use, at low infusion rates of 0.01-0.04 units/min, in patients with refractory shock despite adequate fluid resuscitation and high-dose conventional vasopressors [25].

The Pessimist's View

There is no demonstrated outcome benefit associated with administration of vasopressin in patients with septic shock. Some studies have suggested that while vasopressor agents may increase arterial pressure, some agents are also associated with worsened outcomes [26]. ICU physicians have been too quick to jump on the vasopressin bandwagon, starting to administer vasopressin widely before real evidence of benefit was established. Trials are currently underway to define the potential benefit of administration of low doses of vasopressin in septic shock, but in the meantime, are we again creating an iatrogenic effect?

Oxygen Delivery

The Optimist's View

Dobutamine has taken first place in our list of inotropic agents; we have learned to use it not only in low flow states, but also whenever oxygen delivery may be insufficient. So-called 'pre-optimization', raising oxygen delivery to supranormal values, may be beneficial in high-risk surgical patients, especially when it involves the correction of underlying hypovolemia [27].

The Pessimist's View

The maintenance of supranormal oxygen delivery has not been shown to improve outcomes in critically ill patient populations as a whole, and excessive administration of fluids and inotropic agents may be harmful [28]. Studies on pre-optimization have been usually performed in the United Kingdom but whether the results apply to other settings is largely unexplored.

Early Goal-Directed Therapy

The Optimist's View

The importance of aggressive early and complete resuscitation has been established in severe sepsis/septic shock [29] as in severe trauma. Rivers et al. [29] randomized 263 patients with severe sepsis or septic shock to receive, for the first six hours after admission, either standard resuscitation or early goal-directed therapy in which fluids, vasoactive agents, and red blood cells were given to optimize central venous pressure, arterial pressure and hematocrit and then dobutamine to achieve a target central venous oxygen saturation (ScvO2) of at least 70%. This strategy resulted in markedly lower mortality (30.5% compared to 46.5% in the standard care group, $p = 0.009$), and similar protocols are now implemented in many institutions and are included in recent recommendations regarding optimal management of the patient with severe sepsis [25].

The Pessimist's View

The study by Rivers et al. [29] was a single-center study, performed not in an ICU, but in an emergency department. Before applying such a protocol to all patients, we need to know more about it. Importantly, the reasons for the improvement in outcome seen in this study are not clear; maybe the treatment was simply suboptimal in the control group; perhaps the improved outcomes were related to the choice of target, i.e., $ScvO_2$; possibly they were due to the increased use of fluids and/or dobutamine and/or blood transfusions in the treatment group.

Again, many questions remain and we should not be too keen to jump in until we have at least some of the answers.

Hemodynamic Monitoring

The Optimist's View

Criticism of the pulmonary artery catheter has been met by the development of a number of less invasive monitoring devices, including esophageal Doppler, transesophageal echocardiography, arterial waveform analysis, and thoracic impedance. Using functional hemodynamic monitoring to define responsiveness in the optimization of blood flow improves outcome in cardiac surgery patients [30].

The Pessimist's View

The use of invasive hemodynamic monitoring has certainly been challenged repeatedly in recent years [31-33] and its use has decreased over the last decade. However, although the use of pulmonary artery catheters has not been shown to improve outcome from critical illness, they have not been shown to worsen outcomes either. The development of less invasive monitoring techniques is to be applauded, but can they be shown to improve outcomes? Indeed, has any monitoring device been shown to improve outcomes? Every ICU patient is attached to multiple machines with assorted alarms, but where is the evidence that they decrease mortality? Even if we accept that such monitoring is useful, the assessment of fluid responsiveness by pressure tracing or stroke volume variation has a number of limitations, and is potentially useful only in mechanically ventilated patients, who are well sedated, without arrhythmias, and ventilated with relatively high tidal volumes [34].

Glucose Control

The Optimist's View

Sometimes relatively small and simple strategies can provide big benefits. For example, blood sugar control, maintaining blood glucose at or below 110 mg per decilitre, has been shown to decrease mortality in a mixed group of ICU patients, primarily surgical, many being admitted after cardiac surgery [35]. Although the practicalities of such an approach make it difficult to apply routinely, it is now widely recommended that blood glucose levels should be kept below 150 mg/dl [25].

The Pessimist's View

The beneficial effects of tight glucose control have been shown in only one single-center study, with many postoperative patients after cardiac surgery. Moreover, the associated caloric intake in these patients was quite high. The results still need to be confirmed in large multicenter trials with broader patient populations (large scale studies are ongoing).

Nutritional Support

The Optimist's View

Nutrition has only relatively recently begun to take a key place in ICU patient management, but patients are now fed much sooner and better than in the past with the realization of the importance of good nutrition on outcomes. Indeed, diet can influence both disease development and recovery. Enteral feeding is widely accepted as being superior to parenteral feeding [36, 37] and much has been learnt about dietary requirements including the realization that excessive feeding can be as harmful as inadequate nutrition [38].

The Pessimist's View

Despite improved awareness of feeding issues in the critically ill, we still do not know when to start and how best to feed the patient. Trials of modified solutions, including the so-called immuno-enhancing diets, have not demonstrated improved survival over standard feeding solutions [39-41]. The fact that enteral feeding is preferable to parenteral should not surprise us, being further evidence of a negative iatrogenic event. Even when using the enteral route, overzealous feeding may promote gut ischemia [42, 43], and can result in complications including aspiration with potential increased risks of nosocomial pneumonia. Indeed, we are now being encouraged to consider the concept of 'underfeeding'.

Selective Decontamination of the Digestive Tract

The Optimist's View

The gut may be an important source of microorganisms, which can be involved in the development of nosocomial infection, in particular, VAP. After many years of debate and discussion, selective decontamination of the digestive tract (SDD) was shown to decrease hospital mortality (24% vs 31%, $p=0.02$) in a randomized controlled trial in Holland [44].

The Pessimist's View

SDD certainly decreased mortality rates in this study [44], but it was conducted in a single ICU in a country with low rates of methicillin-resistant *Staphylococcus aureus* (MRSA) and vancomycin resistant enterococci (VRE). Therefore, the results may not immediately apply to other institutions with greater antimicrobial resistance rates [45]. In addition, despite this study and others supporting the use of SDD, it is not widely applied, mainly because of fears of encouraging bacterial resistance, the development of which may not be apparent for months or even years after its introduction.

Hygiene Measures

The Optimist's View

The use of routine hygiene measures, such as hand washing before and after patient contact [46, 47], antibiotic rotation [48], shorter course antibiotic treatments [49] and using barrier precautions when inserting intravascular catheters [50], have all been shown to reduce the incidence of nosocomial infections, and the introduction of infection control protocols can result in sustained reductions in nosocomial infections [51].

The Pessimist's View

The problem of nosocomial infections is getting worse, largely due to the excessive use of antibiotics (especially broad spectrum ones) and the lack of adequate infection control procedures. In particular, it is well recognized that washing hands is a very effective way to prevent the spread of bacteria, but still compliance among personnel is poor [52–54]! Increasingly nosocomial infections are associated with multiresistant organisms with higher morbidity and mortality, which has even led to the temporary closure of some units [55].

Sedation

The Optimist's View

We have swung from an attitude which supported widespread use of large doses of sedative agents to keep patients comfortable, and even to make patient care easier, to a much more conservative approach with the realization that excess sedation can be harmful. Studies have shown that daily interruption of sedative infusions in critically ill patients undergoing mechanical ventilation reduces ICU length of stay and decreases the incidence of complications of critical illness associated with prolonged intubation and mechanical ventilation [56].

The Pessimist's View

The widespread use of sedatives and the realization that more can be too much provides yet more evidence of iatrogenic complications!

Management of Liver Failure

The Optimist's View

The increased use of liver transplantation and improved transplantation techniques and post-operative management has changed outcomes from acute liver disease [57, 58]. The development of extracorporeal systems, such as the molecular adsorbent recirculating system (MARS) system, may further decrease mortality rates [59].

The Pessimist's View

Progress in the field has been related to the development of liver transplantation, including use of living donors, but medically there has been no progress at all. The use of extracorporeal systems is expensive, and although there are promising results from small studies [59], they have not been shown to improve outcomes [60].

Cardiopulmonary Resuscitation

The Optimist's View

Wider availability of defibrillators has changed the outcome from out-of-hospital cardiac arrest (most commonly due to ventricular fibrillation) [61]. Amiodarone has replaced lidocaine in the management of life-threatening ventricular arrhythmias after lidocaine use was associated with increased mortality. Vasopressin has taken its place as a potent and reliable vasoconstrictor in profound hypotension during cardiopulmonary resuscitation (CPR) and is recommended as an alternative to epinephrine in current guidelines [62].

The Pessimist's View

Little progress in cardiopulmonary resuscitation has been achieved, especially in the ICU. Even the superiority of vasopressin over epinephrine has not been shown conclusively [63]. Any progress that has been made is due to simplified guidelines and increased involvement of bystanders in starting effective CPR.

Polytrauma

The Optimist's View

Studies have shown that resuscitation should not necessarily be too aggressive [64], as massive fluid administration may increase bleeding, by increasing intravascular pressures, disrupting clot formation and diluting coagulation factors. The use of factor VIIa may decrease bleeding rates in trauma [65].

The Pessimist's View

The suggestion that too much fluid early in trauma resuscitation can be detrimental [64], again demonstrates our tendency to encourage iatrogenic complications of therapy with overzealous reactions. Furthermore, restricting fluid administration may limit oxygen delivery and contribute to the development of multiple organ failure (MOF). In addition, such an approach is deleterious in the presence of cerebral lesions, where arterial hypotension can have disastrous consequences on brain function. Studies on factor VIIa have shown that this strategy may limit the need for blood transfusions, but no effect on outcome has been demonstrated.

Severe Head Trauma and Cerebral Resuscitation

The Optimist's View

Considerable advances have been made in cerebral monitoring with the development of local brain tissue oxygen monitoring and microdialysis techniques to assess brain metabolic data [66, 67] and mortality rates from severe head trauma have fallen [68, 69]. Induced mild hypothermia may be an option to protect the neurons in hypoxic encephalopathy and has been associated with improved outcomes [70–72].

The Pessimist's View

Despite advances in monitoring, none has actually been shown to improve outcomes and as good markers of cerebral damage are still lacking, the evaluation of cerebral lesions remains largely based on the Glasgow coma score. Evaluation of cerebral blood flow and oxygen availability at the bedside is still difficult, and in terms of new therapies, nothing has been proven. The best established intervention is hyperventilation for intracranial hypertension. But, hyperventilation may reduce cerebral perfusion [73] and thereby worsen outcome, again emphasizing the risk of serious iatrogenic complications of some of our interventions. Inducing hypothermia after cardiac arrest is not easy and has not been shown to reduce mortality rates in a randomized multicenter study

[74], and there is little evidence to support barbiturate therapy either [75]. Steroid therapy, used in head injury patients for years, has recently been shown to worsen outcomes in a multicenter study involving 10,008 patients [76], and craniectomy in severe brain edema may result in increased vegetative states [77].

Stroke

The Optimist's View

Thrombolytic therapy, a treatment that improves outcomes in ischemic stroke, has changed the way we treat thromboembolic stroke [78]. Other pharmacological advances have also been made, with administration of factor VIIa being shown to improve outcome from intracerebral hemorrhage [79]. Improved availability of imaging techniques has also helped in diagnosis and management.

The Pessimist's View

The benefit from thrombolytic therapy is limited to early intervention – within 3 hours of stroke onset – and to patients with ischemic stroke. The study of VIIa in intracerebral hemorrhage [79] is only a phase IIb study, and the limited benefit may not warrant the costs of this therapy.

Renal Failure

The Optimist's View

The development of continuous hemodialysis techniques has allowed us to avoid the 'peak and trough' effect of intermittent dialysis on fluid balance, electrolyte levels, and osmotic shifts. Continuous hemofiltration has evolved into a continuous veno-venous system with relatively complex instruments. We now know that giving diuretics to patients with acute renal failure may increase mortality and worsen renal function [80], especially in the presence of hypovolemia. Low dose dopamine, so-called renal dose dopamine, does not prevent renal insufficiency in critically ill patients [81] and should be abandoned as a routine practice.

The Pessimist's View

So, more evidence that our interventions cause iatrogenic problems; diuretics and low dose dopamine are both harmful pharmacological interventions. And there is no evidence that hemofiltration techniques improve outcomes in critically ill patients.

Blood Transfusions

The Optimist's View

The use of blood transfusions has declined, especially after an important prospective, randomized Canadian study showing a conservative approach may result in somewhat lower mortality rates [82]. Studies are ongoing to determine the optimal transfusion trigger and techniques to better assess and monitor tissue oxygenation are being developed.

The Pessimist's View

Yet more iatrogenicity...!

Other IV Fluids

The Optimist's View

Albumin administration has been controversial for decades, as it is hard to demonstrate beneficial effects and the costs are high. Albumin administration has been suggested to result in high mortality rates [83] but a large Australasian study demonstrated that the use of albumin is safe [84]. Studies are evaluating the potentially beneficial effects of artificial crystalloids and hemoglobin solutions on tissue oxygenation.

The Pessimist's View

The SAFE study showed that for once we have not caused iatrogenic complications! However, although it has been shown to be as safe as saline in the setting of the SAFE study, albumin has not been shown to improve outcomes, and we still do not know if and when to administer it. Hydroxyethyl starch solutions may increase bleeding and alter renal function, gelatin solutions are not very effective and can have allergic reactions, saline solutions may induce hyperchloremic metabolic acidosis, and balanced solutions are hypotonic! And where do hypertonic solutions fit in? There is still a lot to be done to evaluate the best type of i.v. solution.

Process of Care

The Optimist's View

Critical care medicine is better organized now than at its start and many countries now recognize intensive care medicine as a specialty in its own right.

Established treatment protocols for standardization of care have resulted in markedly improved outcomes, reduced costs, and minimized medical errors.

The Pessimist's view

Protocols are developed primarily to avoid iatrogenic problems and to restrict the liberty of the practitioner to make decisions based on their experience.

Medical Emergency Teams

The Optimist's View

The development of medical emergency teams (METs), also known as hospital outreach or rapid response teams, has extended the principles of critical care medicine to a hospital-wide approach, and has been associated with reduced complications after major surgery, reduced ICU admissions, and improved outcomes [85, 86].

The Pessimist's View

METs provide a neat cover up for the lack of emergency medicine training of doctors and nursing staff in the hospital; staff should be better trained rather than replaced.

Conclusions

From an optimist's viewpoint, one could say that the last 50 years has seen great progress in intensive care medicine, perhaps not by any single, tremendous development(s), but by a succession of small steps, which together combine to give us an intensive care service to be proud of, providing quality care for many thousands of patients each year. However, the pessimist would perhaps say that much of the apparent progress in intensive care medicine has come about through the identification and correction of our own iatrogenic effects. It is indeed rather worrisome to realize that that many of our interventions may have had some deleterious effects. This notion has been suggested for mechanical ventilation (especially with high tidal volumes), blood transfusions, and excessive sedation (Table 1). We have increasingly realized that non-invasive is better than invasive and less is better than more. Patients are better treated without endotracheal intubation, with minimal sedation, without excessive use of vasopressor or inotropic agents.

These two viewpoints are both valid, although the true picture perhaps lies somewhere between the two. As with Janus, intensive care medicine has two faces, one looking backwards and the other towards the future. This is not a bad

Table 1. Some potentially harmful iatrogenic interventions

- Excessive antibiotic use
- Iatrogenic fluid overload
- Excessive administration of inotropic agents
- Ventilation with too high tidal volumes
- Excessive sedation
- Use of invasive hemodynamic monitoring
- Unnecessary use of antiarrhythmic agents
- Excessive caloric intake
- Too liberal blood transfusions
- Traumatic effects of endotracheal intubation and airway management

thing and indeed progress has, and can, come from learning from the past and applying those lessons to the future.

Clearly many questions remain unsettled and pose a challenge for the years to come. There is, however, one key point that we have not discussed and that is the role of the intensive care doctor. Here we can only be optimistic: the ICU doctor has made a difference! Closed ICUs under the responsibility of an ICU physician have lower morbidity and mortality rates than open units [87–89]. Proper training of the intensive care doctor must therefore remain a key priority for the future, and with the projected future shortage of ICU physicians [90] we need in addition to develop alternative strategies, such as telemedicine.

References

1. Martin GS, Mannino DM, Eaton S, Moss M (2003) The epidemiology of sepsis in the United States from 1979 through 2000. N Engl J Med 348:1546–1554
2. Milberg JA, Davis DR, Steinberg KP, Hudson LD (1995) Improved survival of patients with acute respiratory distress syndrome (ARDS): 1983–1993. J A M A 273:306–309
3. Navarrete-Navarro P, Rodriguez A, Reynolds N, et al (2001) Acute respiratory distress syndrome among trauma patients: trends in ICU mortality, risk factors, complications and resource utilization. Intensive Care Med 27:1133–1140
4. Moss M, Mannino DM (2002) Race and gender differences in acute respiratory distress syndrome deaths in the United States: an analysis of multiple-cause mortality data (1979–1996). Crit Care Med 30:1679–1685
5. Friedman G, Silva E, Vincent JL (1998) Has the mortality of septic shock changed with time? Crit Care Med 26:2078–2086
6. Nourdine K, Combes P, Carton MJ, Beuret P, Cannamela A, Ducreux JC (1999) Does noninvasive ventilation reduce the ICU nosocomial infection risk? A prospective clinical survey. Intensive Care Med 25:567–573
7. Girou E, Schortgen F, Delclaux C, et al (2000) Association of noninvasive ventilation with nosocomial infections and survival in critically ill patients. J A M A 284:2361–2367

8. Girou E, Brun-Buisson C, Taille S, Lemaire F, Brochard L (2003) Secular trends in nosocomial infections and mortality associated with noninvasive ventilation in patients with exacerbation of COPD and pulmonary edema. JAMA 290:2985–2991
9. The ARDS Network (2000) Ventilation with lower tidal volumes as compared with traditional tidal volumes for acute lung injury and the acute respiratory distress syndrome. N Engl J Med 342:1301–1308
10. Wongsurakiat P, Pierson DJ, Rubenfeld GD (2004) Changing pattern of ventilator settings in patients without acute lung injury: changes over 11 years in a single institution. Chest 126:1281–1291
11. Anzueto A, Baughmann RP, Guntupalli KK, et al (1996) Aerosolized surfactant in adults with sepsis-induced acute respiratory distress syndrome. N Engl J Med 334:1417-1421
12. Taylor RW, Zimmerman JL, Dellinger RP, Straube RC, et al (2004) Low-dose inhaled nitric oxide in patients with acute lung injury: a randomized controlled trial. JAMA 291:1603–1609
13. The ARDS Network (2000) Ketoconazole for early treatment of acute lung injury and acute respiratory distress syndrome: a randomized controlled trial. JAMA 283:1995–2002
14. Guerin C, Gaillard S, Lemasson S, et al (2004) Effects of systematic prone positioning in hypoxemic acute respiratory failure: a randomized controlled trial. JAMA 292:2379–2387
15. Bernard GR, Vincent JL, Laterre PF, et al (2001) Efficacy and safety of recombinant human activated protein C for severe sepsis. N Engl J Med 344:699–709
16. McCloskey RV, Straube RC, Sanders C, Smith SM, Smith CR (1994) Treatment of septic shock with human monoclonal antibody HA-1A. A randomized, double-blind, placebo-controlled trial. CHESS Trial Study Group. Ann Intern Med 121:1–5
17. Angus DC, Birmingham MC, Balk RA, et al (2000) E5 murine monoclonal antiendotoxin antibody in gram-negative sepsis: a randomized controlled trial. E5 Study Investigators. JAMA 283:1723–1730
18. Abraham E, Anzueto A, Gutierrez G, et al (1998) Double-blind randomised controlled trial of monoclonal antibody to human tumor necrosis factor in treatment of septic shock. Lancet 351:929–933
19. Opal SM, Fisher CJ Jr, Dhainaut JF, et al (1997) Confirmatory interleukin-1 receptor antagonist trial in severe sepsis: A phase III, randomized, double-blind, placebo-controlled, multicenter trial. Crit Care Med 25:1115–1124
20. The veterans administration systemic sepsis cooperative study group (1987) Effect of high-dose glucocorticoid therapy on mortality in patients with clinical signs of systemic sepsis. N Engl J Med 317:659–665
21. Annane D, Sebille V, Charpentier C, et al (2002) Effect of treatment with low doses of hydrocortisone and fludrocortisone on mortality in patients with septic shock. J A M A 288:862–871
22. Annane D, Briegel J, Keh D, Moreno R, Singer M, Sprung CL (2003) Clinical equipoise remains for issues of adrenocorticotropic hormone administration, cortisol testing, and therapeutic use of hydrocortisone. Crit Care Med 31:2250–2251
23. Landry DW, Levin HR, Gallant EM, et al (1997) Vasopressin deficiency contributes to the vasodilation of septic shock. Circulation 95:1122–1125
24. Dunser MW, Mayr AJ, Ulmer H, et al (2001) The effects of vasopressin on systemic hemodynamics in catecholamine-resistant septic and postcardiotomy shock: a retrospective analysis. Anesth Analg 93:7–13
25. Dellinger RP, Carlet JM, Masur H, et al (2004) Surviving sepsis campaign guidelines for management of severe sepsis and septic shock. Crit Care Med 32:858–873
26. Lopez A, Lorente JA, Steingrub J, et al (2004) Multiple-center, randomized, placebo-controlled, double-blind study of the nitric oxide synthase inhibitor 546C88: effect on survival in patients with septic shock. Crit Care Med 32:21–30

27. Lobo SM, Salgado PF, Castillo VG, et al (2000) Effects of maximizing oxygen delivery on morbidity and mortality in high-risk surgical patients. Crit Care Med 28:3396–3404
28. Hayes MA, Timmins AC, Yau EH, Palazzo M, Hinds CJ, Watson D (1994) Elevation of systemic oxygen delivery in the treatment of critically ill patients. N Engl J Med 330:1717–1722
29. Rivers E, Nguyen B, Havstad S, et al (2001) Early goal-directed therapy in the treatment of severe sepsis and septic shock. N Engl J Med 345:1368–1377
30. Mythen MG, Webb AR (1995) Perioperative plasma volume expansion reduces the incidence of gut mucosal hypoperfusion during cardiac surgery. Arch Surg 130:423–429
31. Sandham JD, Hull RD, Brant RF, et al (2003) A randomized, controlled trial of the use of pulmonary-artery catheters in high-risk surgical patients. N Engl J Med 348:5–14
32. Richard C, Warszawski J, Anguel N, et al (2003) Early use of the pulmonary artery catheter and outcomes in patients with shock and acute respiratory distress syndrome: a randomized controlled trial. JAMA 290:2713–2720
33. Yu DT, Platt R, Lanken PN, et al (2003) Relationship of pulmonary artery catheter use to mortality and resource utilization in patients with severe sepsis. Crit Care Med 31:2734–2741
34. De Backer D, Heenen S, Piagnerelli M, Koch M, Vincent JL (2005) Pulse pressure variations to predict fluid responsiveness: Influence of tidal volume. Intensive Care Med 31:517–523
35. Van den Berghe G, Wouters P, Weekers F, et al (2001) Intensive insulin therapy in the critically ill patient. N Engl J Med 345:1359–1367
36. Heyland DK, Dhaliwal R, Drover JW, Gramlich L, Dodek P (2003) Canadian clinical practice guidelines for nutrition support in mechanically ventilated, critically ill adult patients. JPEN J Parenter Enteral Nutr 27:355–373
37. Gramlich L, Kichian K, Pinilla J, Rodych NJ, Dhaliwal R, Heyland DK (2004) Does enteral nutrition compared to parenteral nutrition result in better outcomes in critically ill adult patients? A systematic review of the literature. Nutrition 20:843–848
38. Klein CJ, Stanek GS, Wiles CE III (1998) Overfeeding macronutrients to critically ill adults: metabolic complications. J Am Diet Assoc 98:795–806
39. Bower RH, Cerra FB, Bershadsky B, et al (1995) Early enteral administration of a formula (Impact) supplemented with arginine, nucleotides, and fish oil in intensive care unit patients: Results of a multicenter, prospective, randomized, clinical trial. Crit Care Med 23:436–449
40. Caparros T, Lopez J, Grau T (2001) Early enteral nutrition in critically ill patients with a high-protein diet enriched with arginine, fiber, and antioxidants compared with a standard high-protein diet. The effect on nosocomial infections and outcome. JPEN J Parenter Enteral Nutr 25:299–308
41. Atkinson S, Sieffert E, Bihari D (1998) A prospective, randomized, double-blind, controlled clinical trial of enteral immunonutrition in the critically ill. Guy's Hospital Intensive Care Group. Crit Care Med 26:1164–1172
42. Kles KA, Wallig MA, Tappenden KA (2001) Luminal nutrients exacerbate intestinal hypoxia in the hypoperfused jejunum. JPEN J Parenter Enteral Nutr 25:246–253
43. Andel H, Rab M, Andel D, et al (2002) Impact of duodenal feeding on the oxygen balance of the splanchnic region during different phases of severe burn injury. Burns 28:60–64
44. de Jonge E, Schultz MJ, Spanjaard L, et al (2003) Effects of selective decontamination of the digestive tract on mortality and the acquisition of resistant bacteria in intensive care patients. Lancet 362:1011–1016
45. Vincent JL (2003) Selective digestive decontamination: for everyone, everywhere? Lancet 362:1006–1007
46. Pittet D, Hugonnet S, Harbarth S, et al (2000) Effectiveness of a hospital-wide programme to improve compliance with hand hygiene. Infection Control Programme. Lancet 356:1307–1312

47. Swoboda SM, Earsing K, Strauss K, Lane S, Lipsett PA (2004) Electronic monitoring and voice prompts improve hand hygiene and decrease nosocomial infections in an intermediate care unit. Crit Care Med 32:358–363
48. Raymond DP, Pelletier SJ, Crabtree TD, et al (2001) Impact of a rotating empiric antibiotic schedule on infectious mortality in an intensive care unit. Crit Care Med 29:1101–1108
49. Singh N, Rogers P, Atwood CW, Wagener MM, Yu VL (2000) Short-course empiric antibiotic therapy for patients with pulmonary infiltrates in the intensive care unit. A proposed solution for indiscriminate antibiotic prescription. Am J Respir Crit Care Med 162:505–511
50. Raad II, Hohn DC, Gilbreath BJ, et al (1994) Prevention of central venous catheter-related infections by using maximal sterile barrier precautions during insertion. Infect Control Hosp Epidemiol 15:231–238
51. Misset B, Timsit JF, Dumay MF, et al (2004) A continuous quality-improvement program reduces nosocomial infection rates in the ICU. Intensive Care Med 30:395–400
52. Pittet D, Mourouga P, Perneger TV (1999) Compliance with handwashing in a teaching hospital. Infection Control Program. Ann Intern Med 130:126–130
53. Bischoff WE, Reynolds TM, Sessler CN, Edmond MB, Wenzel RP (2000) Handwashing compliance by health care workers: The impact of introducing an accessible, alcohol-based hand antiseptic. Arch Intern Med 160:1017–1021
54. Karabey S, Ay P, Derbentli S, Nakipoglu Y, Esen F (2002) Handwashing frequencies in an intensive care unit. J Hosp Infect 50:36–41
55. Corbella X, Montero A, Pujol M, et al (2000) Emergence and rapid spread of carbapenem resistance during a large and sustained hospital outbreak of multiresistant Acinetobacter baumannii. J Clin Microbiol 38:4086–4095
56. Kress JP, Pohlman AS, O'Connor MF, Hall JB (2000) Daily interruption of sedative infusions in critically ill patients undergoing mechanical ventilation. N Engl J Med 342:1471–1477
57. Bjoro K, Friman S, Hockerstedt K, et al (1999) Liver transplantation in the Nordic countries, 1982–1998: changes of indications and improving results. Scand J Gastroenterol 34:714–722
58. Jain A, Reyes J, Kashyap R, et al (2000) Long-term survival after liver transplantation in 4,000 consecutive patients at a single center. Ann Surg 232:490–500
59. Novelli G, Rossi M, Pretagostini R, et al (2002) MARS (Molecular Adsorbent Recirculating System): experience in 34 cases of acute liver failure. Liver 22 Suppl 2:43–47
60. Khuroo MS, Khuroo MS, Farahat KL (2004) Molecular adsorbent recirculating system for acute and acute-on-chronic liver failure: a meta-analysis. Liver Transpl 10:1099–1106
61. Capucci A, Aschieri D, Piepoli MF, Bardy GH, Iconomu E, Arvedi M (2002) Tripling survival from sudden cardiac arrest via early defibrillation without traditional education in cardiopulmonary resuscitation. Circulation 106:1065–1070
62. European Resuscitation Council (2000) Part 6: advanced cardiovascular life support. Section 7: algorithm approach to ACLS. 7C: a guide to the international ACLS algorithms. Resuscitation 46:169–184
63. Aung K, Htay T (2005) Vasopressin for cardiac arrest: a systematic review and meta-analysis. Arch Intern Med 165:17–24
64. Bickell WH, Wall MJ, Pepe PE, et al (1994) Immediate versus delayed fluid resuscitation for hypotensive patients with penetrating torso injuries. N Engl J Med 331:1105–1109
65. Haas T, Innerhofer P, Kuhbacher G, Fries D (2005) Successful reversal of deleterious coagulopathy by recombinant factor VIIa. Anesth Analg 100:54–58
66. Haitsma IK, Maas AI (2002) Advanced monitoring in the intensive care unit: brain tissue oxygen tension. Curr Opin Crit Care 8:115–120
67. Johnston AJ, Gupta AK (2002) Advanced monitoring in the neurology intensive care unit: microdialysis. Curr Opin Crit Care 8:121–127

68. O'Keefe GE, Jurkovich GJ, Copass M, Maier RV (1999) Ten-year trend in survival and resource utilization at a level I trauma center. Ann Surg 229:409–415
69. Patel HC, Menon DK, Tebbs S, Hawker R, Hutchinson PJ, Kirkpatrick PJ (2002) Specialist neurocritical care and outcome from head injury. Intensive Care Med 28:547–553
70. Marion DW, Penrod LE, Kelsey SF, et al (1997) Treatment of traumatic brain injury with moderate hypothermia. N Engl J Med 336:540–546
71. Jiang J, Yu M, Zhu C (2000) Effect of long-term mild hypothermia therapy in patients with severe traumatic brain injury: 1-year follow-up review of 87 cases. J Neurosurg 93:546–549
72. Polderman KH, Tjong Tjin JR, Peerdeman SM, Vandertop WP, Girbes AR (2002) Effects of therapeutic hypothermia on intracranial pressure and outcome in patients with severe head injury. Intensive Care Med 28:1563–1573
73. Imberti R, Bellinzona G, Langer M (2002) Cerebral tissue PO2 and SjvO2 changes during moderate hyperventilation in patients with severe traumatic brain injury. J Neurosurg 96:97–102
74. Clifton GL, Miller ER, Choi SC, et al (2001) Lack of effect of induction of hypothermia after acute brain injury. N Engl J Med 344:556–563
75. Schwartz ML, Tator CH, Rowed DW, et al (1984) The University of Toronto Head Injury Treatment Study: a prospective, randomized comparison of pentobarbital and mannitol. Can J Neurol Sci 11:434–440
76. Roberts I, Yates D, Sandercock P, et al (2004) Effect of intravenous corticosteroids on death within 14 days in 10008 adults with clinically significant head injury (MRC CRASH trial): randomised placebo-controlled trial. Lancet 364:1321–1328
77. Albanese J, Leone M, Alliez JR, et al (2003) Decompressive craniectomy for severe traumatic brain injury: Evaluation of the effects at one year. Crit Care Med 31:2535–2538
78. The National Institute of Neurological Disorders and Stroke rt-PA Stroke Study Group (1995) Tissue plasminogen activator for acute ischemic stroke. N Engl J Med 333:1581–1587
79. Mayer SA, Brun NC, Begtrup K, et al (2005) Recombinant activated factor VII for acute intracerebral hemorrhage. N Engl J Med 352:777–785
80. Mehta RL, Pascual MT, Soroko S, Chertow GM (2002) Diuretics, mortality, and nonrecovery of renal function in acute renal failure. JAMA 288:2547–2553
81. Bellomo R, Chapman M, Finfer S, Hickling K, Myburgh J (2000) Low-dose dopamine in patients with early renal dysfunction: a placebo- controlled randomised trial. Australian and New Zealand Intensive Care Society (ANZICS) Clinical Trials Group. Lancet 356:2139–2143
82. Hebert PC, Wells G, Blajchman MA, et al (1999) A multicenter, randomized, controlled clinical trial of transfusion requirements in critical care. N Engl J Med 340:409–417
83. Cochrane Injuries Group (1998) Human albumin administration in critically ill patients: systematic review of randomized controlled trials. BMJ 317:235–240
84. Finfer S, Bellomo R, Boyce N, French J, Myburgh J, Norton R (2004) A comparison of albumin and saline for fluid resuscitation in the intensive care unit. N Engl J Med 350:2247–2256
85. Kenward G, Castle N, Hodgetts T, Shaikh L (2004) Evaluation of a medical emergency team one year after implementation. Resuscitation 61:257–263
86. Bellomo R, Goldsmith D, Uchino S, et al (2004) Prospective controlled trial of effect of medical emergency team on postoperative morbidity and mortality rates. Crit Care Med 32:916–921
87. Pronovost PJ, Angus DC, Dorman T, Robinson KA, Dremsizov TT, Young TL (2002) Physician staffing patterns and clinical outcomes in critically ill patients: a systematic review. JAMA 288:2151–2162
88. Blunt MC, Burchett KR (2000) Out of hours consultant cover and case-mix-adjusted mortality in intensive care. Lancet 356:735–736

89. Pronovost PJ, Jenckes MW, Dorman T, et al (1999) Organizational characteristics of intensive care units related to outcomes of abdominal aortic surgery. JAMA 281:1310–1317
90. Angus DC, Kelley MA, Schmitz RJ, White A, Popovich J Jr (2000) Caring for the critically ill patient. Current and projected workforce requirements for care of the critically ill and patients with pulmonary disease: can we meet the requirements of an aging population? JAMA 284:2762–2770

Managing and Leading in Critical Care

W. J. Sibbald

Introduction

Many issues contribute to complexity and uncertainty in health care: technological innovation, funding challenges, concerns about quality and safety, the need to integrate information technology into patient care areas, and intra-professional rivalry. Health care is also on the verge of major organizational changes, such as the regionalization of care, consolidation of services, the flattening of organizational structures, and demands for accountability. This book outlines many of the challenges anticipated for critical care in the next decade, both as a discipline and profession, and thereby emphasizes the need to consider how to prepare for its future.

> *"In order for health care organizations, especially academic health sciences centres, to successfully adapt and flexibly respond to major environmental challenges, it is imperative they improve organizational capabilities in both management and leadership" [1].*

Critical care medicine is particularly in need of developing high-quality physician-manager/leaders. Critical care units consume substantial amounts of hospital budgets relative to other patient care areas. Intensive care units (ICUs) contain expensive technology, employ a multidisciplinary workforce and are frequently a site of tensions among medical disciplines. Accordingly, enlightened management and leadership skills will be needed by future generations of critical care physicians.

> *"Among the most important issues for a successful and effective healthcare system in the future is a sufficient pool of management talent and leadership" [2].*

Leadership and management are not the same thing. When *managing*, physicians are required to plan, allocate, monitor and report on budgeting, participate in clinical governance and deal with human resources. When *leading*, they plan for future activities and assume responsibility for performance in their clinical units. Many experts have concluded that the complexity of today's critical care environment requires that the same individual exert management and leadership skills concurrently.

It is sometimes assumed that a physician nominated to 'lead' a critical care unit department or program will bring management and leadership skills to the position because of previous academic or clinical successes. Although this may occur, competency in health leadership and management should not be assumed simply because a physician has achieved academic or clinical successes. Management and leadership skills are learned traits, and it is increasingly argued that physicians should prepare for management and leadership positions the same way they prepare for research and teaching responsibilities.

> *"The most dangerous leadership myth is that leaders are born – that there is a genetic factor to leadership. This myth asserts that people simply either have certain charismatic qualities or not. That's nonsense; in fact, the opposite is true. Leaders are made rather than born" Warren G Bennis.*

Formal and informal educational processes are essential to physician leaders seeking competencies in the essentials of health leadership and management, such as strategic planning, managing change, communication, conflict resolution, team building and negotiating. Recognizing the importance of health management skills, critical care specialty training committees increasingly require skills preparation in health administration and management. An example of such skills required by one such curriculum (UK Competency program, Section on 'Professionalism') is shown in Table 1 [3].

This chapter will introduce core functions undertaken by managers and leaders, with a special emphasis on translating lessons from non-health care literature to the healthcare environment in general, and critical care in specific. Where appropriate, lessons from the critical care literature will be used to exemplify the appropriateness of lessons from industry. We will borrow from early research about the impact of contemporary leadership and management skills on critical care activities and outcomes. Finally, we will try to identify why success of the future critical care enterprise requires that as much attention is paid to preparing a cohort of trainees as 'clinician *administrators*' as it currently does in preparing other trainees to be 'clinician *teachers*' and 'clinician *researchers*'.

Managing and Management

Introducing concepts such as clinical governance has resulted in a significant shift toward holding physicians accountable for the delivery of quality health care service. In *A First Class Service – Quality in the National Health Service* [4], clinical governance was defined as: "a framework through which NHS organizations are accountable for continuously improving the quality of their services and safeguarding high standards of care by creating an environment in which excellence in clinical care will flourish". Other healthcare systems have also begun a process to engage physician leaders in the accountability framework. Regardless of the nomenclature, many healthcare systems require that physician leaders now formally commit to improving the quality of health care. Examples of how physician leaders can achieve this goal include: developing clinical

Table 1. Management skills required by UK Critical Care Competency Based Training Program

1. Overview: Professionalism implies high standards, commitment to quality, patient care before self-interest, transparent evaluation of service delivered, and the conditional privilege of self-regulation.

2. Knowledge
   - Published standards of care at local, regional and national level
   - Requirements for training
   - Local policies and procedures
   - Methods of audit and translating findings into sustained change in practice
   - Recent advances in medical research relevant to intensive care

3. Skills

   Self-directed learning
   - Enquiring mind, self-prompted search for knowledge
   - Proper use of learning aids where available
   - Contribution to departmental activities
   - Participation in audit
   - Participation in educational activities and teaching other groups appropriate to level of knowledge
   - Maintenance of education and training record
   - Understands research methodology
   - Actively participating in research

   Communication
   - Able to achieve appropriate information transfer.
   - Understands that communication is a two-way process
   - Calls for senior/more experienced help in difficult situations
   - Effective multidisciplinary communication and collaborative practice

   Organization and management
   - Structured approach to developing individual patient care plans
   - Effective member of the ICU team
   - Effective leadership of ICU team
   - Organize multidisciplinary care for groups of patients in the ICU
   - Organize long-term multidisciplinary care for all patients in the ICU
   - Strategic planning of the ICU service within the wider environment
   - Principles of workforce planning
   - Practical application of equal opportunities legislation

4. Attitudes & behavior
   - Caring and compassionate with patients and relatives
   - Ethical behavior
   - Functioning within competence
   - Accepts appropriate advice from other health care professionals
   - Supportive of colleagues
   - Demonstrates initiative in analyzing problems and critically evaluating current practice
   - Professional and reassuring approach
   - Attentive to detail, punctual, clean, tidy, polite and helpful

Table 1. *Continued*

Program
5. Workplace training objectives – Maintain education and training record – Present topics at staff educational meetings – Present topics at regional or national meetings where possible – Active participation in research projects – Experience and discuss staff-relative interactions (e.g.: breaking bad news) – Lead ICU ward round with consultant supervision – Lead ICU ward round without direct supervision - Arrange ICU educational meetings - Attend management meetings as appropriate - Discuss cost-effective care in the ICU - Attendance as observer (with permission from trainee) at SHO training assessments

Table 2. Managerial practices that are used to support *clinical governance*:

- Planning and organizing
- Problem solving
- Monitoring operations and the environment
- Motivating
- Informing
- Clarifying roles and objectives
- Supporting and mentoring
- Consulting and delegating
- Teambuilding and managing conflict
- Networking

risk management and clinical data systems, learning from complaints, making a lifelong commitment to professional development, and involving patients in planning and decision-making. Managerial practices, which support the accountability framework with regards to quality of patient care and efficiency in processes delivering care, are listed in Table 2.

> *"Clinical governance is essentially an organizational concept aimed at ensuring that every health organization creates the culture, the systems and the support mechanisms so that good clinical performance will be the norm and so that quality improvement will be part and parcel of routine clinical practice" (Liam Donaldson, speaking at a conference on Clinical Performance and Priorities in the NHS, at The Queen Elizabeth II Conference Centre, Westminster, November 2, 1999).*

How does this lesson translate into a discussion of the future of critical care? Previously, critical care physicians designated to lead critical care units, programs or departments were generally expected to maintain a good clinical and academic service, but had little in the way of formal accountability with the hospital's administration. As hospital governance is becoming increasingly 'businesslike', physicians appointed to leadership/management positions in any department are being subjected to greater oversight and accountability than in the past. In requiring that physicians also commit to the principles of 'clinical governance', it must be expected that future critical care physicians will be designated to both 'manage' and 'lead' critical care units, programs or departments. Our vision of the future is that in their appointment critical care physician managers/leaders will be required by hospital management to:

- Agree to specific responsibilities that emphasize clinical governance
- Develop objectives for the critical care department or program
- Undertake regular performance reviews

It must also be expected that the critical care physician manager/leader will be held responsible by the hospital for enhancing the unit's efficiency, thus ensuring that resources provided by the hospital are used to provide good quality patient care, at the lowest possible cost.

In looking to the future, it is worthwhile to begin by identifying some of the 'management' principles that the clinical service provided by a critical care department or program will employ.

Responsibilities of the Critical Care Clinical Service

A clinical service, such as a critical care program or department, will need to employ robust evaluation activities to maintain and improve the quality of patient care. The commitment to clinical governance by all physicians will be embodied in hospital bylaws. Thus, the critical care physician-manager will be held responsible for:

1. Creating guidelines for the granting of specific clinical privileges in the ICU;
2. Developing ICU program policies, rules and regulations;
3. Developing recommendations about the need for continuing education programs that are consistent with the type of services offered by critical care and the findings of performance improvement activities; and
4. Overseeing physician staff members' adherence to all of: a) the Medical Staff Bylaws[1], and other pertinent hospital policies; b) sound principles of clinical practice; and c) regulations that promote patient safety.

[1] In North American hospitals, bylaws provide a framework for the medical staff to discharge its responsibilities in matters relating to the quality of medical care, to govern the orderly resolution of issues.

A Critical Care Physician-manager Will have Specific *Roles* and *Functions*

Application of traditional management principles means that physicians undertaking to provide management expertise to critical care will have three primary *roles*:

1. **Interpersonal.** In this role, the ICU physician-manager is a figurehead for the ICU team, meets with stakeholders internal and external to the ICU, and influences decision-making.
2. **Informational.** In this role, the ICU physician-manager monitors activities that are important to the ICU, disseminates knowledge to the ICU team and other relevant stakeholders, and acts as a spokesperson for the ICU.
3. **Decisional.** In the decision-making role, the physician-manager manages conflict, allocates resources to support the ICU's objectives and negotiates with other decision makers inside and outside the hospital.

The physician-manager will also have specific functions, as follows:

- **Planning.** Every physician-manager must ensure their ICU has a plan describing 'where it is going' and 'how it intends to get there'. A completed plan includes objectives, and policies and procedures that guide the critical care program's daily activities. Importantly, the plan becomes a roadmap for managing daily issues and is preparation for dealing with future challenges (because having thought about critical issues in advance provides better responses when they occur).
- **Organizing.** The physician-manager must create a process that identifies what activities should be carried out in specific critical care units, how the activities should be organized and who has the responsibility for carrying them out. The organizing function also involves determining how clinical authority and responsibility are appropriately divided among the different professions that comprise the multidisciplinary critical care team.
- **Staffing and directing.** The physician-manager hires and manages the people for the tasks required by the critical care unit. This function requires the determination of appropriate staffing levels, for example, by aligning nurse and physician resources with patient illness severity. In this function, the physician manager is also reminded to pay attention to the professional development of the critical care workforce, as well as their motivation.
- **Controlling.** As specifically identified by the accountability framework, the physician-manager will be held responsible for ensuring that processes are in place to measure and report on the critical care unit's or service's performance. Accounting, budgeting and utilization management, not currently a significant issue for a majority of critical care leaders, will become an increasingly important aspect of the controlling function. Performance of both specific care units and professionals involved therein, must be measured against accepted benchmarks.
- **Decision-making and problem-solving.** These activities are especially important for the physician-manager. They involve the identification and analysis of situations that require a decision, the development of alternatives, approaches

to implementing solutions in the importance of evaluating the consequences of the specific solution implemented.

Planning For Critical Care

Planning for the critical care service or program is especially important, and deserves brief comment. Planning involves determining the direction of a critical care unit or program through: a) creation of objectives; and b) design and implementation of strategies to achieve those objectives. The critical care physician-manager must commit to a process of planning (both annual and long term). A good long term plan, developed through an iterative process, gives the unit direction, prepares it to deal with change successfully and helps it to prepare for dealing with uncertainty. In anticipating the future, planning involves deciding 'what to do' and 'how to do it'. Good planning requires ongoing surveillance and adaptive change is a prerequisite. By anticipating the future, and comparing findings to present conditions, the ICU physician-leader creates the position to make good decisions about the ICU's direction, its programs and how to deploy and allocate its resources. To summarize, planning for the ICU is important because it:

1. Forces the physician-leader to focus on outputs. All ICU activities should be directed to achieving predefined objectives (or outputs). Optimizing the outputs will dictate the inputs.
2. Enables the ICU manager to develop priorities and make better decisions about the allocation and use of resources. By integrating structures, tasks, technology and people, inputs are converted to outputs.
3. Provides a foundation for resource allocation and control. It enables the ICU physician-manager to measure progress and to determine whether expected results are being achieved.

How Will the Critical Care Physician-Manager's Roles and Functions be Integrated by the Hospital's Management Team?

Appointment of a physician to a management role in critical care will be increasingly accompanied by an explicit job description (Table 3), which will both be aligned with the hospital's goals and objectives and emphasize the accountability agenda previously discussed. Physicians appointed to management roles will have their performance measured on a regular basis; this will not be just 'academic' performance, but also performance related to roles identified in a job description.

Physicians appointed to clinical management roles in critical care also should expect to see an explicit linkage between performance and reward. An increasing body of management research confirms that aligning physician compensation with the achievement of specific objectives (clinical, administrative and academic) is accompanied by enhanced performance. Data from the health literature supports the notion that aligning physician compensation with

Table 3. A model of a job description for critical care physician appointed to lead and manage a critical care unit, program or service integrates roles attributed both to 'management' and 'leadership'

1. Determine the clinically related and administrative activities of the ICU service including, but not limited to, the quality of patient care provided by members of the ICU;
2. Where ICU 'Rules and Regulations' are desired, the physician manager/leader will be accountable for development and implementation of those Rules and Regulations, ensuring that they support the hospital's performance improvement plan that deals with professional medical care in the ICU. With the approval of physician members of the ICU, he/she will submit ICU Rules and Regulations to the Medical Board;
3. Develop and implement ICU programs for orientation of new members, credentials review and privileges delineation for appointment and reappointment, continuing medical education, utilization review, concurrent evaluation of practice, and retrospective evaluation of practice;
4. Transmit to the appropriate authorities the ICU's recommendations concerning appointment, reappointment, delineation of clinical privileges, and disciplinary action with respect to members of the Service;
5. Recommend the criteria for clinical privileges that are relevant to the care provided in the ICU;
6. Assess and recommend to the relevant hospital authority space issues for needed patient care services and technology provided by the ICU;
7. Recommend the qualified and competent physicians required to provide ICU clinical service needs;
8. Determine the qualifications and competence of ICU personnel who are not licensed independent practitioners (example, post graduate trainees) who provide patient care services;
9. Maintain continuing review of the professional performance of physician members with clinical privileges in the ICU, and maintain appropriate documentation;
10. Assist in the development and enforcement of hospital policies and Medical Staff Bylaws, Rules and Regulations, and the requirements and Rules and Regulations in the ICU;
11. Perform such other duties commensurate with his/her office as may from time to time be assigned by the Chief of Staff or the hospital.

specific management objectives is successful, not only with regards to 'typical' managerial tasks, but also for academic productivity [5, 6].

'Good Management' Contributes to 'Performance'

Management research documents that good physician management effectively translates into improved performance with respect to clinical critical care and safety. Based on data collected on almost 18,000 patients in 42 ICUs, Shortell and colleagues reported that superior organizational practices among ICUs were related to a patient-centered culture, strong medical and nursing leadership, effective communication and coordination, and open, collaborative approaches to problem solving and conflict management [7]. Specifically, good caregiver interaction, management co-ordination, and conflict management in the ICU's leadership group was associated with all of the following: a) lower risk-adjusted length of stay, b) lower nurse turnover, and c) a greater ability to meet family member needs.

When compared to ICUs where patient care is provided in an 'open' environment, research also has shown that ICUs which are managed and staffed by trained critical care physicians have better patient outcomes while using fewer resources [8, 9].

Leadership and Leading

Defining physician-*leadership* is more difficult than defining physician-*management*, in part because health leadership research is much less mature than health management research. Yukl stated that "leadership involves influencing processes affecting the interpretation of events for followers, the choice of objectives for the group or organization, organization of work activities to accomplish the objectives, motivation of followers to achieve these objectives, maintenance of co-operative relationships and teamwork, and enlistment of support and co-operation from people outside the group or organization" [10].

Other research emphasizes the importance of good leaders being especially adept at managing through times of change. In managing change, Tichy and Cohen observed that leaders move organizations from where they are to where they need to be [11]. He also felt that good leaders make things happen, are often regarded as revolutionaries, and are adept at facing reality and mobilizing resources to support change.

While a majority of leadership research has occurred in the non-health industries, Shortell and colleagues have begun to evaluate leadership in the health sector. These authors [12] concluded that research about leadership has been too narrow. These authors subsequently argued that high-performance physician leadership depends on key characteristics, namely systems thinking, visioning, facilitating learning, and follower empowerment.

- **Systems thinking.** This stresses that all organizational systems in health are comprised of some common attributes.
- **Visioning.** By visioning, physician leaders lead by 'pulling' not by 'pushing'; good leaders create exciting images of the future and have the ability to sell the vision to colleagues and develop their commitment to it.
- **Facilitating learning.** Changes in healthcare are generally considered revolutionary rather than evolutionary. Thus, creating change requires successful managers who have the commitment and ability to learn and relearn.
- **Empowering followers.** As the essence of leadership is getting things done, Shortell et al. [12] believe that successful physician-leaders understand that their followers are a source of organizational creativity. This means that suc-

cessful physician-leaders understand and create team-orientated approaches for providing patient care and programs to continuously improve quality.

Different Styles of Leadership

While there are different styles of leadership, the successful critical care physician-leader will learn that different approaches are situation-specific, and adapt his/her leadership to the specific situation.

- **Charismatic leadership.** A charismatic leader uses influence based not on tradition or formal authority, but on follower's perceptions that he/she displays exceptional qualities. Charismatic leadership is important when there is an organizational crisis, for example, during a hospital merger. Here, a physician may create a radical vision for change (and survival), and it is the vision presented that attracts followers who believe it will provide stability for them during the crisis.
- **Transformational leadership.** A transformational leader appeals to followers' values and emotions, and mobilizes their energy to re-organize around a task (in contrast, a *transacting* leader motivates followers by appealing to their self-interest). Followers trust, admire and respect the transformational leader, and become motivated to do more than was originally expected of them. The transformational leader motivates followers by making them more aware of the importance of their task outcomes, and convincing them to go beyond their self-interest for the sake of the team.
- **Pragmatic leadership.** The pragmatic physician-leader focuses on the organization, for example, the critical care unit, rather than on the people that comprise the workforce. This leadership approach faces the reality of the environment in which the critical care unit operates. These types of leaders are most effective when an organization is going through rough times.

Effective ICU Physician Leaders Will Use Their Power Judiciously

If an essence of leadership is the ability to influence followers, *power* is the potential to exert influence. 'Power' was defined by Alexander and Morlock [13] as the "ability [or potential] to exert actions that either directly or indirectly cause the change in the behavior and/or attributes of another individual or group". For the ICU physician-leader, power is the probability he/she will be in a position to carry out his/her own will despite resistance from other members of the team. In contrast, 'influence' refers to "actions that, either directly or indirectly, cause change in the behavior and/or attitudes of another individual or group" [13]. Thus, influence is power that is translated into action. Sources of the ICU physician-leader's power are shown in Table 4.

Physician-leaders need to understand the different types of power and be especially aware of their sources of power. Physician managers must also appreciate the need to develop power; this happens by creating opportunities, controlling resources and dealing effectively with contingencies that face the

Table 4. Different types of 'power' exerted by an ICU physician-leader in achieving goals and objectives.

- *Legitimate* power exists when it is derived from a physician leader's position in the hospital.
- *Reward-based* power is the leader's ability to reward desirable behaviors.
- *Coercive* power is based on the leader's ability to prevent someone from achieving rewards they want.
- *Expert* power derives from having knowledge valued by the ICU or hospital, such as expertise in problem solving.
- *Referent* power results when a leader creates admiration and loyalty to the extent that power is gained to influence others.

hospital. Exerting influence should be reserved only for issues of high priority for the ICU, where the greatest benefits will occur from its application. Stated differently, the effective ICU physician leader uses his/her power and influence judiciously.

Effective ICU Physician-leaders are 'Change Managers'

Leading change is considered to be the most important – and difficult – of a physician-leader's responsibilities. Resistance to change, which often includes questioning the need for change, is a natural part of almost all of the physician-manager's projects. Without managing the effect of change proposed on the ICU and its staff's work patterns, the potential benefits of a project may not be achieved. For successful implementation of projects that require change in the behavior of physician colleagues, the physician manager/leader needs to analyze and understand potential resistance, and then create a plan to manage the resistance.

Physician manager/leaders need to learn how to diagnose the forces of change, and then guide successful change. Before beginning any change activity, the ICU physician-leader must have a vision for a better future that is attractive enough to justify the sacrifices and hardship that the change process requires. Guidelines for successful change management are summarized in Table 5 [14].

Over the last decade, research in healthcare has sought to understand how to change clinician behavior, and some good evidence has emerged. Fundamentally, changing physician behavior is most successful with a multi-factorial approach that emphasizes use of 'evidence' rather than focusing on the practice of individual physicians or groups of physicians whose practice is at variance with the majority. The Agency for Healthcare Research and Quality (AHRQ) report *"Making Health Care Safer: A Critical Analysis of Patient Safety Practices,"* [15] summarized strategies which evidence suggests will be effective in changing physician practice, and thus also engage them in processes to improve quality of care (Table 6).

Table 5. Approaches that successful leaders and managers use to implement 'change'.

1. Identify a **change sponsor**, preferably someone who has the authority to begin the change process and the ability to sustain it through to implementation.
2. Create a **clearly defined aim** that can be communicated to all individuals who will be impacted by the change.
3. Insure that you have a **tolerance for ambiguity**: All participants in the change process must understand that ambiguity is a normal part of the change process, but that as the change progresses the ambiguity will decrease and benefits will be identified.
4. Remember that **commitment at all levels** to the project must be maintained through all areas of the ICU that will be affected by the change. Adequate resources must also need to be assigned to the change process.
5. Make sure that **communication is open**: A formal communication plan is an essential, to allow all participants to provide their views and opinions into the change process.
6. Be sure that you have identified an **appropriate change management methodology**, especially when projects are complex, when the cost of failure is high and probability of failure is real because of anticipated resistance to change.

Table 6. 'Evidence based' strategies that are considered the most effective in changing physician practice

- *Mini sabbaticals* that allow clinicians to spend time in other critical care units learning how to practice evidence based healthcare.
- *Personalized feedback* on performance, either in comparison with that of others or against explicit standards, as part of learning process.
- *Computer-assisted decision-making* that provides reminders and easy access to evidence based guidelines and to knowledge itself.
- *On-the-job training* of practical skills.
- Use of *opinion leaders* or 'educational influentials' (colleagues whose performances are respected).

> *"The most important step in facilitating change is to ensure that physicians want to change. The most effective way of encouraging them to change is to help them see evidence based decision-making not as a management imperative, but as an intellectual challenge" [16].*

This aspect of leadership is more completely reviewed in the chapter by Drs Cook and Finfer later in this book.

The Imperative for Using "Evidence" in Decision Making

Physician managers are responsible for making decisions that directly or indirectly impact on the quality of patient care and health care costs. Within a climate of scarce healthcare resources, physician-managers make difficult decisions about complex issues, including the allocation of resources for individual clinical interventions and the organization of the ICU's care processes. Researchers increasingly comment that, much like clinical practice, decision makers do not always use of available research to inform their decision-making. While there are many factors that influence managerial decision-making processes, it can be argued that management decisions in health care should imply 'best available evidence' similar to what is promoted as appropriate for clinical decision-making.

While the initial focus has been directed towards *clinical* decision-making (example, evidence based medicine; EBM), principles of this approach to making decisions are increasingly applied to management and policy decisions. The terminology, 'evidence based health care' adapts the strength of the EBM approach to diverse health care disciplines outside of clinical medicine. By using evidence based health care, Muir Gray [16] argues the physician manager will reduce practice variation by increasing the use of medical interventions of proven effectiveness and by limiting the use of clinical strategies not shown to be effective. As when making a clinical decision, evidence based health care (or evidence based health management) involves a rigorous approach to systematically searching for, finding, critically appraising and applying best evidence to health care management and policy decisions. The four skills required in evidence based health care are similar to those used when searching the clinical literature for diagnostic or treatment options, as outlined in Table 7.

Motivating

Whether working with individuals or teams, the physician-leader needs to motivate his/her colleagues. When successfully motivated, the performance of healthcare workers improves. Motivating is initiated by first understanding

Table 7. The approach to practicing evidence based healthcare for hospital managers and leaders

1. Create an answerable question,
2. Search for evidence to answer the question,
3. Evaluate the evidence retrieved
4. Apply the evidence in making decisions
5. Establish a measurement approach that allows you to evaluate the consequences of the decision

what needs and rewards people view as important. Intrinsic rewards, such as job challenge, opportunities for creativity, responsibility, autonomy and opportunities for growth, motivate some workers; extrinsic rewards, such as job title or pay, motivate others. Successful programs include financial incentives, employee training and goal setting. Combined interventions are more effective than single method approaches and employees respond to different rewards at different times.

Team Building and the Impact of 'Good Teamwork' on Clinical Outcomes and Quality

Given the importance of teamwork to a successful critical care service, team building is a proficiency that must be learned and practiced by the physician-leader. A physician in a team leadership role is most effective when she/he defines the objectives of the task to be performed and then allows team members to contribute to creating solutions. A team is most 'effective' when collaboration (rather than competition) is promoted and team members are encouraged to assume leadership. It is axiomatic that the more inclusive the team, the greater will be the talents and viewpoints available to analyze and deal with problems found in a critical care unit. Gray states the performance [P] of an individual or team is a function of three variables:

$$P = MxC/B$$

where [M] is the level of motivation, [C] is the level of competency and [B] are the barriers needed to be overcome in order to perform well [16].

The impact of good teamwork on ICU clinical outcomes has been well demonstrated. In a public inquiry into patient deaths in the United Kingdom, Professor Ian Kennedy concluded that poor teamwork had a negative effect on clinical performance and patient outcomes [17]. He noted "...in particular, poor teamwork demonstrates a clear lack of effective clinical leadership. Those in positions of clinical leadership must bear the responsibility for this failure." The converse, the positive impact of good teamwork on clinical outcomes, has also been shown. Pronovost and colleagues concluded that when everyone concerned with a patient's care – doctors, residents, nurses, attending physicians, pharmacists and others – participated in rounds together, and created daily goals for care, communication was improved, as was professional job satisfaction [18]. Pronovost's study also noted that better resource use – measured as a one-day decrease in ICU stay – resulted from encouraging good teamwork.

Managing Conflict

Conflict is inevitable in the ICU. Not surprisingly, it impacts negatively on clinical productivity. A common origin of conflict is the uncertainty surrounding patient outcomes, unit planning and daily operations. An example of uncertainty in the ICU is the suddenness of patient admissions and patient related complications. Other conflict points in the ICU include patient care issues when disagreement evolves about the appropriate management of the patient, disagreement between patient families and ICU professionals, differing ethical values relative to patient care decisions, and staff shortages that lead to fatigue.

Although research about conflict issues in the ICU is scant, a recent study described an evaluation of 248 conflicts involving 209 patients. Different types of conflict were described: team-family disputes, intra-team disputes, and intra-family conflict. The leading sources of conflict were disagreements over life sustaining treatments, poor communication, the (lack of) availability of family decision makers and the surrogates' (perceived) inability to make decisions.

"Individual clinicians improve performance by incorporating teamwork, communication and crisis resource management principles into critical care training. Team performance may also be improved by "assessing personality factors when selecting personnel for high-stress areas, explicit assignment of roles, ensuring a common "culture" in the team and routine debriefings" [19].

Conclusion – On becoming a 'Clinician Administrator'

The role of physician-leader-manager in the ICU is becoming increasingly complex. Healthcare systems are imposing demands for accountability and performance that require physician managers to become familiar with new roles and skills. Understanding of epidemiology, statistics, health status and outcomes, mastering information systems and technology are part of the expectations. Physician-managers need to understand and lead quality improvement in a manner that is consistent with new demands for clinical governance. Physician-managers need to learn about health care financing, using budgets for planning, and working within limits and constraints. Problem solving, mentoring and coaching also are required of the new physician-manager. Physician-leaders are expected to be lifelong learners, to provide transformational leadership and create visions to move their ICU in new directions. A summary of the distinction between 'management' and 'leadership' traits/activities is shown in Table 8. This module is only a brief introduction to some of these new skills.

We have previously argued that the chaos characterizing today's healthcare systems, coupled with the stresses critical care will face over the next decade (especially those outlined in this text), will increasingly result in a cohort of critical care physicians undertaking to develop the skills required to become a 'clinician-administrator', as, currently, other trainees will choose to develop expertise as say 'a clinician-researcher' or 'clinician-teacher'. The 'clinician administrator' in critical care will learn through the commitment of professional societies to developing innovative programs that provide training in management and leadership skills.

Accepting the premise that formerly preparing some of our future critical care physicians to be 'clinician administrators' will be as important as preparation to be a 'clinical researcher' or 'clinical educator', what are the attributes and behaviors that will characterize successful ICU physician leaders 10 years from

Table 8. A summary of the different skills required when 'managing' versus 'leading'.

Management and managing	Leadership and leading
Directing	Supporting
Creative thinking	Inspiring creativity
Decision-making	Delegating
Listening	Ensuring understanding
Constructive criticism	Supporting
Problem solving	Resolving conflict
Implementing technology	Humanizing technology

now? A successful critical care physician will be one who understands how to integrate leadership skills into his/her approach to all the unit activities on a daily basis. When leading, the critical care physician will emphasize a vision for the future, and then will create support amongst the critical care stakeholders to move in that direction. Other components of the leadership agenda for successful critical care physicians will emphasize an understanding of how to motivate a multi-professional workforce.

Management research from many sources identifies behavior types in successful leaders, which can be, I believe, easily translated to critical care leadership [20]. This work summarizes that 'best practices' in leadership and management applied to any business, including critical care in our opinion, will include all of the following. The critical care physician-manager will be successful because (s)he [21]:

1. Articulates a clear vision for the critical care unit, program or Department and encourages co-workers to adopt the vision. The leader will identify what the critical care unit stands for and declares this in clear and inspiring terms.
2. Creates priorities and direction to ensure focus.
3. Identifies problems, uses 'evidence' to analyze possible solutions and then translates plans into action.
4. Encourages and supports the critical care staff to commit to lifelong learning, thereby creating an environment that motivates co-workers to commit their talents to pursuit of the critical care objectives.
5. Constantly learns because the environment in which critical care operates is rapidly changing and thus needs a constant infusion of new knowledge to be successful in its many objectives.
6. Balances the interests of all stakeholders.

To summarize, the future of critical care will be bright when existing leaders commit to the development of programs that formerly prepare the next generation of critical care physicians to be 'managers' and 'leaders'. The skills can indeed be learned, and when applied in a consistent and balanced way, result in a critical care system which accepts accountability to the broader governance system, leads in innovation and challenges others in healthcare to adopt the 'best practices' to the benefit of our patients. The writer hopes the trainee in critical care will increasingly search out leadership and management training opportunities, to become part of the new workforce required of the critical care community.

References

1. Monahan PS, Kasperbauer D, McDade SA, et al (1998) Training future leaders of academic medicine: Internal programs at three academic health centers. Acad Med 73:1159–1168
2. Mecklenburg GA (2001) Career performance: How are we doing? J Healthc Manag 46:8–13
3. The Intercollegiate Board for Training in Intensive care Medicine. At: www.ibticm.org. Accessed May 2005
4. Department of Health (1998) A First Class Service – Quality in the National Health Service. HMSO, London
5. Tarquinio GT, Dittus RS, Byrne DW, Kaiser A, Neilson EG (2003) Effects of performance-based compensation and faculty track on the clinical activity, research portfolio, and teaching mission of a large academic department of medicine. Acad Med 78: 690–701
6. Shortell SM, Zazzali JL, Burns LR, et al (2001) Implementing evidence-based medicine: the role of market pressures, compensation incentives, and culture in physician organizations. Med Care 39:I62–78.
7. Shortell SM, Zimmerman JE, Rousseau DM, et al (1994) The performance of intensive care units: does good management make a difference? Med Care 32:508–525
8. Pronovost PJ, Angus DC, Dorman T, Robinson KA, Dremsizov TT, Young TL (2002) Physician staffing patterns and clinical outcomes in critically ill patients: a systematic review. JAMA 288:2151–2162
9. Pronovost PJ, Jenckes MW, Dorman T, et al (1999) Organizational characteristics of intensive care units related to outcomes of abdominal aortic surgery. JAMA 281:1310–1317
10. Yukl G (1994) Leadership in Organizations, 3rd Edition. Prentice Hall, Englewood, p 5
11. Tichy NM, Cohen EB (1997) The Leadership Engine. Harper Business, New York
12. Shortell SM, Kaluzny AD (1996) Organization theory and health services management. In: Shortell SM, Kaluzny AD (eds) Essentials of Health Care Management. Delmar Publishers, Clifton Park, pp 3–33
13. Alexander JA, Morlock LL (1996) Power and politics in health services organizations. In: Shortell SM, Kaluzny AD (eds) Essentials of Health Care Management. Delmar Publishers, Clifton Park, pp 256–285
14. Department of Commerce (2002) Change Management Guideline Art: http://www.oit.nsw.gov.au/Guidelines/4.3.19.a-Change-Man.asp Accessed July 2005
15. Trowbridge R, Weingarten S (2001) Educational techniques used in changing provider behavior. At: http://www.ahrq.gov/clinic/ptsafety/chap54.htm Accessed July 2005
16. Gray JAM (2001) Evidence Based Healthcare. How to Make Health Policy and Management Decisions. Churchill Livingstone, New York
17. The Bristol Royal Infirmary Inquiry. At: http://www.bristol-inquiry.org.uk/index.htm Accessed May 2005
18. Pronovost P, Berenholtz S, Dorman T, Lipsett PA, Simmonds T, Haraden C (2003) Improving communication in the ICU using daily goals. J Crit Care 18:71–75
19. Schull MJ, Ferris LE, Tu JV, Hux JE, Redelmeier DA (2001) Problems for clinical judgement: 3. Thinking clearly in an emergency. CMAJ 164:1170–1175
20. Likert R (1961) New Patterns of Management. McGraw-Hill, New York

21. Starkweather D , Shropshire DG (1994), Managing Effectiveness. In: Taylor RJ, Taylor SB (eds) AUPHA Manual of Health Services Management. Aspen Publishers, Gaithersburg, p 19

Critical Care from 50,000 Feet

D. C. Angus

Introduction

The current book takes on the ambitious task of amassing evidence and opinion about the directions and challenges for critical care in the coming decade. My particular assignment was to provide introductory comments relating to the 'big picture'. In organizing my thoughts, I have started with a conceptual overview of what intensive care 'is', focusing on how it relates to the rest of the healthcare system. With that conceptual model in mind, I have then attempted to summarize how critical care is currently provided, warts and all. From this summary of the current field of play, a number of issues naturally arise that are likely to be of import in the coming decade. It is on how we might tackle these issues that I offer some concluding musings.

A Conceptual Model of Care Delivery for Acute Illness

The Intensive Care Unit

Acute illness may be managed in a variety of settings but traditional measures of the availability of care for acute illness have focused on the intensive care unit (ICU), which is usually the definitive location for stabilization and treatment of acutely ill patients. Although all ICUs share the goal of providing intensive care to the critically ill, they are not uniform. Conceptually, their functional capability is a manifestation of the place, the people, and the product (Fig. 1). The place includes the physical structure, the number of beds, and the technology, such as monitoring capabilities. The people are the ICU staff, and can be defined as the number and type of different staff members (e.g., physicians, nurses, and respiratory therapists), their organizational structure (e.g., mandatory involvement of intensive care physicians in the care of all patients), and the type and quality of leadership, collaboration, and teamwork. The product is the suite of diagnostic strategies and interventions offered by the ICU, and ca be defined by the variety, quality, and quantity of product. There is an obvious interrelationship, or set of internal influences, between the place, people and product. For example, the interventions offered (product) depend on the technologic capabilities available (place) and the training and experience of the staff (people). There are also a number of external factors that influence the ICU. The first external influ-

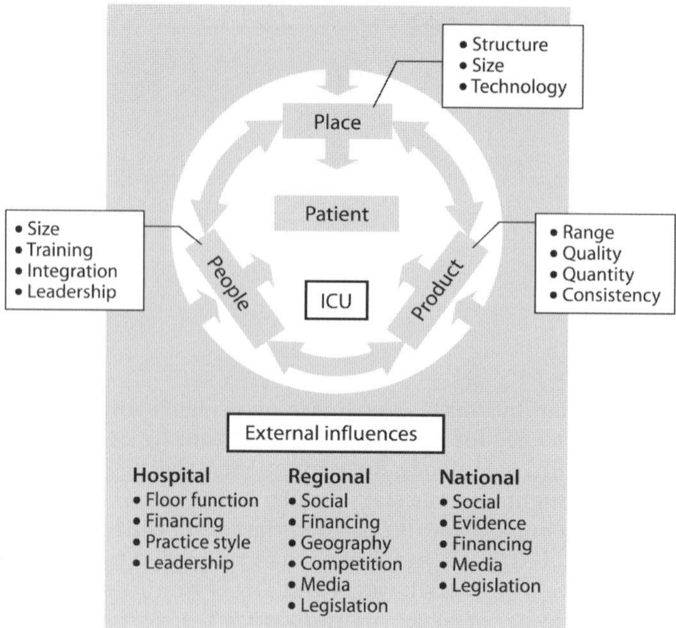

Fig. 1. The functional capability of the intensive care unit (ICU). The ICU functions as a manifestation of the place, the people, and the product. The place includes the physical structure, the number of beds, and the technology, such as monitoring capabilities. The people are the ICU staff, and can be defined as the number and type of different staff members (e.g., physicians, nurses, and respiratory therapists), their organizational structure (e.g., mandatory involvement of intensive care physicians in the care of all patients), and the type and quality of leadership, collaboration, and teamwork. The product is the suite of diagnostic strategies and interventions offered by the ICU, and can be defined by the variety, quality, and quantity of product. However, three levels (hospital, regional, and national) of external entities also influence the functional capability of the ICU.

ence is the hospital in which the ICU is located. Factors such as the capability of the hospital floors to handle sick patients will influence who is transferred and when, both into and out of the ICU. Financial pressures faced by the hospital will have trickle-down effects on the provision of ICU services. And, the prevailing professional culture may have strong influences on who is admitted to the ICU and how the ICU is staffed.

The hospital operates within a region, and a number of regional variables influence ICU function. A sparsely-populated mountain region places different demands on acute care services than a large, urban community. The surgical/trauma ICU at LDS Hospital in Salt Lake City, Utah serves as a regional referral center for patients developing acute illness hundreds of miles away and thus requires an efficient long distance inter-hospital referral and transport system that works in all weather conditions. In contrast, the surgical/trauma ICU at Los Angeles County hospital serves a predominantly poor, densely-populated part of Los Angeles riddled with high crime and unemployment. In this instance, priorities include providing expert care for a high volume of penetrating trauma on limited public funds while complex inter-hospital transport systems are less important.

Regional characteristics can lead to change in acute care services provision over time. For example, in the United States, local competition from other hospitals may lead hospital administrators to build or upgrade ICUs in an effort to market technologic superiority. In the United Kingdom, regional health board funding decisions can have profound impact on the provision of ICU services. Swings in the strength of the local economy and labor market will also impact funding and staffing over time. Finally, local news stories, especially if suggestive of poor care, can sway public opinion, engage local politicians, and pressure hospital administrators to change the provision of services.

National factors also affect ICU delivery. Obvious factors include overall healthcare policy and funding decisions. There is usually close interaction between funding agencies, such as government health departments, and national professional organizations and accreditation bodies. These different agencies and organizations are responsible for implementing standards for training and certification and may also determine the number of training positions and work hours, which influence current and future supply of acute care health providers. In addition to these factors, there are a number of less obvious national influences, such as the overall financial health of the nation and its commitment to healthcare spending, the prevailing cultural values, legislative and judicial processes both directly and indirectly related to healthcare, and media representation of acute illness. For example, in the United States, the Leapfrog group, a national consortium of Fortune 500 companies, is currently pressuring hospitals to staff ICUs with full-time intensivists. Leapfrog believes current ICU staffing is inadequate and hopes external pressure can lead to improved healthcare quality, reduced healthcare costs, and, ultimately, reduced health insurance premiums for the workforce employed by its member companies. Leapfrog is promoting change through public awareness, and has been remarkably successful in gaining high profile media coverage, and through financial incentives to health insurance companies to force provider compliance.

Another recent example was the sudden, large increase in resources for intensive care by the UK government. While the rationale was multifactorial, the considerable media coverage that highlighted an apparent lack of availability of ICU beds seemed to play a key role.

The Episode of Care for the Acutely Ill

Care for the acutely ill clearly extends beyond the walls of the ICU (Fig. 2). An episode of acute illness can require care at a number of different points, and be influenced by a number of different characteristics. While the ICU serves as a simple demonstration of the complexity and hierarchy of influences on acute care delivery, the reality is further complicated by the number of different elements in the care process, and changes at any point in the chain of care may have important consequences for the patient's outcome. For example, Cook et al. dis-

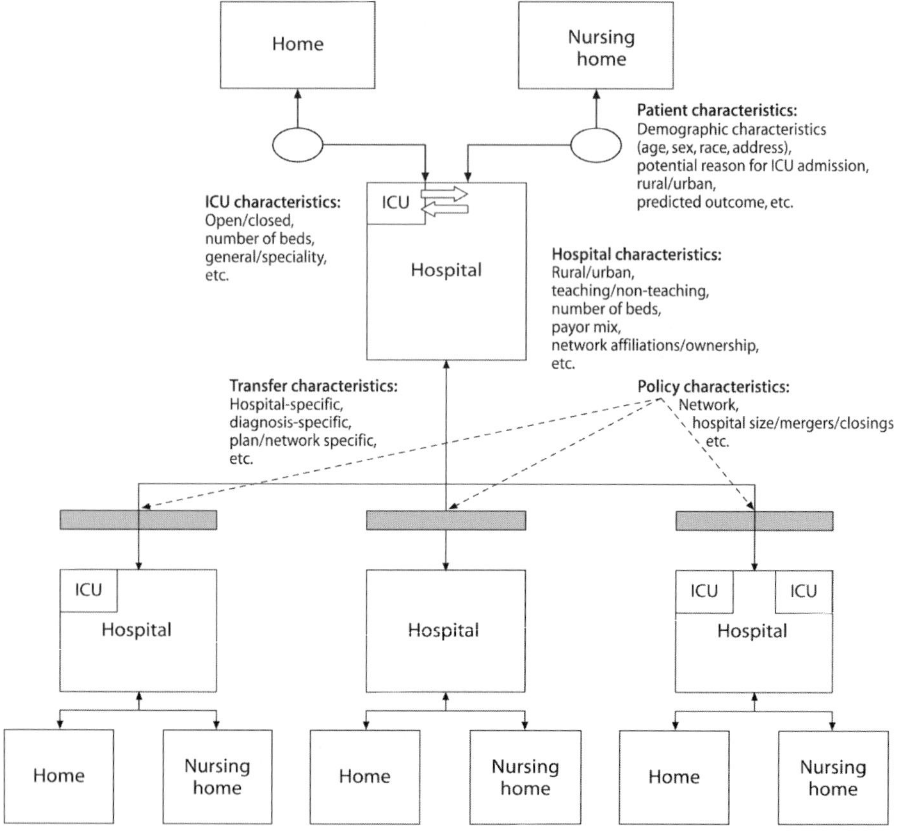

Fig. 2. The chain of care for the critically ill. The care for a critically ill patient extends beyond the specific ICU that takes care of him or her. It is a chain of actions stretching from the location where the critical illness first occurred (e.g., home) to the location where the critical illness has resolved (from [64] with permission).

cussed how the ICU might 'outreach' to affect care on the floor (e.g., through the use of medical emergency teams (METs)), finding acutely deteriorating patients sooner, and thus hopefully improving outcomes. [1].

One side-effect of embracing the complexity of extended acute care at multiple time-points by multiple providers is that we complicate measurement, feedback, and behavior modification. This is because there are now a number of different clinician groups to target, optimal strategies for improvement may differ across groups, and determining what the output of the care is that should be measured, and when, is less clear. For example, should adjustment for severity of illness be assessed before ICU admission? If so, how soon? Should the outcome be at hospital discharge? If so, and outcome improves, was it due to changes in pre-ICU or intra-ICU care?

The Current Provision of Care for the Acutely Ill

Although a relatively young field, intensive care has grown rapidly in recent decades. For example, in the United States, there are approximately 6,000 ICUs in the 4,000 acute care hospitals caring for 5–6 million Americans, or 2% of the population, each year. Nominally, the reasons for ICU care are to provide physiologic monitoring and life support as needed to patients who are either acutely ill or at risk of acute deterioration. In other countries, the same level of care may be provided elsewhere in the hospital, such as on the regular floor or in a high dependency unit. The common theme, however, is that a place in the hospital is dedicated to care of the acutely ill. The evidence that creating such a place improves outcomes is scant at best. There are early studies supporting the value of admitting patients post myocardial infarction to a coronary care unit for cardiac monitoring and defibrillation when indicated [2–4], and anecdotal reports of improved outcomes for trauma and burns patients when cared for in specialized ICUs.[5–8] However, there are no large, contemporary trials of specialized care environments, such as an ICU, for acutely ill adults. Furthermore, a large population-based study of ICU care comparing western Massachusetts in the US to the province of Alberta in Canada found 2–3 times higher provision of ICU services in western Massachusetts but no difference in outcome [9].

There is an empiric argument for creating a place dedicated to the provision of acute care. The staff working in that place can be trained specifically for management of acute illnesses and gain further expertise through constant practice. This argument is analogous to the contention that surgery is better performed at high volume centers [10, 11]. There is also circumstantial evidence in support of specialized acute care services. Goldfrad and Rowan demonstrated that patients discharged prematurely from ICUs due to bed pressure incurred a significantly higher hospital mortality.[12] If ICU care was not beneficial, then early discharge to the hospital floor should not have affected outcome. Similarly, the UK collaborative extracorporeal membrane oxygenation (ECMO) trial found that babies transferred to regional ECMO centers, where there was a higher level of specialized acute care services, had markedly improved outcomes that extended even to the babies that did not receive ECMO [13]. Nathens and Turkovich recently reported that statewide trauma systems in the US, with referral of the sickest patients to centers of expertise, significantly improved outcomes [14].

As noted above, not all ICUs are equivalent. Many studies have suggested that ICU staffing may affect patient outcome. In the United States in particular, many ICUs do not have dedicated intensivist physician staffing. Yet, numerous studies suggest that intensivist-staffed ICUs have lower mortality rates, and possibly more efficient use of resources [15]. Recently, Tarnow-Mordi et al also highlighted the importance of nurse staffing in the ICU, reporting that patients were significantly more likely to die when cared for in the ICU during periods of peak occupancy, when nurses were overloaded with work [16]. Importantly, the magnitude of differences in outcome associated with these staffing patterns is as large, and often larger, than that reported for many drugs and devices used in the acutely ill.

Organizing care for the acutely ill in a particular place can also have a number of unintended, harmful consequences. For example, the necessities of round-the-clock acute care lead to significant noise and light pollution in the ICU, which may have a variety of consequences for the patient, including sleep deprivation and psychological disturbances [17]. Treatment for these sequelae is often increased use of sedative and neurotropic agents, which themselves may have both short and long-term consequences, including prolonged mechanical ventilation with increased risk of nosocomial infection, chemical dependency, extrapyramidal symptoms, social isolation from relatives and staff, and residual neuropsychological impairment [18–21]. The ICU may also promote a culture of overly aggressive use of diagnostic and interventional strategies, many of which may have harmful side-effects, such as the increased risk of pulmonary embolus with pulmonary artery catheterization [22]. Such a care strategy, especially for a patient unable to communicate his or her treatment preferences, may lead to unwanted care, angry relatives, and, for those patients who die, poor end-of-life care.

Some of the studies quoted above suggest that regionalizing care of the acutely ill may offer significant advantages. Scarce, expensive resources can be consolidated in a single center where their use can be optimized and the staff can gain the most concentrated training and expertise. Regionalization today exists in four main areas of acute illness: neonatal intensive care, trauma care, burn care, and certain specialized surgical services. There is evidence in each of these areas that outcomes are improved with regionalization [13, 14, 23]. However, there are many barriers to regionalization and even these acute care services are often only partially regionalized. For example, in the United States, 40% of all neonates who are ventilated and die do so without transfer to a tertiary care center.[24] There are many potential barriers to regionalization. The requisite communications and referral infrastructure may be missing or inadequate, patients and families may be unwilling to travel for care, and their local caregivers may be reluctant to cede control to the regional center.

These sobering facts should, of course, be balanced with consideration of the many positive aspects of intensive care. Huge technologic and scientific advances have been made in our understanding of critical illness and the ways in which we can best care for it. Over the last few years, there has been a profusion of large, high quality randomized clinical trials shedding light on the optimal way to care for ICU patients. We now have high quality evidence informing us on optimal ventilator management and weaning [25], prevention of ICU complications such as pneumonia [26, 27], stress ulcers [28], and deep venous thromboses [29], and treatment of ICU syndromes, such as severe sepsis [30–32]. In addition, there are now several collaborations, such as the Canadian Critical Care Trials Group (CCCTG), the Australian and New Zealand Intensive Care Society (ANZICS) trial group, and the NIH ARDS Network, that are continuing to conduct large, high quality randomized trials that will shed further light on how best to provide critical care.

There are also many large scale private, academic, and government efforts to monitor and improve the quality of intensive care delivery. Examples from the US include the Leapfrog Group initiative to promote intensivist staffing in non-rural ICUs [33–36], development and assessment of ICU quality measures by the Joint Commission on Accreditation of Hospitals Organization (JCAHO) [37], regional and statewide severity-adjusted outcomes reporting [38, 39], and the VHA Inc. effort to promote and measure use of evidence-based care bundles for ventilated patients and patients with severe sepsis [40]. Similar efforts are underway in Europe, Canada, Australia and elsewhere. Thus, both the intensive care specialties and the stakeholder groups that pay for, or use, intensive care are becoming increasingly active in addressing a number of the key barriers to optimal, high quality intensive care.

Future Demand for Care of the Acutely Ill

Regardless of our level of satisfaction with current services, we must plan for changes. The post-World War II 'baby boom' populations of Europe and the United States are entering their sixth and seventh decades, peak ages for incurring acute illnesses. In the United States, there are currently no plans to increase the number of training positions for intensivists. Thus, based on demographic changes alone, a person's likelihood of receiving intensivist-led ICU care is anticipated to decrease considerably in the next 10–20 years [41]. Furthermore, it is unrealistic to believe that the only demand for ICU services will be driven by demographic change. Since 1990, with only a small change in population characteristics, ICU use has grown in the US by almost 30% [42–44]. Despite the oft-quoted belief that technologic advance would lead to reduced healthcare resource consumption, new advances consistently drive up our demand for health services [23, 45]. In the United Kingdom, where there was a fixed cap on the provision of ICU services during the 1990s, demand for ICU care resulted in a three-fold increase in the number of premature discharges [12]. Thus, it seems likely that we must actively plan to provide acute care to more people, and find efficient ways to do so given the limited healthcare budget.

Ideal Characteristics of an Acute Care Delivery System

I posit that the ideal system would have the following features. First, we would retain the ICU as a focused location for the provision of acute care services to the sickest patients. This approach has the conceptual advantage of concentrated expertise and technologic support. However, better standardization of the capabilities of an ICU is essential. In addition, the transition into and out of the ICU must be better delineated both to ensure efficient use of resources and to provide a better continuum of care. Systems such as METs may help standardize and improve pre-ICU care[46–48] while post-ICU follow-up clinics are one example of a more gradual 'hand-off' of the sequelae of critical illnesses to the primary care providers [49, 50]. Although 24/7 staffing by intensivists is desirable, this seems impractical, given workforce and funding constraints. Thus, some sort of levels of ICU are necessary, such as those proposed recently by the American College of Critical Care [51]. The best use of different levels of ICUs is obviously triage of the sickest patients to the highest level ICUs, which is *de facto* regionalization.

Distributing ICU Services Optimally Across Regions and Systems

Currently, there is no systematic approach to ensure which patients are admitted to ICUs and when. In the absence of such a system, a patient who may benefit from ICU care may or may not receive that care simply based on the hospital in which she receives care. This almost certainly means a suboptimal matching of ICU services to population needs. Furthermore, it is possible that different ICUs have different levels of expertise, as proposed by the American College of Critical Care Medicine [52]. Yet, there is no system to triage patients to different levels, based on need. In contrast, the introduction of regionalized ICU care for neonates and for trauma victims has demonstrated a clear improvement in overall outcomes [13, 53]. Although the introduction of regionalized care for all adult ICU use is somewhat daunting, and associated with significant barriers, it seems that such an approach will be essential if ICU services are to be used most efficiently and most optimally.

To ensure regionalization works, I would encourage estimates of the need for a certain number of ICUs of different levels for a given community. Then, there must be standard entry criteria and an appropriate communications and referral system. Creating and enforcing such a system is not straightforward. Trauma systems have the following advantageous characteristics. Their creation was mandated and funded at the state government level; triage is aided by a simple classification of injury severity, the Injury Severity System [54], which can be calculated in the field by paramedics, and the allocation of all cases can be routed through a regional radio command post.

In comparison, a broad ICU triage and regionalization system has the following problems. First, there is no regional or national mandate or funding for regionalized care. Indeed, in many markets, hospitals competing against each other will seek to duplicate services. As an example, in 1994 32% of ECMO cases were >20 miles, and 22% were >40 miles, away from the regional ECMO centers in California [24]. Almost half of these centers performed only ≥5 ECMO runs per year, even though the ELSO recommends 12 per year as a minimum standard [55]. Second, we do not currently have any broad patient classification system that determines need for ICU care. Indeed, ICU severity adjustment systems typically calculate risk of death after ICU admission [56–59]. Finally, patients developing acute illness do so in a variety of settings, including the operating room and the hospital floor. There is no common communications system that will know of all these patients in time to triage their care. Furthermore, the correct decision might be to limit certain surgical procedures to institutions that have the appropriate ICU services should complications develop. This requires major systems changes that are unlikely to happen without the appropriate political will.

Recruiting and Maintaining the Optimal ICU Workforce

Currently, most ICU patients are not cared for by physicians trained in intensive care. Likewise, ICUs across the country face difficulties recruiting and retaining nursing staff. The difficulties will increase as an aging population creates increased demand for ICU services. Although the number of training positions could be increased, these positions may not be filled, and the expansion in positions required if this were to be the only solution seems unrealistically high. Therefore, a multipronged approach with alternative staffing models seem essential. For the physician shortage, collaborative care models with hospitalists and emergency medicine physicians should probably be explored. Physician extender models, such as use of nurse practitioners or physician assistants [60], may also be helpful. And, the use of telemedicine, as demonstrated in a pilot study by Rosenfeld et al [61], holds promise. The nursing challenge may be even more difficult to meet. In all areas of healthcare, it has been increasingly difficult to maintain a nursing workforce. Numerous efforts to protect the workforce have already been employed in recent years, yet the problem continues. The crux is that a career in nursing is simply less attractive than it once was. For physician and nursing staff, the keys will be to determine adequate levels of training and capabilities required for staff working in the ICU and to adequately fund the appropriate initiatives.

Providing Critical Care Outside the ICU

Even though there will be challenges providing adequate staffing within the ICU, we are also going to have to confront the need to provide adequate care for the critically ill outside the ICU. Rivers et al. have demonstrated the importance of early, aggressive resuscitation prior to ICU admission [31], several groups have demonstrated the value of METs leaving the ICU to stabilize and treat hospital floor patients who have acute crises [47, 62], and others have also demonstrated that involvement of ICU staff in the care of patients after ICU discharge appears to improve outcome [46]. Determining how to systematically and efficiently deliver critical care in these settings will be an important safety and quality goal in the future.

Harnessing Insight into the Pathophysiology of Critical Illness

Although there has been great insight into the pathophysiology of injury, response to injury, and organ dysfunction, the payoff in terms of changed care paradigms has been small thus far. We still have no reliable markers of the host response to injury that can be used to guide therapy. A recent study of antibiotic therapy tied to procalcitonin yielded very promising results [63], but much work remains in this area. Similarly, the only specific agent approved by the U.S. FDA for severe sepsis is recombinant activated protein C, while many other promising agents have so far failed to improve survival in randomized trials. It is attractive to consider the possibility that we will eventually have a wider array of therapies in our armamentarium to be used in a titrated fashion, tailored to augment an individual's response to injury.

Engaging Patients and Families in the Care Process

Intensive care is one of the most technologic and de-humanizing parts of medicine. Patients are frequently incompetent and unable to communicate and often require considerable pharmacologic and mechanical support; the ICU is often a harsh environment, with considerable noise and light pollution; and families are under considerable stress because of uncertainty over the fate of their loved one. It is essential that we tackle these issues head on. There are several challenges. For example, we need drugs that control pain and agitation without inducing coma or delirium. We need to promote better communication skills in ICU staff. We need better decision support tools that allow patients, families and staff to better understand prognosis and the change in prognosis associated with alternative care strategies. And, we need to find ways to build and run ICUs that are less harsh, perhaps with open visiting hours, rooms that are more private and attractive, and life support and monitoring techniques that are less invasive.

Promoting Public Awareness of Intensive Care

Despite the huge impact critical care now has on health, it remains outside the public consciousness. This is almost certainly an important handicap. Great advances in medicine have come through better partnering of the healthcare system with the public and patients. For example, until just a few years ago, treatment decisions for prostatic hypertrophy were based on measurements of micturition. However, once a better understanding of patients' preferences was elicited, the entire paradigm of care changed such that treatment is now based primarily on a patient's choice after weighing the trade-offs of incontinence and impotence. It is highly likely that a variety of ICU care decisions might be made differently if we knew more about how to titrate care options to meet a patient's or family's preferences. Of course, this requires a greater understanding by the general public of intensive care, when it is required, and what it provides. Otherwise, intensive care will continue to be provided to patients often unable to communicate their preferences and families often unprepared to make carefully considered decisions. A greater understanding by the public will also help forge and promote research priorities and standards of care in intensive care.

Conclusion

Intensive care has become an important part of the healthcare system. However, it is still provided in a very heterogeneous, and likely suboptimal, fashion. Future challenges will include providing an adequate workforce, ensuring critical care is delivered to the right patients at the right time, converting advances in our understanding of the biology of critical illness into improved care and outcomes, and partnering successfully with patients, families, and society in forging the critical care of the future.

References

1. Cook DJ, Montori VM, McMullin JP, Finfer SR, Rocker GM (2004) Improving patients' safety locally: Changing clinician behaviour. Lancet 363:1224–1230
2. Bosch X, Verbal F, Lopez de Sa E, et al (2004) [Differences in the management and prognosis of patients with non-ST segment elevation acute coronary syndrome according to the department of initial admission]. Rev Esp Cardiol 57:283–290
3. Bosch X, Perez J, Ferrer E, et al (2003) [Clinical characteristics, management, and prognosis of patients with acute myocardial infarction not admitted to the coronary care unit. Usefulness of an intermediate care unit as the initial admission site]. Rev Esp Cardiol 56:262–270
4. Silva P, Galli M, Campolo L (1993) Prognostic significance of early ischemia after acute myocardial infarction in low-risk patients. IRES (Ischemia Residua) Study Group. Am J Cardiol 71:1142–1147
5. Marmarou A, Anderson RL, Ward JD, Choi SC, Young HF (1991) NINDS traumatic coma date bank: intracranial pressure monitoring methodology. J Neurosurg 75(Suppl):S21–S27
6. (1984) Guidelines for initial management after head injury in adults. Suggestions from a group of neurosurgeons. Br Med J (Clin Res Ed) 288:983–985
7. Park CA, McGwin GJ, Smith DR, et al (2001) Trauma-specific intensive care units can be cost effective and contribute to reduced hospital length of stay. Am Surg 67:665–670
8. Herruzo-Cabrera R, Fernandez-Arjona M, Garcia-Torres V, Martinez-Ratero S, Lenguas-Portero F, Rey-Calero J (1995) Mortality evolution study of burn patients in a critical care burn unit between 1971 and 1991. Burns 21:106-109
9. Rapoport J, Teres D, Barnett R, et al (1995) A comparison of intensive care unit utilization in Alberta and western Massachusetts. Crit Care Med 23:1336–1346
10. Birkmeyer JD, Siewers AE, Finlayson EVA, et al (2002) Hospital volume and surgical mortality in the United States. N Engl J Med 346:1128–1137
11. Dudley RA, Johansen KL, Brand R, Rennie DJ, Milstein A (2000) Selective referral to high-volume hospitals: Estimating potentially avoidable deaths. JAMA 283:1159–1166
12. Goldfrad C, Rowan K (2000) Consequences of discharges from intensive care at night. Lancet 355:1138–1142
13. UK Collaborative ECMO Trial Group (1996) UK collaborative randomised trial of neonatal extracorporeal membrane oxygenation. Lancet 348:75–82
14. Nathens AB, Jurkovich GJ (2000) The effect of organized systems of trauma care on motor vehicle crash mortality. JAMA 283:1990–1994
15. Pronovost PJ, Angus DC, Dorman T, Robinson KA, Dremsizov TT, Young TL (2002) Physician staffing patterns and clinical outcomes in critically ill patients. A systematic review. JAMA 288:2151–2162
16. Tarnow-Mordi WO, Hau C, Warden A, Shearer AJ (2000) Hospital mortality in relation to staff workload: a 4-year study in an adult intensive-care unit. Lancet 356:185–189
17. Cooper AB, Thornley KS, Young GB, Slutsky AS, Stewart TE, Hanly PJ (2000) Sleep in critically ill patients requiring mechanical ventilation. Chest 117:809–818
18. Hopkins RO, Weaver LK, Pope D, Orme JF, Bigler ED, Larson-Lohr V (1999) Neuropsychological sequelae and impaired health status in survivors of severe acute respiratory distress syndrome. Am J Respir Crit Care Med 160:50–56

19. Hudson LD, Lee CM (2003) Neuromuscular sequelae of critical illness. N Engl J Med 348:745–747
20. Ibrahim EH, Ward S, Sherman G, Kollef MH (2000) A comparative analysis of patients with early-onset vs late-onset nosocomial pneumonia in the ICU setting. Chest 117:1434–1442
21. Rello J, Quintana E, Ausina V, et al (1991) Incidence, etiology, and outcome of nosocomial pneumonia in mechanically ventilated patients. Chest 100:439–444
22. Sandham JD, Hull RD, Brant RF, et al (2003) A randomized, controlled trial of the use of pulmonary-artery catheters in high-risk surgical patients. N Engl J Med 348:5–14
23. McClellan M (1996) Are the returns to technological change in health care declining? Proc Natl Acad Sci USA 93:12701–12708
24. Angus DC, Linde-Zwirble WT, Griffin M, Clermont G, Clark RH (2001) Epidemiology of neonatal respiratory failure in the US: Projections from California and New York. Am J Respir Crit Care Med 164:1154–1160
25. Ely EW, Baker AM, Dunagan DP, et al (1996) Effect on the duration of mechanical ventilation of identifying patients capable of breathing spontaneously. N Engl J Med 335:1864–1869
26. The ARDS Network (2000) Ventilation with lower tidal volumes as compared with traditional tidal volumes for acute lung injury and the acute respiratory distress syndrome. N Engl J Med 342:1301–1308
27. Drakulovic MB, Torres A, Bauer TT, Nicolas JM, Nogue S, Ferrer M (1999) Supine body position as a risk factor for nosocomial pneumonia in mechanically ventilated patients: a randomised trial. Lancet 354:1851–1858
28. Cook DJ, Reeve BK, Guyatt GH, et al (1996) Stress ulcer prophylaxis in critically ill patients. Resolving discordant meta-analyses. JAMA 275:308–314
29. O'Grady NP, Alexander M, Dellinger EP, et al (2002) Guidelines for the prevention of intravascular catheter-related infections. Centers for Disease Control and Prevention. MMWR Recomm Rep 51:1–29
30. Bernard GR, Vincent JL, Laterre PF, et al (2001) Efficacy and safety of recombinant human activated protein C for severe sepsis. N Engl J Med 344:699–709
31. Rivers E, Nguyen B, Havstad S, et al (2001) Early goal-directed therapy in the treatment of severe sepsis and septic shock. N Engl J Med 345:1368–1377
32. Annane D, Sebille V, Charpentier C, et al (2002) Effect of treatment with low doses of hydrocortisone and fludrocortisone on mortality in patients with septic shock. JAMA 288:862–871
33. Galvin R, Milstein A (2002) Large employers' new strategies in health care. N Engl J Med 347:939–942
34. Birkmeyer JD, Dimick JB (2004) Leapfrog patient safety standards 2003: The potential benefits of universal adoption. At: http://leapfroggroup.org/media/file/Leapfrog-Birkmeyer.pdf, Accessed July 2005
35. Pronovost PJ, Needham DM, Waters H, et al (2004) Intensive care unit physician staffing: Financial modeling of the Leapfrog standard. Crit Care Med 32:1247–1253
36. Young MP, Birkmeyer JD (2000) Potential reduction in mortality rates using an intensivist model to manage intensive care units. Eff Clin Pract 3:284–289
37. JCAHO (2004) National Patient Safety Goals. At: http://www.jcaho.org/accredited+organizations/patient+safety/04+npsg/index.htm. Accessed July 2005
38. Sirio CA, Shepardson LB, Rotondi AJ, et al (1999) Community-wide assessment of intensive care outcomes using a physiologically-based prognostic measure: Implications for critical care delivery from Cleveland Health Quality Choice. Chest 115:793–801
39. (2003) Michigan begins initiative to improve ICUs. Critical Connections 1.
40. Pronovost PJ, Berenholtz SM (2004) Improving Sepsis Care in the Intensive Care Unit: An Evidence-Based Approach. VHA Health Foundation, Irving

41. Angus DC (2001) Demands of an aging population for critical care and pulmonary service: In reply to letters to the editor. JAMA 285:1018
42. Halpern NA, Pastores SM, Greenstein RJ (2004) Critical care medicine in the United States 1985–2000: An analysis of bed numbers, use, and costs. Crit Care Med 32:1254–1259
43. Kersten A, Milbrandt EB, Rahim MT, et al (2003) How big is critical care in the US? Crit Care Med 31 (Suppl):A8 (abst)
44. Rahim MT, Milbrandt EB, Dremsizov TT, et al (2003) Pricing critical care: An updated Russell equation. Crit Care Med 31 (Suppl):A8 (abst)
45. Fuchs VR (1999) Health care for the elderly: how much? Who will pay for it? Health Aff (Millwood) 18:11–21
46. Angus DC, Carlet J, on behalf of the 2002 Brussels Roundtable Participants (2003) Surviving intensive care: A report from the 2002 Brussels Roundtable. Intensive Care Med 29:368–377
47. Bellomo R, Goldsmith D, Uchino S, et al (2003) A prospective before-and-after trial of a medical emergency team. Med J Aust 179:283–287
48. Bellomo R, Goldsmith D, Uchino S, et al (2004) Prospective controlled trial of effect of medical emergency team on postoperative morbidity and mortality rates. Crit Care Med 32:916–921
49. Young C, Millo JL, Salmon J (2002) Reduction in post-ICU, in-hospital mortality following the introduction of an ICU nursing outreach service. Crit Care 6 (Suppl 1):S117 (abst)
50. McMullin J, Cook DJ (2003) Changing ICU behavior to focus on long-term outcomes. In: Angus DC, Carlet J (eds) Surviving Intensive Care: Update in Intensive Care and Emergency Medicine No. 39. Springer-Verlag, Berlin, p 287–296
51. Task Force of the American College of Critical Care Medicine, Society of Critical Care Medicine (1999) Guidelines for intensive care unit admission, discharge, and triage. Crit Care Med 27:633–638
52. Haupt MT, Bekes CE, Brilli RJ, et al (2003) Guidelines on critical care services and personnel: Recommendations based on a system of categorization of three levels of care. Crit Care Med 31:2677–2683
53. Nathens AB, Jurkovich GJ, Maier RV, et al (2001) Relationship between trauma center volume and outcomes. JAMA 285:1164–1171
54. Baker SP, O'Neill B, Haddon WJ, Long WB (1974) The injury severity score: A method for describing patients with multiple injuries and evaluating emergency care. J Trauma 14:187–196
55. Extracorporeal Life Support Organization (1997) ELSO Guidelines for Neonatal ECMO Centers. At: http://www.elso.med.umich.edu/guide.htm. Accessed July 2005
56. Knaus WA, Draper EA, Wagner DP, Zimmerman JE (1985) APACHE II: A severity of disease classification system. Crit Care Med 13:818–829
57. Knaus WA, Wagner DP, Draper EA, et al (1991) The APACHE III prognostic system. Risk prediction of hospital mortality for critically ill hospitalized adults. Chest 100:1619–1636
58. Lemeshow S, Teres D, Klar J, Avrunin JS, Gehlbach SH, Rapoport J (1993) Mortality Probability Models (MPM II) based on an international cohort of intensive care unit patients. JAMA 270:2478–2486
59. Le Gall JR, Lemeshow S, Saulnier F (1993) A new Simplified Acute Physiology Score (SAPS II) based on a European/North American multicenter study. JAMA 270:2957–2963
60. Snyder JV, Sirio CA, Angus DC, et al (1994) Trial of nurse practitioners in intensive care. New Horiz 2:296–304
61. Rosenfeld BA, Dorman T, Breslow MJ, et al (2000) Intensive care unit telemedicine: Alternate paradigm for providing continuous intensivist care. Crit Care Med 28:3925–3931
62. Bellomo R, Goldsmith D, Uchino S, et al (2004) A prospective controlled trial of the effect of the medical emergency team on post-operative morbidity and mortality. Crit Care Med 32:916–921

63. Christ-Crain M, Jaccard-Stolz D, Bingisser R, et al (2004) Effect of procalcitonin-guided treatment on antibiotic use and outcome in lower respiratory tract infections: cluster-randomised, single-blinded intervention trial. Lancet 363:600–607
64. Angus DC, Black N (2004) Improving care of the critically ill: Institutional and health-care system approaches. Lancet 363:1314–1320

Expectations Around Intensive Care – 10 Years On

K. Hillman

"What is the future, after all, but a structure of hopes and expectations? Its residence is in the wind; it has no reality....... "
What is marvellous about the present is that we have succeeded......."

J.M. Coetzee, Nobel Prize for literature.

Introduction

The future of the specialty of Intensive Care will be determined as much by the expectations of society and governments as by the discovery of new drugs and ventilatory modes. Societal expectations currently are based around rapid advances in all aspects of medicine, which can alienate dying as a failure to our management rather than a national and normal part of life. Managing expectations around what intensive care medicine can realistically offer will increasingly involve our profession instigating and being part of a discourse with governments and our society.

Intensive care emerged in the early 1950s and, over a relatively short time, has developed into a medical and nursing specialty, taking its place among other specialties in most large and even many smaller hospitals.

The role of intensive care medicine has expanded rapidly, largely as a result of the changing nature of acute hospitals. Before the 1950s, most acute hospitals were much the same in what they had to offer. There were no antibiotics; no chemotherapy; no therapeutic or diagnostic endoscopy; little in the way of radiography; no nuclear medicine; little cardiac and neurosurgery; few specialized anesthetic or recovery units to support operative services; and no means of supporting organ failure such as dialysis and artificial ventilation.

Hospitals were often places where patients were cared for when convalescing after surgery or being nursed while the disease took its own course, such as with tuberculosis or other serious infections. While the medical profession may not have always been completely transparent about what little they had to offer, the community had few expectations and usually realized the real meaning of the euphemisms around the disease prognosis and the widespread acceptance of dying.

The development of intensive care coincided with the need for patients to be temporarily supported during a life-threatening phase of their illness while the potentially treatable component was managed with the increasing availability of complex procedures and powerful drugs. We became competent at sustaining life with interventions such as artificial ventilation, dialysis and inotropes, supported by sophisticated monitoring and expert nursing. These life-sustaining skills coincided with rapid developments by other medical specialties, which required temporary support in an intensive care unit (ICU). We no longer had to actively look for business. Intensive care was an essential adjunct to widespread advances in complex therapies. We kept the patients alive while they recovered from their procedures or waited for the effect of the drugs. The level of intensive care provided in a hospital now determines the role of acute hospitals as much as the ICU is determined by the function of the acute hospital [1].

Community Expectations

Expectations have developed around the role of intensive care and acute hospitals. The community is constantly deluged with reports of miracles around what health care can offer. Rarely does a week go by when we do not read or hear about life-saving drugs and procedures in the lay media. The medical research industry attracts good minds and seemingly endless funding. Increasing numbers of medical journals are published in order to report all these advances. The result is that patients admitted to hospital now usually expect to be cured in one way or another; no matter how old or sick they are. The community, governments, the research industry, the media, and the health care industry itself are complicit around this image. Aging and dying are no longer naturally accepted as an inevitable part of life. There is little motivation to challenge this image of modern health care. Government and funders of health care would be accused of simply wanting to save money; private industry would not benefit from a more realistic portrayal of the limitations of health care; and the community wants to believe that most diseases can now be cured. Finally, it probably enhances the self-image of the medical profession to be positive about what can be offered, rather than emphasize its limitations. Moreover, many of our medical colleagues do not understand the limitations of intensive care. They observe miracle cures as a result of intensive care when previously patients died. Because of increasing specialization, our colleagues understand little about what we do and what our limitations are.

Many of our colleagues have had no training in, or education around, intensive care medicine and see it as an area where their sickest patients go and hopefully are returned to their care, cured. We are now faced with the reality that many patients are now admitted to hospital when they are seriously ill, whether they have a treatable or curable disease or not. As intensivists we are pressured to take an increasing proportion of these patients into intensive care. Approximately 70% of total health care costs in our society are spent during the last three months of people's lives.

I would like to think that my specialty will, within 10 years, initiate and facilitate the community debate which needs to occur around these issues. There are no easy answers but intensivists are in the unique position to understand what ICUs can offer but also where their limitations are. The ICU in 10 years will also have a more honest and transparent dialog with other hospital specialists as well as prospective patients and their carers. Their clinical experience backed up by research will enable them to resist pressures to simply prolong dying. We will increasingly become the experts on dying and the limits of futile treatment in acute hospitals. Our specialty will become more actively consulted on these issues, rather than being simple technicians, indiscriminately applying their technologies. I can see that the specialty of palliative care will also become more involved in the dying processes in acute hospitals and we will work more closely with these specialists to establish guidelines and policies around futile care.

Hospital Safety Expectations

The community is also increasingly expecting a consistent and high standard of care in acute hospitals. Large studies have demonstrated high levels of preventable hospital deaths [2, 3]. Many of these patients suffer a slow unrecognized deterioration whilst in hospital [4-6]. At-risk patients are recognized late and often cared for by medical staff not trained or experienced in acute medicine [7]. Moreover we know that delayed admission to the ICU adversely affects outcome [8, 9] and that late resuscitation, even if it is aggressive and goal orientated is not effective [10, 11], whereas early resuscitation of seriously ill patients results in improved outcomes [12].

Intensive care clinicians are increasingly involved in systems aimed at improving patient safety outside the walls of their own ICUs [13-15].

Expectations Around the Boundaries of Intensive Care

While we needed the security of the four walls of ICU to nurture our specialty, it will become increasingly obvious that the geography of an ICU does not determine the needs of the seriously ill.

Already in many countries there are systems such as the Medical Emergency Team (MET), developed and run by intensive care clinicians specifically designed to recognize at-risk patients early and to provide rapid stabilization and resuscitation. Outreach teams from ICUs provide expert opinion on the seriously ill as well as educational support [16].

Staff from intensive care are often involved in many other activities in sites outside their own units [15]. These include acute resuscitation in emergency departments; being integral members of trauma teams; providing a hospital central line service; maintaining a parenteral nutrition service; and running outpatients to follow-up patients who have been managed in ICUs. Obviously extra funding is necessary to provide such services from the ICU. The ICU in 10 years will increasingly become the center of such activities.

The nature of acute hospitals will also drive many of these changes. The hospital population will become older with more co-morbidities. Staff from ICUs in 10 years time will be involved with, and consulted about, how to manage the seriously ill in acute hospitals. The boundaries of the ICU will become less distinct as we consider optimal care regardless of whether the patient is within the ICU or not. Number of ICU beds will be greater and high dependency units (HDUs) managed by trained and experienced intensivists will be more numerous. Patients will be admitted earlier into ICU/HDU in order to stabilize them before serious cellular damage occurs. Instead of being discharged as soon as they are extubated, patients will remain in a more appropriate HDU environment until it is safe to place them in a general ward environment. Expectations of the community and health care providers for greater safety of at-risk patients in acute hospitals will drive much of this process.

Expectations around patient safety will change the role of the intensivist. In 10 years time they will have a higher profile as acute care physicians in hospitals. This trend will increase as a result of increasing specialization by our medical colleagues, who are often not trained or experienced in acute medicine and yet are responsible for overall patient care in a hospital population who are not only increasingly at-risk but also have multiorgan problems. The single organ specialist will have a more limited role caring for ambulant outpatients rather than seriously ill patients [1].

The expectations of government and those responsible for health care provision will reflect the community's expectations around standards of patient safety in acute hospitals with increasing pressures for more ICU and HDU beds and more involvement of intensivists in the seriously ill and at-risk patients outside the ICU.

There will come a point where intensive and expensive treatment in an ICU during the last few days of life will be questioned, if only on the basis of cost and scarcity of resources alone. However, I believe the ICU in 10 years will be larger; often with HDUs attached. Both will be managed by nurses and doctors specifically trained in acute medicine within a multiorgan perspective. There will be a greater number of intensivists and more round the clock presence of intensive care specialists, both within ICUs and in systems designed to care for seriously ill patients across the hospital.

Expectations of Intensive Care Nursing Staff

The expectations of intensive care nursing staff may also change within 10 years. In order to overcome nursing shortage challenges, the role of the specialist nurse will probably change. They will be performing a greater range of functions with less direct input from the medical profession, accompanied by less involvement of junior medical staff apart from their role as trainees. Routine care of the seriously ill will be increasingly evidence based, conducted according to protocols and performed by nursing staff, e.g., ventilator and dialysis management; fluid challenges; rates of inotrope support; levels of sedation; stress ulcer prophylaxis; control of blood sugar; and feeding.

Procedures such as intravenous and intra-arterial cannulization and performing routine pathology could also be conducted by nursing staff, leaving the role of intensive care medical specialists to address more complex medical issues and overall medical management direction.

Expectations of Intensive Care Medical Staff

Expectations around the long hours on duty and on-call by intensivists may also change, resulting in a greater number of intensivists to share the workload as well as a change in their role as outlined above in relation to the change in the nursing role.

Whether physicians agree or not, they will have greater involvement in how their ICU is managed and along with a high clinical workload will be expected to contribute increasingly to the administration of the ICU. The ICU will not only have more beds in 10 years time, it will have increased support staff and space in order to manage a complex and high cost environment.

The expectations of medical staff may not necessarily coincide with those of the community and neither of these expectations may coincide with expectations of health care funders. The intensivist will play an increasingly important role in the discourse and debate around resolving the dilemma of higher cost care with resources that are not infinite. Our specialty could drain a large and increasing percentage of a country's gross national product. It would be a brave politician who will cap our expenditure if it involves the immediate shortening of someone's life.

Conclusion

Within 10 years, our ICU will be the source of greater discussions with the community about limits of therapy and futile care. The intensivist of the future will be involved with increasing numbers of patients having end-of-life care, even if it is to arbitrate and consult on the potential benefit of ICU admission. If trends continue, the standards of excellence we have provided will be demanded by most people in our society just in case a miracle can be performed and a few extra days of life extracted. Our units will need to arbitrate community expectations with our own expectations of what we can achieve. The ICU's role will increasingly need to encompass the function as acute palliative care physicians in order to be responsible about how we allocate resources and how we do not become complicit with society's expectations around what modern medicine can offer. Perhaps our ICUs will have specialized rooms where dying can occur in a more dignified fashion; rooms where we can say to carers that there is nothing more in the way of curative care that we can offer but we can guarantee excellent care during the dying process.

References

1. Hillman K (1999) The changing role of acute-care hospitals. Med J Aust 170:325-328
2. Brennan TA, Leape LL, Laird N, et al (1991) Incidence of adverse events and negligence in hospitalised patients: result of the Harvard medical Practice Study I. N Engl J Med 324:370-376

3. Wilson R, Runciman WB, Gibbert RW, Harrison BT, Newby L, Hamilton JD (1995) The quality in Australian health care study. Med J Aust 163:458-471
4. Hillman KM, Bristow PJ, Chey T, et al (2001) Antecedents to hospital deaths. Inter Med J 31:343-348
5. Schein RM, Hazday N, Pena M, Ruben BH, Sprung CL (1990) Clinical antecedents to in-hospital cardiopulmonary arrest. Chest 98:1388-1392
6. Goldhill DR, White SA, Sumner A (1999) Physiological values and procedures in the 24 h before ICU admission from the ward. Anaesthesia 45:529-534
7 McQuillan P, Pilkington S, Allan A, et al (1998) Confidential inquiry into quality of care before admission to intensive care. BMJ 316:1853-1858
8. Rapport J, Teres D, Lemeshow S, Harris D (1990) Timing of intensive care unit admission in relation to ICU outcome. Crit Care Med 18:1231-1235
9. Dragsted L, Jorgenson J, Jensen N-H et al (1989) Interhospital comparisons of patient outcome from intensive care: Importance of lead time bias. Crit Care Med 17:418-422
10. Hinds C, Watson D (1995) Manipulating hemodynamics and oxygen transport in critically ill patients. N Engl J Med 333:1074-1075
11. Gattinoni L, Brazzi L, Pelosi P (1995) A trial of goal-oriented hemodynamic therapy in critically ill patients. N Engl J Med 333: 1025-1032
12. Rivers E, Nguyen B, Havstad S, et al (2001) Early goal-directed therapy in the treatment of severe sepsis and septic shock. N Engl J Med 345:1368-1377
13. Lee A, Bishop G, Hillman KH, Daffurn K (1996) The medical emergency team. Anaesth Intensive Care 23:186-186
14. Hourihan F, Bishop G, Hillman KM, Daffurn K, Lee A (1995) The medical emergency team: a new strategy to identify and intervene in high risk patients. Clin Intensive Care 6:269-272
15. Hillman K (2002) Critical care without walls. Curr Opin Crit Care 8:594-599
16. Leary T, Ridley S (2003) Impact of an outreach team on re-admissions to a critical care unit. Anaesthesia 58:328-332

The Safety and Quality Agenda in Critical Care Medicine

T. Dorman

Introduction

Despite data that appear to support that fact that healthcare induces harm through acts of commission and omission, providers, in general, have been either unwilling or unable to admit their role in the observed and unobserved events that were occurring, even when they happened right in front of them. A major reason for this indifference seems to be that providers only had two groups to blame for these events, themselves or the patients. Given that many providers view themselves as infallible, the events had to be the patients' fault and, as such interventions were considered unlikely to be beneficial. In the fast-paced, high-stress intensive care unit (ICU) environment, the likelihood of events occurring secondary to these acts of commission and omission logically increases exponentially. Several wake up calls regarding the need to address these acts and events finally created the right pressures so that safety and quality programs across healthcare in general and in the ICU in particular have been crafted. The payors, recognizing the opportunity to control costs entered the arena and are now promulgating pay for performance programs [1]. As additional forces, such a horizontal and vertical integration, medical emergency response teams, genomic and proteomic medicine, and technological solutions affect healthcare delivery in the ICU a logical question arises. Will there be a need for a safety and quality agenda in 2015 and if so will it be a focus of our attention?

What is the Safety and Quality Agenda?

Safety is at the forefront of all service driven industries where errors cause harm to people or where they have the potential to cause harm to people. The method of championing safety in healthcare has historically used blame as a catalyst for change. In other industries where great harm is possible, industries like aviation and nuclear power, the concept of safety is addressed by implementing a no-fault or limited fault approach [2]. This approach is designed to address systems and not just people. As a component of their systems approaches, both industries mentioned also established programs designed to report and learn from errors and near misses in order to improve safety and prevent harm.

Systems approaches to event investigation are logical based upon the principles of safety science. These core principles of safety science include:

- We will make mistakes
- We need to create a culture where mistakes are identified
- We must focus on systems rather than people
- Leaders control the potential to change systems

"We will make Mistakes"

Since almost all aspects of care to varying degrees are dependent on humans, events will happen. Seems like an obvious statement given the fact that as humans we are all fallible. Unfortunately, the clear recognition of this fact is vital to the safety and quality movement. If we assume humans will get it right all the time then we do not addresses issues related to the complexity of the task or process that have clear potential as failure modes. Why address them if they cannot and will not occur because our human team will never miss anything at anytime? Our experience in healthcare parallels that in other safety-focus industries: humans will miss things and systems must be designed with this principle in mind. Common system design methodologies that have shown utility include reducing complexity and independent redundancy. Let us examine each of these and start with reducing complexity. The likelihood of getting a process correct without any event can be calculated from the simple mathematical formula of ($\%^n$) x 100. The % is the percent likelihood of getting each step correct and the n is the number of independent steps. If we assume that getting each step correct occurs with a probability of 0.95 and that there are 50 steps in the process then we are likely to get it perfectly correct about 0.95^{50} or 8% of the time. If we increase our performance at each step to 0.99 then will get it completely right about 61% of the time. Although I cannot speak for all hospitals and ICUs, at our institution when we did a flow map of all of the steps from the decision to give an antibiotic through to its actual administration we found that the process included more than 70 steps. Stated otherwise, we had a system designed such that failure had to happen. The questions was not if but when and to whom? I hope it is now easy to see how all of our systems need to be reexamined and that we need to remove complexity wherever possible.

The second attenuation strategy is independent redundancy. The best example of this comes from the field of anesthesiology. Adequate oxygenation during an anesthetic is considered so vitally important that numerous redundant steps are in place to avoid this life-threatening event from occurring. These steps include identifying all oxygen related tubing, wall plates, etc as the same color, green. On top of this is a pin index system so that someone should not be able to attach the oxygen tubing to some other gas source such as nitrous oxide. Unfortunately, human ingenuity being what it is, industrious individuals figured out how to get around the pin index system so we added oxygen analyzers to the system. This addressed the human work around failure mode as well as addressing events where maintenance workers had inadvertently hooked up the system wrong inside the walls or at the gas source. Providers under times of duress sometimes turned the knobs on the wrong flow meter effectively administering hypoxic gas mixtures. Consequently, the knobs were reconstructed so that the tactile feel of the oxygen knob was different than the other gases and in addition a fail safe mode was created where the flow meters interdigitate in a manner where if the oxygen is turned down the other gases fall to maintain the same gas ratio. All of these were not deemed redundant enough so pulse oximetry was the next layer created. Despite these and additional redundancies not discussed here hypoxic gas mixtures are still delivered to patients, albeit at a greatly reduced rate. This demonstrates how starting with the premise that we will make mistakes helps us focus on both the entire process (the system) and each individual step. It also demonstrates how despite reducing complexity and adding redundancy we may still only attenuate episodes of harm but not eliminate them. These redundancies though do help reduce the rate of administering hypoxic gases by preventing it completely in some cases whereas in others it is recognized before patient harm is induced, i.e., the provider intervenes when the oxygen saturation is falling but before hypoxemia occurs.

"We Need to Create a Culture where Mistakes are Identified"

Medicine has grown as a hierarchical culture. Although this 'captain of the ship' approach, on the surface, seems to be required to prevent chaos in decision making it has an unintended consequence that sets up the environment for undesirable events to occur. Safety science does not argue that having a team leader is bad, in fact leadership is required for high level team functioning, and no matter how one looks at it, care is a team process. Safety science studies have shown that a hierarchical structure can impede information transfer [2]. This is not an inherent aspect of hierarchies but their implementation in relative autocratic fashion. Unfortunately, all too commonly the structure is overtly or covertly intended to be autocratic stemming from the belief that without such structure chaos will ensue in crisis situations. The data, however, seem to show that when the structure is set up in an autocratic fashion an impediment is created for communication. Consequently, events occur despite someone recognizing that the system and the patient are on a pathway to harm. The individual who recognizes the events though feels as though they cannot speak up. They seem to feel this way for many reasons that include fear of reprisal, the perception that they are not wanted or expected to speak up, the perception that their opinion is not respected so why bother speaking up, and the perception that the 'captain' is infallible so questioning is not necessary and in fact can only be seen as insulting. Sometimes the reason seems to be as superficial as they do not want to bother the person above them. These autocratic hierarchical systems are also commonly endowed with the notion that finding an individual to blame is a useful and necessary component of repair. This culture of blame only serves to reinforce the barriers to effective team communication. This effective team communication is vitally important to the avoidance of events or the attenuation of events. Programs aimed at full team training have consequently been created and have been shown in other industries and now within healthcare to enhance performance, enhance job satisfaction, enhance employee retention, and to be associated with fewer errors and events [3]. It appears that a useful member of these teams includes institutional executives. They not only can better respond to safety needs in the clinical environment, but they can also bring to bear institutional resources and by routine participation they demonstrate the institutional commitment to a more open communication structure [4]. We have done an informal review of all malpractice claims at out institution over a couple year period and have discovered that in about 80% of the cases someone not only recognized the events as they were unfolding and may have documented that recognition, but the 'message' never made it to the appropriate individual or commonly the message was apparently ignored. It should be noted that in some circumstances it seems that the individuals who recognized the events and were being ignored were the family and friends.

"We Must Focus on Systems Rather Than People"

This principle serves multiple purposes. It helps insulate those involved in the event from blame and quite frankly the system is at fault. A useful concept is that 'every system is perfectly designed to achieve the results it does'. Read that sentence again, it is that important. It does not mean that the individual (or individuals) is absolved of all responsibility. In fact, that assumption is not only wrong but obviously quite dangerous. People do make mistakes and do need interventions to improve their performance. Having a process in place so that education and training occur cyclically is the health system's responsibility. Taking responsibility for one's actions and demonstrating competency is the individual's responsibility.

Let us briefly examine a clinical scenario to see how a systems view can be enlightening. In one of our ICUs a patient, despite being allergic, received penicillin for clinical features consistent with sepsis. The physician forgot they were allergic. The nurse had been taught that the earlier antibiotics were administered the better the outcome and so they borrowed another patient's dose. They borrowed the dose because they had learned from experience that the turn around time for drugs from pharmacy was highly variable. The patient received the dose and suffered an anaphylactic arrest. In this scenario, the physician clearly contributed by writing the antibiotic order and not rechecking for allergies and the nurse also did not check for allergies and used a work-around, although extremely well intentioned, that eliminated the ability of the pharmacy to check allergies. The older blame view would then lead to these individuals being reprimanded, but the system still would contain all of the flaws that either caused the problem or permitted them to happen without attenuation. For instance, the unit directors have ensured the staff were educated on the value of early antibiotics but contributed by not ensuring they had a system in place to address a practice that everyone knew was a common occurrence (e.g., drug borrowing). The hospital contributed as the system of using facsimile to pharmacy had been a broken system for years and so the staff had built work-arounds that were well known. The health system contributed by not having computer physician order entry in place and during an episode of restructuring a year earlier the institution had removed the pharmacy "runners" that ensured more timely delivery of medications to the point of care.

James Reason has taught us that system failures lead to adverse events and that these system failures typically have three important aspects for consideration:

- They often arise from managerial and organizational decisions (or lack of decisions) that shape working conditions.
- They often result from production pressures.
- The damaging consequences may not be evident until a "triggering event" occurs [5].

"Leaders Control the Potential to Change Systems"

Importantly, leaders not only control the financial strings, they control the potential to change systems. Some easy steps include:

- Commit to no harm
  - We need to revolutionize how we think about our desired outcomes. At present we tend to focus on benchmark values of performance. Unfortunately, benchmarks rarely equal best practice, but more typically represent average practice. Our goal must become zero harm realizing that harm will occur (we will make mistakes) but that does not mean our goal should not be a performance level of no harm. Occasionally someone who hears this will say that that goal is a set up for a culture of failure. Of course, when asked what they personally expect the goal to be from their care providers it is not benchmark performance but no harm.
- Encourage open communication
  - This means we need to focus on systems not people. When we focus on people blame rises quickly to the surface. Leaders can partner with staff to help train and build better teams. Leaders can attend team training, participate in follow-up rounds on a frequent basis (e.g., executive walk rounds), and lead by example not fiat. Team training that includes situational awareness training is required. Training in adequate disclosure is just being addressed in initial attempts to enhance openness.
- Celebrate safety
  - We should identify and celebrate workers when appropriate as heroes. Two simple old adages apply:
  - People who feel good about themselves, produce good results
  - Help people reach their full potential, catch them doing something right.

When creating safe systems we all need to remember that we must measure to improve. Everyone believes they are providing high quality care, but repeatedly the data show this to be much less true than expected. As part of the measurement approach we must educate all that measurement is for learning and testing, not for judgment. This is about continuous improvement not blame. Finally, and maybe the hardest of all is that data do not improve processes, people do. We need to be willing to manage people or no progress can be made.

Although much of what I have focused on has been the science of safety, it is clear that quality is often tightly linked to safe practices. They are not synonymous and it is possible to improve safety in one area while inducing harm elsewhere. This is another reason why it is critical that we measure both outcomes and process measures iteratively.

Why Do We Need a Safety and Quality Agenda Today?

There are many reasons, which range from those tightly coupled to data to the issue of public trust. In simple terms, our patients are sick enough and at risk enough that we do not need to induce additional risk needlessly. The Institute of Medicine has attempted to quantify the amount of induced harm [6]. Many disagree with their calculations, but reports from several countries seemingly validate their numbers. Of even more concern though is that these projects look for and identify acts of commission (e.g., giving an antibiotic to an allergic patient) and they make no estimates of the harm induced through acts of omission (e.g., failure to administer beta blockers after a myocardial infarction), even though acts of omission appear to occur almost five time more frequently. The Rand Corporation has published that physicians are slow to adopt evidence-based practices (typically takes 7-15 years) and in their last review of care to the elderly noted that physicians only provide evidence-based therapies about 50% of the time [7]. Finally, from a published data perspective, it has been stated that on average, every patient in the ICU suffers on average one event every day.

An eye opening exercise is to sit down with staff and ask how they will harm the next patient. Every single time we have done this, staff describe a litany of practices that put patients at risk (and please remember we ourselves are or will be patients). Given these issues we clearly need a safety and quality agenda in today's medicine. Furthermore, over the last decade or so there has been a slow erosion of public trust in health care. Focusing on safety and quality in a logical and scientifically sound manner is required in order to rebuild that public trust.

What Forces are Causing Changes in the ICU in General?

These are so numerous that it is not possible or practical for me to attempt to list or describe all of them. They include processes that range from the unit structure, to specific technological aspects of care, through changes in the educational and research systems. Finally, advances in genomic and proteomics hold the promise of improving decision-making and thus care, but will need to be deployed following the principles established within this manuscript.

Will These Forces and their Outcomes Change the Need for a Safety and Quality Agenda by 2015?

No!

Healthcare has a centuries old culture of autocracy without communication that utilizes blame as a primary means to address events. The safety and quality movement has its roots from years ago, but really has only taken hold in the last few years and it is unlikely that all cultures will be changed that quickly or that all harm will be eliminated by 2015. In fact, in US ICUs, 30% or less of the patients have care delivered by the evidence-based intensivist-directed multiprofessional team model. When a patient dies in one of the units without the evidence-based model no physician or administrator explains to the patient's family that part of the reason for death was an act of omission, the omission of the presence of an intensivist. In these centers that lack utilization of the intensivist-directed model, powerful individual physicians still have the ability to prevent progress to a scientifically proven safer and higher quality model. The Leapfrog Group initiated its standard in 2000 and in areas of penetration has seen an increase in use of the intensivist model from about 17% to close to 30%. At that rate of growth it is likely to take the full decade to get to full implementation. Our safety and quality program is growing one state at a time. An example of the steps that we have found to be useful can be seen in Table 1. We should remember that as we eliminate certain risks, new ones will rise to the top of the list and will require attention. More important than any of these issues and numerous others is that just as physicians are students of medicine for life, we will always have room to improve.

Conclusion

Patients are being harmed by acts of commission and acts of omission at rates that are unacceptable. The safety and quality agenda is sorely needed today and

Table 1. Components of the Comprehensive Unit Safety Program (CUSP)

- Cultural survey
- Educate staff on the science of safety
- Identify staff safety concerns
- Executive walk rounds
- Implement improvements
- Document results
- Disseminate results and share stories
- Resurvey staff

will continue to be needed in 2015. The forces at play in healthcare are unlikely to diminish the need for the safety and quality agenda to remain a significant driver. In order to maintain progress we need to: a) create the will to change at levels of the health care team; b) improve team training in communication, measurement, and people management; and c) execute the vision of a care system dedicated to no harm.

References

1. Goldfield N, Burford R, Averill R, et al (2005) Pay for performance: an excellent idea that simply needs implementation. Qual Manag Health Care 14:31–44
2. Pronovost PJ, Thompson DA, Holzmueller CG, et al (2005) Defining and measuring patient safety. Crit Care Clin 21:1–19
3. Carlisle C, Cooper H, Watkins C (2004) "Do none of you talk to each other?" The challenges facing the implementation of interprofessional education. Med Teacher 26:542–552
4. Colias M (2004) Making the rounds. Stanford's Martha Marsh says she believes in getting to know hospitals she runs from bottom up. Mod Healthc 34:30–31
5. Reason JT, Carthey J, de Leval MR (2001) Diagnosing "vulnerable system syndrome":an essential prerequisite to effective risk management. Qual Health Care 10 (Suppl2):ii21–25
6. Kohn LT, Corrigan JM, Molla S (1999) To Err Is Human: Building a Safer Health System (1999) Committee on Quality of Health Care in America, The Institute of Medicine, National Academy Press, Washington
7. Mc Glynn EA, Asch SM, Adams J, et al (2003) The quality of health care delivered to adults in the United States. N Engl J Med 348:2635–26458.

The Challenge of Emerging Infections and Progressive Antibiotic Resistance

S. M. Opal

"If we do not change our direction, we are likely to end up where we are headed"

ancient Chinese proverb

Introduction

Our collective vulnerability to the threat of emerging microbial pathogens remains disturbingly evident as we enter the twenty-first century. Despite two centuries of knowledge about the germ theory of disease, breaking the genetic code, and sequencing the genomes of virtually every major bacterial and viral pathogen capable of causing disease in humankind, we still find ourselves susceptible to infectious diseases. Densely concentrated cities with interconnected human societies linked by international aviation put us at continued risk from future epidemics that will inevitably occur [1]. The ever expanding population growth of our species will force environmental change as we venture into sparsely inhabited rainforests, populate remote ecosystems and cultivate natural habitats to support our voracious human appetite for goods and services. Global warming, environmental degradation and land development along with human upheavals and natural calamities will create new outbreaks with novel pathogens and renew the spread of ancient scourges like cholera [2] and plague [3].

Numerous examples of intercontinental spread of microbial pathogens within the last five years alone give notice of the susceptibility of human populations to emerging infectious diseases (Table 1) [4–20]. This is perhaps best exemplified by the tragic events set into motion in late 2002 when a previously unidentified, obscure, animal coronavirus (now known as severe acute respiratory syndrome [SARS]-CoV) was first introduced into an unsuspecting human population in Southern China [9]. Current molecular evidence indicates that a food handler in an exotic food 'wet market' in Guangdong Province probably first became infected by an animal coronavirus from a civet cat. This newly derived animal virus was adapt at infecting humans and was efficiently spread person-to-person by infected aerosol [10]. An ill Chinese physician from the affected region traveled to Hong Kong to attend a wedding. While spending a single night in Amoy Garden Hotel in the city, this infected individual appeared to spread the virus to at least 12 other hotel guests. Over the next several days these people returned to their homes in five different countries incubating the SARS-CoV pathogen in their respiratory secretions. Over the next 3–4 months, this newly acquired coronavirus spread to over 27 countries worldwide and caused over 8000 cases of SARS resulting in nearly 800 deaths in early 2003 [9]. Through a global effort from a large number of very diligent public health officials and laboratory scientists, the outbreak ended within a year and has yet to be seen again, except for occasional laboratory-acquired accidents [9].

A diverse array of pathogens has produced recent outbreaks and concerns for our vulnerability to pathogens within the global village we occupy and share with other flora, fauna and microorganisms (Table 1). The spread of mosquito-

Table 1. Emerging infectious disease threats in the 21st century

Disease	Causative Organism	Cause and Outcome
Avian influenza [4-7]	Influenza A (H_5N_1)	Risk of pandemic influenza; sporadic human cases of avian flu in Asia -mortality rates>70%
Severe acute respiratory syndrome (SARS) [8–10]	SARS associated coronavirus	Risk of spread of zoonotic viruses; outbreak from a southern China to world-wide epidemic in 2003 – 8000 cases and 800 deaths
Monkey pox [11]	Orthopox virus	Risk of exotic pet trade; outbreak in wild rodents and humans in Mid-Western USA from sale of Gambian Giant rats from Africa
West Nile Virus (WNV) [12, 13]	Mosquito-borne flavivirus	Risk of international spread; WNV from Africa to New York in 1999, thousands of cases and hundreds of deaths in North America over next 5 years
Inhalational anthrax [14, 15]	Intentional release of *Bacillus anthracis* spores in USA mail system	Vulnerability to bioterrorism; 11 cases, 5 fatalities in Oct-Nov 2001, perpetrator never identified
Hemorrhagic fever outbreaks [15, 16]	Ebola virus – Zaire (filovirus)	Disruption of ecosystems; repeated outbreaks in Gabon and Congo rainforests in 2001–2004
Antibiotic resistant bacteria, viruses, fungi [17–20]	Vancomycin-resistant *S. aureus* Oseltamivir-resistant influenza Azole-resistant *Candida spp.*	Misuse of antimicrobials promote spread of resistance genes – community outbreaks now occur

borne West Nile virus in North America [12, 13], prion-related food-borne variant Creutzfeldt-Jakob Disease [21], and hemorrhagic fever viruses [16] are a constant reminder of our susceptibility to pathogens that naturally reside in other animal species. The omnipresent fear of the next pandemic of influenza has been heightened by recent evolutionary changes in virulence and transmissibility of avian flu viruses [22].

Standard chemotherapeutic regimens for infectious diseases may not reliably rescue persons with severe infections in the new millennium. Community and nosocomial outbreaks of multidrug resistant pathogens as evidenced by methicillin and vancomycin resistance [17] in *Staphylococcus aureus* and resistance to the new anti-viral neuraminidase inhibitors [18, 19] by recent influenza isolates are cause for real concern. The care of hospitalized, critically ill patients is likely to fundamentally change if current trends in the progressive emergence of antimicrobial resistance to commonly prescribed antibiotics are not significantly altered in the near future. Regrettably, there is little evidence that the situation is likely to change unless concerted efforts are taken on several fronts to reverse the current trajectory of increasing antibiotic resistance [17, 20].

The Genetics of Antibiotic Resistance

The fitness of a microorganism is dependent upon its capacity to genetically adapt to rapidly changing environmental conditions. Antimicrobial agents exert strong selective pressures on microbial populations, favoring those organisms that are capable of resisting them. Genetic variability may occur by a variety of mechanisms. Point mutations may occur in a nucleotide base pair, which is referred to as *micro-evolutionary change* [23]. These mutations may alter the target site of an antimicrobial agent, altering with its inhibitory capacity.

Point mutations inside or adjacent to the active sites of existing beta-lactamase genes (e.g., genes for TEM-1, SHV-1) have generated a remarkable array of newly recognized extended-spectrum beta-lactamases [23]. Beta-lactam antibiotics have been known for almost 80 years and their widespread use has created selection pressures on bacterial pathogens to resist their inhibitory actions. At least 267 different bacterial enzymes have now been characterized that hydrolyze beta-lactam antibiotics [24]. The hydrolyzing enzymes exist in four basic molecular classes and are classified as listed in Table 2. The enzymes are either serine hydrolases (class A, C, and D) or zinc containing metalloenzymes with a zinc-binding thiol group its active site (class B enzymes). The microevolutionary events that account for the differential activities of this array of beta-lactamases have been carefully studied, and these bacterial enzymes now even have their own internet website devoted specifically to their molecular properties (http://www.lahey.org/studies/webt.htm).

Beta-lactamase activity has become so ubiquitous among bacterial populations that it has prompted the development of specific beta-lactamase inhibitor compounds (clavulanate, tazobactam and sulbactam) in an effort to combat this common bacterial resistance mechanism. This has been countered by the generation of inhibitors of these beta-lactamase inhibitors by multidrug-resistant

Table 2. The functional classification scheme for beta-lactamases

Group	Enzyme Type	Clavulanate inhibition	Molecular Class	Common Examples
1	Cephalosporinase	No	C	*Enterobacter cloacae* P99
2a	Penicillinase	Yes	A	*Staphylococcus aureus*
2b	Broad-spectrum	Yes	A	SHV-1, TEM-1
2be	Extended-spectrum	Yes	A	*Klebsiella oxytoca* K1
2br	Inhibitor-resistant	Diminished	A	TEM-30 (IRT-2)
2c	Carbenicillinase	Yes	A	AER-1, PSE-1, CARB-3
2d	Cloxacillinase	Yes	A or D	OXA-1
2e	Cephalosporinase	Yes	A	*Proteus vulgaris*
2f	Carbapenemase	Yes	A	IMI-1, NMC-A, Sme-1
3	Carbapenemase metalloenzymes	No	B	*Stenotrophomonas maltophilia* L1, IMP-1
4	Penicillinase	No		*Burkholderia cepacia* , SAR-2

(see references [23, 24])

bacteria [23] in the ongoing conflict between pathogens and chemotherapeutic strategies to eradicate these microorganisms.

Recently it has been demonstrated that at least some bacterial populations have the capacity to increase their mutation rates during times of environmental stress such as exposure to an antibiotic. This stress response is known as the 'SOS' response or transient hypermutation [25]. It is highly advantageous for the organism to increase the rate of genetic variation at times of unfavorable environmental conditions. It is possible for bacteria to upregulate the pace of evolution in an attempt to develop a clone that can resist the action of an antibiotic. The DNA polymerase in such organisms has reduced fidelity of replication and subsequently an increased rate in the mutational occurrences as a result of excess nucleotide mispairing. The recombination system of bacteria (the *recA* system) becomes less restrictive in the degree homology between DNA sequences before a crossover event is permitted to occur. A flurry of mutational events occur in stressed bacteria in a final attempt to generate a resistant subpopulation of bacteria in the presence of an environmental challenge such as the presence of a new antibiotic. This process has even been phenotypically linked with alterations in growth rate and biofilm formation in some strains of *Pseudomonas aeruginosa* [26].

A second level of genomic variability in bacteria is referred to as a *macro-evolutionary* change and results in whole-scale rearrangements of large segments of DNA as a single event. Such rearrangements may include inversions, duplications, insertions, deletions, or transposition of large sequences of DNA from one location of a bacterial chromosome or plasmid to another. These whole-scale rearrangements of large segments of the bacterial genome are frequently created by specialized genetic elements known as *transposons* or *insertion sequences*, which have the capacity to move independently as a unit from the rest of the bacterial genome [23].

Acquisition of foreign DNA sequences from the extracellular environment may be taken up by naturally competent bacteria (e.g., some streptococci and neisserial organisms) by transformation. These sequences can then become integrated into the host genome into homologous sequences by the generalized recombination and DNA repair system bacteria. Inheritance of these foreign DNA elements further contributes to the organism's ability to cope with selection pressures imposed upon them by antimicrobial agents [23].

A third level of genetic variability in bacteria is created by the acquisition of foreign DNA carried by plasmids and bacteriophages. These extrachromosomal DNA elements provide ready access to disposable yet potentially highly advantageous genes including antibiotic resistance genes from plasmids or phage particles. These elements are autonomously self-replicating, and they can remain unattached in the cytoplasm of bacterial cells or integrate directly into the chromosome of the bacterial host. They have the capacity to replicate and move independently from the chromosome adding further variability to the entire bacterial genomic DNA. Evidence from whole genome sequencing projects indicates that these genomic rearrangements, bacteriophage sequences and insertion sequences are commonplace in bacterial chromosomes [27].

These genetic variations provide bacteria with the seemingly limitless system to alter their genomes, rapidly evolve and develop resistance to virtually any antimicrobial agent. Recent examples of vancomycin-resistance in enterococci [23], *S. aureus* [27], and extended spectrum beta-lactamases [23], carbapenemase production [28] and transferable quinolone resistance in *P. aeruginosa* and enterobacteria [23] attest to the capacity of microorganisms to adapt to environmental stresses induced by antibiotic exposure. Viruses [19] and fungi [20] are also quite capable of rapid antimicrobial resistance development and these resistance capacities pose additional threats in the management of ICU patients with serious infections from a variety of potential pathogens [29].

The Origins of Antibiotic Resistance Genes and Mechanisms of Resistance

Antibiotic resistance genes probably arose from detoxifying enzymes or synthetic enzymes with altered substrate specificity by critical mutations or recombination events resulting in the formation of mosaic genes with entirely new functions [30]. Altered penicillin binding proteins that mediate beta-lactam resistance in multiple bacterial genera (e.g., methicillin-resistant *S. aureus* [MRSA], penicillin-resistant streptococci and pneumococci, chromosomal resistance in gonococci) may have evolved from gene fusions for penicillin binding proteins involved in bacterial cell wall synthesis [23]. Another common resistance strategy is a change in the regulation of metabolic activity of an enzyme system that is affected by the antibiotic. Increasing the rate of folate precursor synthesis, for example, can overcome the inhibitor effects of sulfa drugs and trimethoprim [30].

Many common antibiotic resistance genes were accidentally acquired ('stolen') from antibiotic producing bacteria. Streptomyces and related soil bacteria are the source of many standard antimicrobial agents in use in clinical medicine today. These bacteria have co-evolved the capacity to synthesize antibiotics along with the necessary resistance genes to protect their own metabolic machinery from the very antibiotic they produce. The resistance genes from these antibiotic producing bacteria provide a ready genetic blueprint to resist the target antibiotic if susceptible bacteria can acquire these resistance genes. Recent evidence confirming that this does indeed occur was found by Yokoyama and colleagues in Japan during an investigation of a sudden outbreak of *P. aeruginosa* with high-level resistance to essentially all the clinically available aminoglycosides [31]. These investigators discovered that the resistant strain had acquired a new methylase gene that blocked the binding site for inhibition by aminoglycosides on a specific sequence on 16S ribosomal RNA. This identical mechanism and highly homologous gene is found in aminoglycoside-producing strains of Streptomyces and related bacteria.

Detoxifying Enzymes

At least seven distinctive mechanisms of antibiotic resistance have been described in bacteria and are summarized on Table 3. Detoxifying enzymes are used to degrade beta-lactams [24], and modify aminoglycosides so they no longer enter bacterial membranes and attach to their ribosomal target. There are over 30 such enzymes identified that can inhibit aminoglycosides by one of three general reactions: *N*-acetylation, *O*-nucleotidylation, and *O*-phosphorylation [23]. Detoxifying enzymes are also one of the resistance mechanisms against chloramphenicol, and are rarely utilized by certain bacterial strains to inactivate macrolides, lincosamides, tetracyclines and streptogramins.

Decreased Permeability

It was recognized early in the history of antibiotic development that penicillin is effective against Gram-positive bacteria but not against Gram-negative bacteria [23]. This difference in susceptibility to penicillin is due in large part to the outer membrane, a lipid bilayer that acts as a barrier to the penetration of antibiotics into the cell. Situated outside the peptidoglycan cell wall of Gram-negative bacteria, this outer membrane is absent in Gram-positive bacteria. The outer portion of this lipid bilayer is composed principally of lipopolysaccharide (LPS) made up of tightly bound hydrocarbon molecules that impede the entry of hydrophobic antibiotics, such as penicillins or macrolides.

The passage of hydrophilic antibiotics through this outer membrane is facilitated by the presence of porins, proteins that are arranged so as to form water-

Table 3. Mechanisms of antibacterial resistance by major drug class

	β–lactam	Amino-glycoside	Sulfa/TMP	Quino-lone	Macro-lide	Glyco-peptide	TCN
Enzymatic inactivation	+++	+++	–	–	+ (Gram-neg)	–	+
Im-permeable	+ (Gram-neg)	+ (Gram-neg)	+ (Gram-neg)	+ (Gram-neg)	++ (Gram-neg)	++ (Gram-neg)	+
Efflux	+	+	–	+	++	–	+++
Altered target site	++	++	+++	+++	+++	+++	+
Protected target site	–	–	–	+	–	–	++
Excess target	–	–	++	–	–	+	–
Bypass process	–	–	+	–	–	–	–

Gram-neg: Gram-negative bacteria; TMP: trimethoprim; TCN: tetracycline; +++: most common mechanism; ++: common; +: less common, –: not reported (see reference [23])

filled diffusion channels through which antibiotics may traverse [23]. Bacteria usually produce a large number of porins with differing physiochemical properties, permeability characteristics and size; approximately 10^5 porin molecules/cell for *Escherichia coli*. Bacteria are able to regulate the relative number of different porins in response to the osmolarity of their microenvironment. In hyperosmolar conditions, *E. coli* represses the synthesis of larger porins (OmpF) while continuing to express smaller ones (OmpC) [32].

Mutations resulting in the loss of specific porins can occur in clinical isolates and determine increased resistance to beta-lactam antibiotics. Resistance to aminoglycosides and carbapenems emerging during therapy has also been associated with a lack of production of outer membrane proteins. In *P. aeruginosa*, resistance to imipenem appears to be due to an interaction between chromosomal beta-lactamase activity and a loss of a specific entry channel, the D2 porin [33].

The rate of entry of aminoglycoside molecules into bacterial cells is a function of their binding to a usually non-saturable anionic transporter, whereupon they retain their positive charge and are subsequently 'pulled' across the cytoplasmic membrane by the internal negative charge of the cell. This process requires energy and a threshold level of internal negative charge before significant transport occurs *(proton motive force)* [34]. These aminoglycoside-resistant isolates with altered proton motive force may occur during long-term aminoglycoside therapy. These isolates usually have a 'small colony' phenotype due to their reduced rate of growth.

Drug Efflux

Active efflux of antimicrobial agents is increasingly utilized by bacteria and fungi as a mechanism of antibiotic resistance. Some strains of *E. coli, Shigella*, and other enteric organisms express a membrane transporter system that leads to multidrug resistance by drug efflux [35]. Specific efflux pumps also exist that promote the egress of single classes of antimicrobial agents. Efflux mechanisms are the major mechanism of resistance to tetracyclines in Gram-negative bacteria. Some strains of *S. pneumoniae, S. pyogenes, S. aureus*, and *S. epidermidis*, use an active efflux mechanism to resist macrolides, streptogramins, and azalides [23]. This efflux mechanism is mediated by the *meF* (for macrolide efflux) genes in streptococci and *msr* (for macrolide streptogramin resistance) genes in staphylococci. A similar efflux system, encoded by a gene referred to as *mreA* (for macrolide resistance efflux), has been described in group B streptococci. This mechanism of resistance may be more prevalent in community-acquired infections than was generally appreciated. Dissemination of these resistance genes among important bacterial pathogens constitutes a major threat to the continued usefulness of macrolide antibiotics [36].

Active efflux mechanisms may also contribute to the full expression of beta-lactam resistance in *P. aeruginosa*. Multidrug efflux pumps in the inner and outer membrane of *P. aeruginosa* may combine with periplasmic beta-lactamases and membrane permeability components for full expression of antibiotic resistance [37]. Active efflux of fluoroquinolones by specific quinolone pumps or multidrug transporter pumps has also been detected in enteric bacteria and staphylococci [23].

Alter Target Sites

Resistance to a wide variety of antimicrobial agents, including tetracyclines, macrolides, lincosamides, streptogramins and the aminoglycosides, may result from alteration of ribosomal binding sites. The MLS_B-determinant has the genes that produce enzymes to dimethylate adenine residues on the 23-S ribosomal RNA of the 50-S subunit of the prokaryotic ribosome, disrupting the binding of these drugs to the ribosome.

Resistance to aminoglycosides may also be mediated at the ribosomal level. Mutations of the S12 protein of the 30-S subunit have been shown to interfere with binding streptomycin to the ribosome. Ribosomal resistance to streptomycin may be a significant cause of streptomycin resistance among enterococcal isolates. Ribosomal resistance to the 2-deoxystreptamine aminoglycosides (gentamicin, tobramycin, amikacin) appears to be uncommon and may require multiple mutations in that these aminoglycosides bind at several sites on both the 30S and 50S subunits of the ribosome [23].

Vancomycin and other glycopeptide antibiotics such as teicoplanin bind to D-alanine-D-alanine, which is present at the termini of peptidoglycan precursors. The large glycopeptide molecules prevent the incorporation of the precursors into the cell wall. Resistance of enterococci to vancomycin has been classified as A–G based upon the genotype, type of target site modification and level of resistance to vancomycin and teicoplanin [38]. Strains of *E. faecium* and *E. faecalis* with high-level resistance to both vancomycin and teicoplanin have class A resistance. Class A resistance is mediated by the *vanA* gene cluster found on an R plasmid. This protein synthesizes peptidoglycan precursors that have a depsipeptide terminus (D-alanine-D-lactate) instead of the usual D-alanine-D-alanine. The modified peptidoglycan binds glycopeptide antibiotics with reduced affinity, thus conferring resistance to vancomycin and teicoplanin. The other classes of vancomycin resistance genes vary in level of resistance, species distribution and specific cell wall alterations [23, 38].

Vancomycin-intermediate strains of resistant *S. aureus* (VISA) have been isolated with heterogeneous resistance patterns. VISA strains express unusually thick peptidoglycan cell walls that are less completely cross-linked together. The cell wall in some strains of VISA contains non-amidated glutamine precursors that provide an increased number of false binding sites to vancomycin [39]. The vancomycin molecules are absorbed to these excess binding sites thereby reducing vancomycin concentrations at the growth point of peptidoglycan synthesis along the inner surface of the cell wall. The arrival of high level vancomycin resistance from vanA expressing *S. aureus* [17] has created a renewed sense of urgency in the need to develop novel strategies to combat multi-drug resistant bacterial pathogens.

Beta-lactam antibiotics inhibit bacteria by binding covalently to penicillin-binding proteins (PBPs) in the cytoplasmic membrane. These target proteins catalyze the synthesis of the peptidoglycan that forms the cell wall of bacteria. In Gram-positive bacteria, resistance to beta-lactam antibiotics may occur by a decrease in the affinity of the PBP for the antibiotic or with a change in the amount of PBP produced by the bacterium [23]. These low affinity binding PBPs may be inducible where their production is stimulated by exposure of the microorganism to the beta-lactam drug [40]. The structural gene *(mecA)* that determines the low-affinity PBP of MRSA shares extensive sequence homology with a PBP of *E. coli*, and the genes that regulate the production of the low-affinity PBP have considerable sequence homology with the genes that regulate the production of staphylococcal penicillinase [23].

The PBPs of beta-lactamase–negative penicillin-resistant strains of *N. gonorrhoeae, N. meningitidis*, and *Haemophilus influenzae* have shown reduced penicillin-binding affinity [41]. Their PBPs appear to be encoded by hybrid genes containing segments of DNA scavenged from resistant strains of related species, similar to penicillin-resistant pneumococci [23].

DNA gyrase (also known as bacterial topoisomerase II) is necessary for the supercoiling of chromosomal DNA in bacteria in order to have efficient cell division [23]. Another related enzyme, topoisomerase IV is also required for segregation of bacterial genomes into two daughter cells during cell division. These enzymes consist of two A subunits encoded by the *gyrA* gene and two B subunits encoded by the *gyrB* gene (or parC and parE for topoisomerase IV. Although spontaneous mutation ot the A- subunit of the *gyrA* locus is the most common cause of resistance to multiple fluoroquinolones in enteric bacteria, B-subunit alterations may also affect resistance to these drugs.

DNA gyrase (topoisomerase II) is the primary site of action in Gram-negative bacteria whereas topoisomerase IV is the principal target of quinolones in Gram-positive bacteria. Mutations in a variety of chromosomal loci have been described that resulted in altered DNA gyrases resistant to nalidixic acid and the newer fluoroquinolones in Enterobacteriaceae and *P. aeruginosa*. Many of these mutations involve the substitution of single amino acids at key enzymatic sites (located between amino acids 67–106 in the gyrase A subunit) that are involved in the generation of the DNA gyrase–bacterial DNA complex [42].

There are two common genes that mediate resistance to sulfa drugs in a wide variety of pathogenic bacteria. These are known as *sul1* and *sul2*. These genes give rise to altered forms of the target enzyme for sulfonamide, dihydropteroate synthase (DHPS) [43]. The altered DHPS enzymes mediated by the sulfonamide resistance genes no longer bind to sulfa yet continue to synthesize dihydropteroate from para-aminobenzoic acid substrate.

Trimethoprim is a potent inhibitor of bacterial dihydrofolate reductase (DHFR). A large number of altered DHFR enzymes with loss of inhibition by trimethoprim have been described from genes found primarily on R plasmids. These altered DHFR genes are widespread in Gram-negative bacteria and are also found in staphylococci (the *dfrA* gene) [44].

Protection of the Target Site

Tetracycline resistance may be mediated by a mechanism that interferes with the ability of tetracycline to bind to the ribosome. The ubiquitous *tetM* resistance gene and related tetracycline resistance determinants protect the ribosome from tetracycline action. The tetM gene generates protein with elongation factor-like activity that may stabilize ribosomal transfer RNA interactions in the presence of tetracycline molecules [45].

Excess Synthesis of the Inhibited Target

Sulfonamides compete with para-aminobenzoic acid to bind the enzyme dihydropteroate synthase, and thereby block folic acid synthesis necessary for nucleic acid synthesis. Sulfonamide resistance may be mediated in some bacteria by the over production of the synthetic enzyme dihydropteroate synthase. The gene responsible for DHPS is *felP* and strains of bacteria that produce excess DHPS can overwhelm sulfa inhibition [43]. Trimethoprim resistance may also occur in a similar fashion, by making excess amounts of dihydrofolate reductase from the bacterial chromosomal gene *folA* [44].

Bypass Mechanism of Resistance

An unusual mechanism of resistance to specific antibiotics is by the development of auxotrophs, which have specific growth factor requirements not seen in wild-type strains. These mutants require substrates that normally are synthesized by the target enzymes, and thus if the substrates are present in the environment, the organisms are able to grow despite inhibition of the synthetic enzyme by an antibiotic. Bacteria that lose the enzyme thymidylate synthetase are 'thymine dependent'. If they can acquire exogenous supplies of thymidine to synthesize thymidylate via salvage pathways from the host, they are highly resistant to sulfa drugs and trimethoprim [23].

The Transmission of Resistance Genes Between Bacterial Species

Once an antibiotic resistance gene evolves, the resistance determinant can disseminate among bacterial populations by transformation, transduction, conjugation, or transposition. Favored clones of bacteria then proliferate in the flora of patients who receive antibiotics. Antibiotic-resistance genes were found among bacteria even in the pre-antibiotic therapy era [23]. However, selection pressures placed upon microbial populations by a highly lethal antimicrobial compound create an environment in which individual clones that resist the antibiotic are markedly favored. These resistant populations then proliferate and rapidly replace other susceptible strains of bacteria. While some antibiotic resistance genes place a metabolic 'cost' on bacteria, many microorganisms have evolved strategies to limit this cost by limiting expression, alternate gene products or phase variation. These mechanisms allow favorable but sometimes 'costly' genes that mediate antibiotic resistance to persist in the absence of continued antibiotic selection pressure and yet be rapidly expressed upon re-exposure to antibiotics [46].

Plasmids

Plasmids are particularly well adapted to serve as agents of genetic evolution and R-gene dissemination. Plasmids are extrachromosomal genetic elements that are made of circular double-stranded DNA molecules that range from less than 10 to greater than 400 kilobase pairs and are extremely common in clinical isolates of bacterial pathogens. Although multiple copies of a specific plasmid or multiple different plasmids, or both, may be found in a single bacterial cell, closely related plasmids often cannot coexist in the same cell. This observation has led to a classification scheme of plasmids based upon incompatibility groups [23].

Plasmids may determine a wide range of functions besides antibiotic resistance, including virulence and metabolic capacities. Plasmids are autonomous, self-replicating genetic elements that possess an origin for replication and genes that facilitate its stable maintenance in host bacteria. Conjugative plasmids require additional genes that can initiate self-transfer.

The transfer of plasmid DNA between bacterial species is a complex process, and thus conjugative plasmids tend to be larger than non-conjugative ones. Some small plasmids may be able to utilize the conjugation apparatus of a co-resident conjugative plasmid. Many plasmid-encoded functions enable bacterial strains to persist in the environment by resisting noxious agents, such as heavy metals. Mercury released from dental fillings may increase the number of antibiotic-resistant bacteria in the oral flora. Hexachlorophene and other topical bacteriostatic agents in the environment may actually promote plasmid-mediated resistance to these agents and other antimicrobial agents [47].

Transposable Genetic Elements

Transposons are specialized sequences of DNA that are mobile and can translocate as a unit from one area of the bacterial chromosome to another. They can also move back and forth between the chromosome and plasmid or bacteriophage DNA. Transposable genetic elements possess a specialized system of recombination that is independent of the generalized recombination system that permits recombination of largely homologous sequences of DNA by crossover events (the *rec*A system of bacteria). The *rec*A-independent recombination system ('transposase') of transposable elements usually occurs in a random fashion between non-homologous DNA sequences and results in whole-scale modifications of large sequences of DNA as a single event [23].

There are two types of transposable genetic elements, *transposons* and *insertion sequences.* These mobile sequences probably play an important physiologic role in genetic variation and evolution in prokaryotic organisms. Transposons differ from insertion sequences in that they mediate a recognizable phenotypic marker such as an antibiotic-resistance trait. Either element can translocate as an independent unit. Both elements are flanked on either end by short identical sequences of DNA in reverse order *(inverted repeats).* These inverted-repeat DNA termini are essential to the transposition process. Transposons and insertion sequences must be physically integrated with chromosome, bacteriophage, or plasmid DNA in order to be replicated and maintained in a bacterial population. Some transposons have the capability to move from one bacterium to another without being transferred within a plasmid or bacteriophage. These *conjugative* transposons are found primarily in aerobic and anaerobic Gram-positive organisms and can rapidly and efficiently spread antibiotic resistance genes [30, 48].

Transposition, like point mutation, is a continuous and ongoing process in bacterial populations. Transposons are also essential in the evolution of R plasmids that contain multiple antibiotic-resistance determinants [47]. High-level vancomycin resistance (vanA) in enterococci is mediated by a composite transposon that encodes a series of genes needed to express vancomycin resistance [38]. Single transposons may encode multiple antibiotic-resistance determinants within their inverted-repeat termini as well [23].

Genetic exchange of antibiotic-resistance genes occurs between bacteria of widely disparate species and different genera. Identical aminoglycoside-resistance genes can spread between Gram-negative and Gram-positive bacteria and between aerobic and anaerobic bacteria [49]. Given the highly variable environmental selection pressures created by a wide variety of antibiotics and the plasticity of bacterial genomes, the ongoing evolution of multi-drug resistant bacterial organisms is probably inevitable [23].

DNA Integration Elements

The structural genes that mediate antibiotic resistance are often closely linked and may exist in tandem along the bacterial chromosome or plasmid. Genetic analysis of sequences of DNA adjacent to resistance genes has identified unique integration units near promoter sites [50]. These integration regions are known as *integrons*, and they function as convenient recombinational 'hot spots' for site-specific recombination events between largely non-homologous sequences of DNA. The integron provides its own integrase function [94] with a common attachment and integration site for acquisition of foreign DNA sequences.

Integrons are widespread in bacterial populations and provide a convenient site for insertion of multiple different resistance genes from foreign DNA sources. There are four classes of integrons with type I integrons being the most common in pathogenic microorganisms [23]. Integrons also serve as efficient expression cassettes for resistance genes. Integrons possess a promoter site in close proximity to the 5'end of the newly inserted DNA sequence. Numerous clusters of different resistance genes have been linked into integrons through specific insertion sites. Integrons may have as many as five resistance genes linked in sequence and flanked between specific 59 base-pair spacer units [50, 51]. Integron-mediated multiple resistance gene cassettes have been flanked by transposons, mobilized to plasmids, and then transferred between bacterial species by conjugation. By these systems of genetic exchange, widespread dissemination of multiple antibiotic resistance genes is accomplished in a rapid and frighteningly efficient manner [50].

Are We Approaching The End of the Antimicrobial Era?

For some time concerned scientists have been warning about the possibility of widespread antibiotic resistance leading to the loss of effectiveness of antibiotics in clinical medicine [49–52]. These warnings have largely been ignored as it was assumed that this human need and the profit motive of free enterprise would stimulate pharmaceutical companies to continuously develop new antibiotics. If we could discover new targets for future antimicrobial drugs it may be possible to keep pace or even exceed the rate of antibiotic resistance gene development by microbial pathogens. For a number of disconcerting reasons, humans may be losing ground rather than gaining on pathogens in the 21st century.

A recent survey of new pharmaceutical products in 2002 found only five new antibiotics out of the 506 new molecular entities in the research and development pipeline [52]. The pace of new antibiotic discovery is turning into a trickle and drying up compared to what it was even 20 years ago [53]. The market reality is regrettably set against the development of new antibiotics in favor of more lucrative options with greater market profit from drugs for chronic illnesses with less risk and longer revenue streams [52–54]. The reimbursement and return on investments are unfavorable for antibiotics and the market system is not meeting the needs of society with respect to new antibiotic development. Some far reaching and bold initiatives are desperately needed if a crisis in loss of antibi-

Table 4. Disincentives for new antibiotic drug development

Disincentives	Possible Solutions
Expense (800 million US dollars/ new molecular entity) forces companies into broad-spectrum antibiotic market	Shorten regulatory process; extend patent life; government protection from liability claims; speed development with genomics and high throughput screening process
Specific narrow-spectrum antibiotics are small markets – 'niche' product – difficult to regain development costs	Not-for-profit drug companies; government funding of small market-narrow spectrum drugs; move research and development to low income status countries
Restricted use and short duration of treatment limits profits (antibiotic treatment is for days-weeks not years)	Improve patent position of antibiotics; extend 'orphan' drug status to new antibiotics
Antibiotic resistance development limits lifespan of drug market	Ban non-medical use of antibiotics; good antibiotic stewardship
Regulatory difficulties with combination therapies (must test each individual component first before combination)	Change regulatory requirements; not-for-profit companies with multiple partners; anti-trust law exemptions
Use of 19th century diagnostic methods (culture and susceptibility tests) to treat 21st century diseases encourages empiric broad-spectrum antibiotic drug use	Employ real-time PCR, genomics, proteomics to identify pathogens, and resistance genes; target and treat specific infections with narrow spectrum drugs

PCR: polymerase chain reaction

otic effectiveness is to be avoided [52, 53]. The disincentives for new antibiotic development and some proposed solutions are listed in Table 4.

The Future of Antibiotic Use in Clinical Medicine

Bacterial strains contain complex aggregations of genes that may be linked together to combat the inhibitory effects of antibiotics. Since prokaryotic organisms all contribute to a common 'gene pool', favorable genes mediating antibiotic resistance may disseminate among bacterial diverse microbial genera and species. Increasing evidence of multiple antibiotic resistance mechanisms within the same bacterium against a single type of antibiotic, and cooperation between bacterial populations within biofilms attest to the remarkably ingenuity and flexibility of bacterial populations [23, 29, 30]. Thus the use of one antibiotic may select for the emergence of resistance to another. Mobile genetic elements and rapidly evolving integron cassettes with multiple antibiotic resistance genes endow bacteria with a remarkable capacity to resist antibiotics [50]. Although the development of antibiotic resistance may be inevitable, the rate at which it develops can be reduced by the rational use of antibiotics.

The wider accessibility to molecular techniques and computer technology to rapidly identify the specific microorganisms, their resistance potential, and track their spread between patients within the hospital and or the community will be of considerable benefit in the control of antibiotic resistance. The need to utilize empiric, broad-spectrum antibiotics for days and even weeks while samples are being sent for culture and susceptibility testing needs to stop. We need specific information in real time to assure patients with specific infections are being treated with effective, narrow-spectrum drugs [23].

The use of antibiotics for non-medical uses should be entirely banned. Up to 50% of antibiotic use today is for non-medical use in agriculture, food preparation, and other industrial uses [52]. This adds to environmental contamination with low levels of antibiotics. Sub-inhibitory concentrations of antibiotics foster the development of resistant clones of bacteria that can cause infections in humans. The use of non-antibiotic approaches to the management of infectious diseases needs to be supported and developed. The use of plasma-based antibody therapies and anti-bacterial, anti-viral and anti-fungal vaccines should be encouraged in the future [55–57].

The management of common invasive pathogens such as staphylococcal infections has become very complicated given the rapid spread of simultaneous beta-lactam, aminoglycoside, and quinolone-resistant isolates [58]. Recent reports of vancomycin-resistant *S. aureus* in Japan and the United States suggest that common, invasive, microbial pathogens may become refractory to any chemotherapeutic agent in the future [17, 23, 58].

New drug discoveries have allowed us to be one step ahead of the bacterial pathogens for the latter half of the twentieth century. It is unlikely we will continue this record of remarkable success against microbial pathogens in the new millennium. The rapid evolution of resistance has limited the duration of the effectiveness of antibiotics against certain pathogens. The best hope for the future is the continued development of new antibiotic strategies [53]. In order to retain the antimicrobial activity of existing and new antibiotics, clinicians can assist through careful antibiotic stewardship and tightened infection control measures. Antimicrobial agents have had a substantial impact in decreasing human morbidity and mortality rates and have served us well over the antimicrobial era. It behooves us to improve our diagnostic and surveillance efforts and to exercise caution in administering antibiotics if we are to maintain their continued efficacy.

References

1. Hufnagel L, Brockmann D, Geisel T (2004) Forecast and control of epidemics in a globalized world. Proc Natl Acad Sci 101:15124–15129
2. Briand S, Khalifa H, Peter CL et al (2003) Cholera epidemic after increased civil conflict-Monrovia, Liberia, June–Sept 2003. MMWR 52:1093–1095
3. Galimand M, Guiyoule A, Gerbaud G, et al (1997) Multidrug resistance in *Yersinia pestis* mediated by a transferable plasmid. N Engl J Med 337:677–680
4. Guan Y, Poon LL, Chang CY, et al (2004) H5N1 influenza: a protean pandemic threat. Proc Natl Acad Sci USA 101:8156–8161

5. Cheung DY, Poon LL, Lau AS, et al (2002) Induction of proinflammatory cytokines in human macrophages by influenza A (H5N1) wiruses: a mechanism for the unusual severity of human disease? Lancet 360:1831–1837
6. Kobasa D, Takada A, Shinya K, et al (2004) Enhanced virulence of influenza A viruses with the haemagglutinin of the 1918 pandemic virus. Nature 431:703–707
7. Gamblin SJ, Haire LF, Russell RJ, et al (2004) The structure and receptor binding properties of the 1918 influenza hemagglutinin. Science 303:1838–1842
8. Cheng PKC, Wong DA, Tong LKL, et al (2004) Viral shedding patterns of coronavirus in patients with probable severe acute respiratory syndrome. Lancet 363:1699–1700
9. Weinstein RA (2004) Planning for epidemics – The lessons of SARS. N Engl J Med 350:2332–2334
10. Svoboda T, Henry B, Shulman L, et al (2004) Public health measures to control the spread of the severe acute respiratory syndrome during the outbreak in Toronto. N Engl J Med 350:2352–2361
11. Melski J, Reed K, Stratman E, et al (2003) Multistate outbreak of monkeypox- Illinois, Indiana, Wisconsin, 2003. MMWR Morb Mortal Wkly Rep 52:537–540
12. Petersen LR, Hayes EB (2004) Westward HO? – The spread of West Nile virus. N Engl J Med 351:2257–2258
13. Knudsen TB, Andersen O, Kronborg G (2003) Death from the Nile crosses the Atlantic: The West Nile fever story. Scand J Infect Dis 35:823–825
14. Borio L, Inglesby T, Peters CJ, et al (2002) Hemorrhagic fever viruses as biological weapons. JAMA 287:2391–2405
15. Borio L, Frank D, Mani V, et al (2001) Death due to bioterrorism-related anthrax: Report of two patients. JAMA 286:2554–2559
16. Georges-Coubot MC, Lu CY, Lansoud-Soukate J, Leroy E, Baize S (1997) Isolation and partial molecular characterization of a strain of Ebola virus during a recent epidemic of viral haemorrhagic fever in Gabon. Lancet 349:181
17. Centers for Disease Control and Prevention (2002) *Staphylococcus aureus* resistant to Vancomycin—United States, 2002. MMWR Morb Mortal Wkly Rep 51:565–567
18. Moscona A (2004) Oseltamivir-resistant influenza? Lancet 364:733–734
19. Kiso M, Mitamura K, Sakai-Tagawa Y, et al (2004) Resistant influenza A viruses in children treated with oseltamivir: descriptive study. Lancet 364:759–765
20. White TC, Holleman S, Dy F, Mirels LF, Stevens DA (2002) Resistance mechanisms in clinical isolates of *Candida albicans*. Antimicrob Agents Chemother 46:1704–1713
21. Johnson RT, Gibbs CJ Jr (1998) Creutzfeldt-Jakob Disease and related transmissible spongiform encephalopathies. N Engl J Med 339:1994–2004
22. Center for Disease Control and Prevention (2004) Outbreaks of avian influenza A (H5N1) in Asia and interim recommendations for evaluation and reporting of suspected cases – United States, 2004. MMWR Morb Mortal Wkly Rep 53:97–100
23. Opal SM, Mederios AA (2005) Mechanisms of Antibiotic Resistance. In: Mandell GL, Bennett JE, Dolin R (eds) Principles and Practice of Infectious Diseases, 6th edition. Elsevier, Philadelphia, pp 236–253
24. Bush K, Jacoby GA, Medeiros AA (1995) A functional classification scheme for β-lactamases and its correlation with molecular structure. Antimicrob Agents Chemother 39:1211–1233
25. Tompkins JD, Nelson JL, Hazel JC, et al (2003) Error-prone polymerase, DNA polymerase IV, is responsible for transient hypermutation during adaptive mutation in *Escherichia coli*. J Bacteriol 185:3469–3472
26. Drenkard E, Ausubel FM (2002) Pseudomonas biofilm formation and antibiotic resistance are linked to phenotypic variation. Nature 416:740–743
27. Chang S, Sievert DM, Hageman JE, et al (2003) Infection with vancomycin-resistant *Staphylococcus aureus* containing the vanA resistance gene. N Engl J Med 348:1342–1347

28. Senda K, Arakawa Y, Nakashima K, et al (1996) Multifocal outbreaks of metallo-β-lactamase-producing *Pseudomonas aeruginosa* resistant to broad-spectrum β-lactams, including carbapenems. Antimicrob Agents Chemother 40:349–353
29. Fridkin SK, Gaynes RP (1999) Antimicrobial resistance in intensive care units. Clin Chest Med 20:303–316
30. Hawkey PM (1998) The origins and molecular basis of antibiotic resistance. BMJ 317:657–660
31. Yokoyama K, Doi Y, Yamane K, et al (2003) Acquisition of 16S rRNA methylase gene in *Pseudomonas aeruginosa*. Lancet 362:1888–1893
32. Hasegawa Y, Yamada H, Mizushima S (1976) Interactions of outer membrane proteins 0–8 and 0–9 with peptidoglycan sacculus of *Escherichia coli* K–12. J Biochem (Tokyo) 80:1401–1409
33. Livermore DM (1992) Interplay of impermeability and chromosomal beta-lactamase activity in imipenem-resistant *Pseudomonas aeruginosa*. Antimicrob Agents Chemother 36:2046–2048
34. Mates SM, Eisenberg ES, Mandel LJ, et al (1982) Membrane potential and gentamicin uptake in *Staphylococcus aureus*. Proc Natl Acad Sci USA 79:6693–6697
35. Williams JB (1996) Drug efflux as a mechanism of resistance. Br J Biomed Sci 53:290–293
36. Levy SB (2002) Active efflux, a common mechanism for biocide and antibiotic resistance. J Appl Microbiol 92 (Suppl):65S–71S
37. Srikumar R, Li XZ, Poole K (1997) Inner membrane efflux components are responsible for β-lactam specificity of multidrug efflux pumps in *Pseudomonas aeruginosa*. J Bacteriol 179:7875–7881
38. McKessar SJ, Barry AM, Bell JM, et al (2000) Genetic characterization of vanG, a novel vancomycin resistance locus for *Enterococcus faecalis*. Antimicrob Agents Chemother 44:3224–3228
39. Cui L, Murakami H, Kuwahara-Arai K, Hanaki H, Hiramatsu K (2000) Contribution of a thickened cell wall and its glutamine nonamidated component to the vancomycin resistance expressed by *Staphylococcus aureus* M450. Antimicrob Agents Chemother 44:2276–2285
40. Fontana R, Grossato A, Rossi L, et al (1985) Transition from resistance to hypersusceptibility to beta-lactam antibiotics associated with loss of a low-affinity penicillin-binding protein in a *Streptococcus faecium* mutant highly resistant to penicillin. Antimicrob Agents Chemother 28:678–683
41. Mendelman PM, Chaffin DO, Kalaitzoglou G (1990) Penicillin-binding proteins and ampicillin resistance in *Haemophilus influenzae*. J Antimicrob Chemother 25:525–534
42. Schmitz FJ, Higgins P, Meyer S, Fluit AC, Dalhoff A (2002) Activity of quinolones against gram-positive cocci: mechanisms of drug action and bacterial resistance. Eur J Clin Microbiol Infect Dis 21:647–659
43. Enne VI, King A, Livermore DM, Hall MC (2002) Sulfonamide resistance in *Haemophilus influenzae* mediated by acquisition of *sul2* or a short insertion in chromosomal folP. Antimicrob Agents Chemother 46:1934–1939
44. Huovinen P (1987) Trimethoprim resistance. Antimicrob Agents Chemother 31:1451–1456
45. Morse SA, Johnson SR, Biddle JW, Roberts MC (1986) High-level tetracycline resistance in *Neisseria gonorrhoeae* is result of acquisition of streptococcal tetM determinant. Antimicrob Agents Chemother 30:664–670
46. Massey RC, Buckling A, Peacock SJ (2001) Phenotypic switching of antibiotic resistance circumvents permanent costs in *Staphylococcus aureus*. Curr Biol 11:1810–1814
47. Foster TJ (1983) Plasmid-determined resistance to antimicrobial drugs and toxic metal ions in bacteria. Microbiol Rev 47:361–409

48. El Solh N, Allignet J, Bismuth R, et al (1986) Conjugative transfer of staphylococcal antibiotic resistance markers in the absence of detectable plasmid DNA. Antimicrob Agents Chemother 30:161–169
49. Papadopoulou B, Courvalin P (1988) Dispersal in *Campylobacter* spp. of aphA-3, a kanamycin resistance determinant from gram-positive cocci. Antimicrob Agents Chemother 32:945–948
50. Recchia GD, Hall RM (1997) Origins of the mobile gene cassettes found in integrons. Trends Microbiol 5:389–394
51. Hall MAL, Block HEM, Donders RT, et al (2003) Multidrug resistance among enterobacteriaceae is strongly associated with the presence of integrons and is independent of species or isolate origin. J Infect Dis 187:251–259
52. Spellberg B, Powers JH, Brass EP, Miller LG, Edwards JE (2004) Trends in antimicrobial drug development. Clin Infect Dis 31:1279–1286
53. Nathan C (2004) Antibiotics at the crossroads. Nature 431:899–902
54. Service RF (2004) Orphan drugs of the future? Science 303:1798
55. Nicholson KG, Colegate AE, Podda A, et al (2001) Safety and antigenicity of non-adjuvanted and MF59-adjuvanted influenza A/Duck/Singapore/97 (H5N3) vaccine; a randomized trial of two potential vaccines against H5N1 influenza. Lancet 357:1937–1943
56. Heath PT, Booy R, Azzopardi HJ, et al (2000) Antibody concentration and clinical protection after Hib conjugate vaccination in the United Kingdom. JAMA 284:2334–2340
57. Mbelle N, Huebner RE, Wasas AD, et al (1999) Immunogenicity and impact on nasopharyngeal carriage of a nonavalent pneumococcal conjugate vaccine. J Infect Dis 180:1171–1176
58. Lowy FD (2003) Antimicrobial resistance: the example of *Staphylococcus aureus*. J Clin Invest 111:1265–1273

Technology Assessment

J. Bakker and P. Verboom

Introduction

Intensive care medicine is the department where life-supporting technologies bare the promise of survival and restoration of quality of life. As intensive care medicine uses a disproportional part of hospital budgets (1–10% of the hospital beds using up to 35% of the hospital budget [1]), efficient use of resources is warranted. Intensive care societies and governments recognize 'health technology assessment' as a process aimed to improve patient care. Many organizations deal with health technology assessment and have websites that contain abundant information on all aspects of health technology assessment (Table 1).

Technology in the intensive care unit (ICU) is usually considered to reflect the many devices commonly present in the vicinity of the critically ill patient. However, this technology is more than these devices alone, it also includes drugs, procedures and the organizational and support systems. Therefore, intensive care medicine itself can be viewed as a technology. Given the limited number of quality studies showing efficiency of intensive care technology, some even ask for a rigorous assessment as did McPherson in 2001: "In the end, intensive care

Table 1. Some relevant websites

Canadian Coordinating Office of Health Technology Assessment	www.ccohta.ca
Therapeutics Initiative	www.ti.ubc.ca
NHS Health Technology Assessment Program	www.hta.nhsweb.nhs.uk
National Institute for Clinical Excellence	www.nice.org.uk
Clinical Information Directory: Agency for Health Care Research and Quality	www.ahcpr.gov/clinic
National Board of Health Denmark	www.sst.dk
International Network of Agencies for HTA	www.inahta.org
Clinical Trials Site	www.clinicaltrials.gov
National Research Register national	www.update-software.com/

provision at the margin of possible benefit simply has to be assessed by random allocation like everything else about which there is legitimate doubt" [2].

In this chapter, we will briefly describe the basics of health technology assessment and its current place in the clinical practice of intensive care medicine in relation to different technologies frequently used. Finally we will discuss what place health technology assessment should have in 10 years from now.

Health Technology Assessment: Principles

Health technology assessment has been defined as the careful evaluation of a medical technology for evidence of its safety, efficacy, feasibility, indications for use, costs, and cost-effectiveness and its ethical and legal implications, both in absolute terms and in comparison with other competing technologies [3, 4]. Several key features distinguish health technology assessment from health related research [5]. First, the goal of health technology assessment is to deliver data that support policy-making. Health technology assessment does not only support policy-making of governmental bodies or healthcare insurance companies but also hospital decision-makers and individual health care workers. Second, health technology assessment typically integrates efforts of multiple disciplines by synthesizing information, examining databases and by generating primary data. The audience of a health technology assessment is, unlike the results of research, usually not limited to other research workers. The results of health technology assessment should typically be distributed among different bodies to facilitate decision and policy-making. Health technology assessment therefore addresses, safety, efficacy, effectiveness and efficiency of technologies used in patient care.

Safety

Authorities generally regulate the safety of technologies such that the technology is manufactured to a standard resulting in electrical safety, compliance to environmental specifications, etc. However, compliance to these safety standards does not guarantee that the device will do no harm when used in the treatment of patients. For instance, a diagnostic technology (such as the pulmonary artery catheter) is safe in itself but can increase both morbidity and mortality in critically ill patients when complications occur during introduction of the device or when data delivered by the device are incorrectly interpreted, applied in therapeutic protocols, etc. Since the recent report of the Institute of Medicine [6] much attention has been paid to the prevention of medical errors during the process of care. Although our goal should be perfect safety for our patients, preventive measures, safety programs, decision support systems, etc., all have their costs. Initial improvements in safety usually decrease total costs rapidly whereas costs increase significantly for a marginal increase in benefit when we want to reach total safety [7]. Patient safety practice has been defined as: "A process or structure whose application reduces the probability of adverse events resulting from exposure to the health care system across a range of diseases and procedures" [8]. Therefore a rigorous assessment of safety programs is appropriate but hardly present in the literature.

In addition, requests for maximal safety may have side effects in that they may stall progress [9].

Efficacy versus Effectiveness

Efficacy studies typically address the question of whether the technology can be of benefit to the patient under ideal circumstances (well controlled study with clear entry criteria and end-points in well utilized facilities). Effectiveness, on the other hand is the assessment of the technology in the real world, usually by a pragmatic approach as to whether the technology does result in clinical benefit in this situation. This is a relevant distinction as centers participating in large multicenter studies are usually specialized hospitals able to recruit significant number of patients with well-equipped departments and adequate intensive care staffing. These factors all have been found to influence patient outcome [10–14] and may thus influence effectiveness of these technologies when used in other hospitals.

Efficiency

Assessment of the efficiency addresses the costs and the consequences of implementing the technology and thus helps to resolve the question of whether the technology studied should be implemented in clinical practice. The quality of an economic evaluation depends heavily on the data-quality of the costs measured or calculated. In Table 2 some definitions used in economic evaluations are described.

Two methods of cost calculation are frequently used in intensive care medicine. First, top-down costing is a retrospective method that apportions costs into different subgroups where the mean cost per patient day is the total costs divided by the total number of patient days. This rough calculation does not permit detailed studies in specific patient groups and thus limits its use. However, this method is useful for a broad-based assessment of different technologies. Second, the bottom-up costing method summates all the different resources used by individual patients to build the total costs of patient care. This much more accurate method is labor intensive and thus requires use of data management systems for long-term collection of costing data. This method is more suitable to compare the cost-effectiveness of different technologies especially when detail is important (e.g., is the use of strict blood glucose control cost-effective in patients with sepsis).

Although many proxies for cost calculation are used validation of these proxies is hardly available. On the other hand some measures of outcome have a direct relationship with costs so that a decrease in intensive care and hospital stay has been used as a proxy for a decrease in total costs of care [15].

Table 2. Definitions in costing technology

Direct versus indirect costs	Direct costs relate to the health care process (e.g., drugs, personnel, interventions, disposables, blood and blood products). Indirect costs are generated outside the health care process (e.g., loss of production as long as the patient is unable to work)
Fixed versus variable costs	Fixed costs do not change with changes in production over a short period of time (rent, salaries, lease of equipment). Variable costs vary with the level of production (e.g., drugs, fluids, disposables). Total costs refer to the costs of producing a particular quantity of output and is the summation of the fixed and variable costs.
Marginal costs	Total costs related to a change in production by one unit
Incremental costs	Difference in total costs when comparing different alternatives
Discounting	As both costs and benefits are valued differently in the present time and future time these have to be discounted to generate long-term costs and benefits.

Different types of economic evaluations are used in health technology assessment. A *cost-minimization analysis* studies whether an alternative technology can replace the current technology but at lower costs. An important additional analysis in a study like this is the change in risk with the alternative technology as the analysis implicitly assumes the benefits of both technologies are equal. A *cost benefit analysis* takes into account all costs and benefits, both calculated in equivalent monetary units.

A *cost-effectiveness analysis* takes into account all costs and benefits but uses different terms to describe them. Costs are usually expressed in monetary units whereas the benefits of the technology studied are expressed in non-monetary outcomes. Preferably, these non-monetary outcomes should be easily comparable between different technologies. Therefore, the most valid non-monetary outcome used is the number of life years gained. However, intermediate outcomes can also be used (decrease in ventilator days). If used these intermediate outcomes should have a generally accepted relationship to survival. The results of these analyses are often expressed as a ratio: the number of life years gained per amount of money. A cost-effective analysis results in an incremental cost-effectiveness ratio. The difference in costs of the alternatives is then divided by the difference in effectiveness. An incremental cost effectiveness analysis can have four possible outcomes as depicted in Figure 1. By running simulations and defining acceptable thresholds [16] one can support decision-making: should we use the new technology?

A *cost-utility analysis* is used when there is no, or only a minor, impact on survival but a major impact on morbidity or when the technologies studied do not have equivalent outcomes. The costs are similar to the cost-effective analysis

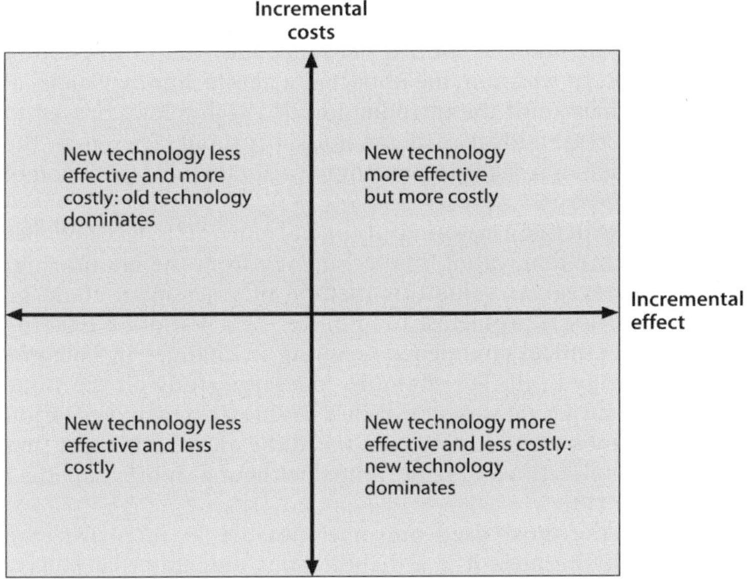

Fig. 1. Possible outcomes of an incremental cost effectiveness analysis of two technologies.

however the outcome measures used attempt to capture intermediate states of health, morbidity, and quality of life to produce a more complete assessment. An outcome measure frequently used in this analysis, which combines survival benefit and quality of life, is the quality adjusted life year (QALY).

Other Measures of Outcome

As mentioned in the previous section an economic outcome measure is frequently used in health technology assessment. However, other outcomes could help to assess new technologies in intensive care medicine:

- Resource utilization
- Safety
- Mortality
- Clinical comfort
- Accuracy of diagnosis

To value the benefit from an intervention one first needs to define the scope of the analysis. Introducing a new diagnostic test that helps to exclude the diagnosis of sepsis could reduce use of antibiotics and decrease the incidence of resistant bacteria without affecting clinical outcome. This would be of no direct benefit for our patients in the ICU but would be of great benefit for society, hospital organization, and even future patients [17]. As clinicians require proof of a meaningful outcome to start using the technology its diffusion into clinical practice is not only dependent on the proof of cost-effectiveness. Therefore, the clinicians' perception of the magnitude and the clinical relevance may limit diffusion of cost-effective technologies. In addition, the impact of a new technology on local (ward, hospital) budgets may limit the introduction of a technology proven to be cost-effective when increased local costs are not substituted. Therefore, the addition of a budget-impact analysis is important to facilitate local diffusion of the technology.

It is even more difficult to define a meaningful clinical outcome in technologies already in use. Although the removal of this technology from the monitoring/ therapeutic arsenal may reveal its value this method of assessment could be limited by practical and ethical problems. In addition, removal of an existing technology may decrease clinical confidence resulting in changes in outcome not related to the technology itself. For example, in a large study on the value of pulse oximetry during surgery it was shown that having data on oxygenation increased the number of interventions and convinced the anesthesiologist that major life threatening complications were prevented without a significant effect on morbidity or mortality [18].

Mortality is probably the most used outcome measure in intensive care medicine studies. Not only because it is a dichotomous outcome that is easy to count and not subject to much discussion about the distinction, but also because it is one of the best meaningful outcome measures in a department with significant baseline mortality. In addition, we should use an outcome measure that is a genuine result of the technology studied. Thus, when assessing a monitoring technology, a different outcome measure should be used as the monitor will trigger a procedure rather than affect outcome by itself. Much of the discussion on the efficacy of the pulmonary artery catheter is troubled by the use of inadequate end-points for the technology itself. When using mortality as an end-point in assessing monitoring technology one should assess the procedure triggered (treatment protocol) rather than the monitor itself [19].

Funding of Health Technology Assessment

Apart from assessment of drugs, not much is regulated for new or existing technologies in intensive care medicine when it comes to efficiency and cost-effectiveness. Assessment is mostly funded by industry and the costs of these studies are passed on to the consumer. However, while the profits in drug technology may be large, return of investment in device and diagnostic technologies may be much less. This usually results in less rigorous studies when these technologies are assessed. Assessment of process technology is even more difficult and usually only possible with significant government funding [20, 21]. Costs of assessments could be reduced if industry, hospitals and government worked together. A collaboration like this would also improve agreement on methodologies and approaches to health technology assessment in intensive care [22]. Many examples already exist where government and hospitals/clinicians work together to provide the intensive care community with assessments of different technologies commonly used in intensive care medicine [23–27].

Technology Assessment: Current Place in Intensive Care

Intensive care medicine is an environment rich in diagnostic, monitoring, therapeutic, life support and informatics technologies. Some technologies even have combined monitoring, diagnostic and therapeutic effects. Even in relatively simple cases a vast array of technologies is part of standard treatment. In a straightforward case of pneumococcal septic shock more than 40 technologies could be used (Table 3). From the example given in Table 3 it is clear that many technologies have not been assessed and probably many will not undergo rigorous health technology assessment in the future. Nevertheless, many clinicians believe technologies they use on a regular basis have been shown to be effective by properly conducted randomized controlled clinical trials when in fact these technologies have not been properly studied [28]. As mentioned before, clinicians also have problems correctly addressing the nature of the technology. Diagnostic, monitoring and prevention technologies are sometimes seen as being therapeutic

Table 3. Review of technologies used in pneumococcal septic shock

Diagnosis: Pneumonia	Treatment: Infection	Monitoring
History taking	Antibiotics	Pulse oximetry
Physical examination		Capnometry
X-ray	**Treatment: Shock**	Temperature
Laboratory investigation	Hemodynamic optimization (ER)	Heart rate – EKG
Blood culture	Admission to intensive care	Blood pressure
Sputum culture	Fluids	Central venous pressure
Protected specimen brush	Vasoactive agents Steroids	Pulmonary pressures
		Cardiac output
Diagnosis: Shock	**Treatment: Supportive**	Mixed venous oxygenation
Blood pressure	Mechanical Ventilation (invasive – noninvasive)	Pulse pressure variation
Fluid resuscitation	Prone positioning	Intrathoracic blood volume
Measure of adequate fluid resuscitation	Renal replacement therapy	Extravascular lung water
	Glucose control	Right ventricular ejection fraction-volumes
Diagnosis: Severity of disease	Selective decontamination gut	Echocardiography
APACHE II-III	Prophylactic heparin	Urine output
SOFA	Enteral feeding	Skin temperature-color-perfusion index
	Nursing care	Gastric retention
	Sedatives-pain medication	Sedation-pain score
	Rotation therapy	SOFA score
	Continuous subglottic suctioning	TISS-score
	Tracheostomy	Laboratory
	Weaning	Follow-up cultures
	Physiotherapy	
	Prayers	

EKG: electrocardiogram; SOFA: sequential organ failure assessment, TISS: therapeutic intervention scoring system technologies [28]. This confusion could lead to incorrect perception of the technology and its clinical utility and thus result in disuse in clinical practice.

As intensive care medicine originates from major specialties like anesthesiology, internal medicine and surgery, utilization drift has been responsible for the diffusion of many technologies. For instance, mechanical ventilation as applied in the operating room (10–15 ml/kg tidal volume and zero positive end-expiratory pressure) without apparent harm to patients, was utilized in the ICU in similar settings. It required years and numerous studies to produce convincing evidence that these modes of ventilation when applied to ICU patients for longer periods of time actually increase morbidity and mortality [29, 30].

Currently, many monitoring, diagnostic and information technologies disseminate into clinical practice before they are sufficiently evaluated. Especially in Europe, governments rarely require proof of effectiveness let alone cost-effectiveness for these technologies. The CE-marking required to market throughout Europe without additional approval of individual countries is a technical label rather than a functional one. Most importantly, obtaining a CE-mark does not require the involvement of clinicians at any stage. In the United States the FDA does require some proof of efficacy of these technologies.

The Future

Health technology assessment is an established field within our health care system with solid fundaments in many countries. However, although the main purpose of health technology assessment is to facilitate policymaking and support decision-making the vast majority of studies performed resulting in explicit policies has not changed practice. The implementation of guidelines resulting from assessments is variable [31]. The adoption of guidelines depends on the level of professional support, an adequate evidence base, the economic effects of the guidelines, the presence of a guideline implementation system in the organization and coherence in the group of clinicians. These factors can guide us into the future of health technology assessment in intensive care medicine, where not only drugs have to go through rigorous assessment but also other technologies will be assessed before their introduction in the clinical arena.

Professional Support

Assessment of new or existing technologies should become the joint effort of all stakeholders. Therefore clinicians and professional societies should be involved early in the process of assessment and the development of standards. National societies, government and industry could develop national assessment centers. This would have several advantages. First, funding of these centers would be a joint effort and thus less expensive to the individual participants. Second, different centers (national and international) could join efforts to assess technologies in subgroups of ICU patients with a low incidence. Thirdly, the costs of technology would ultimately decrease and the time needed to perform an assessment could decrease substantially. National societies should promote and diffuse the results of health technology assessment to their members being aware of its possible legal implications [32]. In order for health technology assessment to evolve from simple dissemination to complex interactive communication [5] it is important that it is implemented into the educational programs of medical students and specialists and in the training programs of intensivists.

Adequate Evidence Base

A growing concern is expressed regarding the association between the source of funding of studies and the conclusions drawn from these studies [33–35]. Performing assessments in a joint structure as described above could overcome these concerns that may greatly limit the diffusion of new technologies into clinical practice. The process of health technology assessment should be transparent and clear for those who should use it for policy-making. In many studies in intensive care medicine the costing methodology is highly variable and sometimes the most important cost components are not reported [36].

In addition, assessment of specific groups of technology (diagnostic, therapeutic) could follow a standardized framework evaluating how technology works in the laboratory, its range of uses and diagnostic accuracy, and its impact on clinicians' practices and patients' outcomes [17, 37, 38]. Structured assessment and reporting of results by national and international assessment centers could change the mindset of the clinicians to adopt guidance rather than submit themselves to guidance.

Special attention should be paid to the relevance of different clinical outcome measures. Traditionally, morbidity and mortality are accepted meaningful clinical endpoints for the clinician. Both policy-makers and clinicians should accept quality of life, improvement in physical functioning, and relief of anxiety and stress etc. as relevant end-points in health technology assessment. As these endpoints are already accepted clinical goals, incorporating these in health technology assessment could help clinicians to see themselves as 'doers' as well as 'users' of the assessments [39].

Economic Effects

Diffusion of new technologies into clinical practice is dependent on coverage by government or health insurance companies even if rigorous health technology assessment has shown cost-effectiveness. As an example, the use of activated Protein C (Xigris®) is about 8 times higher in Belgium when compared to The Netherlands. Part of this huge difference can be explained from the coverage present in Belgium and almost absent in The Netherlands. It is therefore important to link coverage to an assessment. In addition this could also strengthen the available evidence by increasing the pool of participants in a trial and broadening the venues of care to ensure their application to community-based practice or to limit their provision to centers of excellence [39].

In addition, intensive care departments should be proactive in the assessment of the local implications of implementation. Preferably this should be a multidisciplinary process where clinicians, managers and hospital administrators join efforts to value new technologies in a local setting and seek additional funding to implement them.

Conclusion

Health technology assessment is an important and recognized field of research in today's health care system. Health technology assessment should be a continuing process where re-evaluation of existing technologies is as important as the first evaluation of a new technology. Intensive care departments of the near future should be the 'doers' and the 'users'. Organized efforts in which professional autonomy is respected are likely to have long-term success. Technology assessment in the intensive care of the near future should not be simply more research but should be a way of thinking of the 'new' intensivists.

References

1. Jacobs P, Noseworthy TW (1990) National estimates of intensive care utilization and costs: Canada and the United States. Crit Care Med 18:1282–1286
2. McPherson K (2001) Safer discharge from intensive care to hospital wards. BMJ 322:1261–1262
3. Perry S, Eliastam M (1981) The National Cancer for Health Care Technology. JAMA 245:2510–2511
4. European Society of Intensive Care, Section on Technology Assessment (1999) Health Technology Assessment In Intensive Care Medicine: The Current Status In Clinical-Industry Workshop. European Society of Intensive Care Medicine, London
5. Battista RN, Hodge MJ (1999) The evolving paradigm of health technology assessment: reflections for the millennium. CMAJ 160:1464–1467
6. Kohn LT, Corrigan JM, Donaldson MS (2000) To Err Is Human: Building a Safer Health System. Institute of Medicine. National Academy Press, Washington
7. Warburton RN (2005) Patient safety--how much is enough? Health Policy 71:223–232
8. Shojania KG, Duncan BW, McDonald KM, Wachter RM (2002) Safe but sound: patient safety meets evidence-based medicine. JAMA 288:508–513
9. Loefler I (2004) Evidence based medicine. BMJ 328:842
10. Pronovost PJ, Angus DC, Dorman T, Robinson KA, Dremsizov TT, Young TL (2002) Physician staffing patterns and clinical outcomes in critically ill patients: a systematic review. JAMA 288:2151–2162
11. Baldock G, Foley P, Brett S (2001) The impact of organisational change on outcome in an intensive care unit in the United Kingdom. Intensive Care Med 27:865–872
12. Cross DT 3rd, Tirschwell TL, Clark MA, et al (2003) Mortality rates after subarachnoid hemorrhage: variations according to hospital case volume in 18 states. J Neurosurg 99:810–817
13. Birkmeyer JD, Stukel TA, Siewers AE, Goodney PP, Wennberg DE, Lucas FL (2003) Surgeon volume and operative mortality in the United States. N Engl J Med 349:2117–2127
14. Aiken LH, Clarke SP, Cheung RB, Sloane DB, Silber JH (2003) Educational levels of hospital nurses and surgical patient mortality. JAMA 290:1617–1623

15. Sedrakyan A, Van der Meulen J, Lewsey J, Treasure T (2004) Video assisted thoracic surgery for treatment of pneumothorax and lung resections: systematic review of randomised clinical trials. BMJ 329:1008
16. Angus DC, Linde-Zwirble WT, Clermont G, et al (2003) Cost-effectiveness of drotrecogin alfa (activated) in the treatment of severe sepsis. Crit Care Med 31:1–11
17. Gattas DJ, Cook DJ (2003) Procalcitonin as a diagnostic test for sepsis: health technology assessment in the ICU. J Crit Care 18:52–58
18. Moller JT, Pedersen T, Rasmussen LS, et al (1993) Randomized evaluation of pulse oximetry in 20,802 patients: I. Design, demography, pulse oximetry failure rate, and overall complication rate. Anesthesiology 78:436–444
19. Reinhart K, Radermacher P, Sprung CL, Phelan D, Bakker J, Steltzer H (1997) PA catheterization–quo vadis? Do we have to change the current practice with this monitoring device? Intensive Care Med 23:605–609
20. Stiell IG, Wells GA, Field BJ, et al (1999) Improved out-of-hospital cardiac arrest survival through the inexpensive optimization of an existing defibrillation program: OPALS Study Phase II. JAMA 281:1175–1181
21. Technology Subcommittee of the Working Group on Critical Care, Ontario Ministry of Health (1991) The assessment of technology in Ontario's critical care system. CMAJ 144:1613–1615
22. Sibbald WJ (2003) Introduction: theme articles on technology assessment in critical care. J Crit Care 18:38–40
23. Heyland DK, Cook DJ, Marshall J, et al (1999) The clinical utility of invasive diagnostic techniques in the setting of ventilator-associated pneumonia. Canadian Critical Care Trials Group. Chest 115:1076–1084
24. Stewart TE, Meade MO, Cook DJ, et al (1998) Evaluation of a ventilation strategy to prevent barotrauma in patients at high risk for acute respiratory distress syndrome. Pressure- and Volume-Limited Ventilation Strategy Group. N Engl J Med 338:355–361
25. Cook DJ, Brun-Buisson C, Guyatt GH, Sibbald WJ (1994) Evaluation of new diagnostic technologies: bronchoalveolar lavage and the diagnosis of ventilator-associated pneumonia. Crit Care Med 22:1314–1322
26. Technology Subcommittee of the Working Group on Critical Care, Ontario Ministry of Health (1991) Hemodynamic monitoring: a technology assessment. CMAJ 145:114–121
27. Technology Subcommittee of the Working Group on Critical Care, Ontario Ministry of Health (1992) Noninvasive blood gas monitoring: a review for use in the adult critical care unit. CMAJ 146:703–712
28. Ferreira F, Vincent JL, Brun-Buisson C, Sprung C, Sibbald W, Cook D (2001) Doctors' perceptions of the effects of interventions tested in prospective, randomised, controlled, clinical trials: results of a survey of ICU physicians. Intensive Care Med 27:548–554
29. Hickling KG, Walsh J, Henderson S, Jackson R (1994) Low mortality rate in adult respiratory distress syndrome using low-volume, pressure-limited ventilation with permissive hypercapnia: a prospective study. Crit Care Med 22:1568–1578
30. The Acute Respiratory Distress Syndrome Network (2000) Ventilation with lower tidal volumes as compared with traditional tidal volumes for acute lung injury and the acute respiratory distress syndrome. N Engl J Med 342:1301–1308
31. Sheldon TA, Cullum N, Dawson D, et al (2004) What's the evidence that NICE guidance has been implemented? Results from a national evaluation using time series analysis, audit of patients' notes, and interviews. BMJ 329:999
32. Damen J, van Diejen D, Bakker J, van Zanten AR (2003) Legal implications of clinical practice guidelines. Intensive Care Med 29:3–7
33. Miners AH, Garau M, Fidan D, Fischer AJ (2005) Comparing estimates of cost effectiveness submitted to the National Institute for Clinical Excellence (NICE) by different organisations: retrospective study. BMJ 330:65
34. Lexchin J, Bero LA, Djulbegovic B, Clark O (2003) Pharmaceutical industry sponsorship and research outcome and quality: systematic review. BMJ 326:1167–1170

35. Als-Nielsen B, Chen W, Gluud C, Kjaergard LL (2003) Association of funding and conclusions in randomized drug trials: a reflection of treatment effect or adverse events? JAMA 290:921–928
36. Gyldmark M (1995) A review of cost studies of intensive care units: problems with the cost concept. Crit Care Med 23:964–972
37. Cook DJ, Hebert PC, Heyland DK, et al (1997) How to use an article on therapy or prevention: pneumonia prevention using subglottic secretion drainage. Crit Care Med 25:1502–1513
38. Keenan SP, Guyatt GH, Sibbald WJ, Cook DJ, Heyland DJ, Jaeschke RZ (1999) How to use articles about diagnostic technology: gastric tonometry. Crit Care Med 27:1726–1731
39. Eisenberg JM (1999) Ten lessons for evidence-based technology assessment. JAMA 282:1865–1869

Trends in Pediatric and Neonatal Critical Care in the Next 10 Years

R. C. Tasker

Introduction

The specialty of pediatric intensive care provides medical treatments for the most critically ill infants and children, most of whom will be mechanically ventilated. It therefore requires highly trained specialist staff. Fortunately – or unfortunately, depending on your perspective – pediatric intensive care is a low volume, high cost service that cannot be provided in every locality. However, in the modern world, the ideal is that it should be available to all children who need it regardless of where they live [1]. The scope of this review will be to set the stage for 10 years from now – what are the issues in pediatric intensive care, and can we determine what will be required for infants and children of the future?

An Historical Perspective of Pediatric and Neonatal Critical Care

Intensive care units (ICUs) and critical care medicine were founded on treatments for the severely ill [2]. There is a European history of neonatal care that dates back to the early 1900s. However, in the modern era of pediatrics, a quantum change to our thinking did not really start until the polio epidemic in Copenhagen, 1952. Since then our specialty has been fashioned by three major forces. First, the disease and predicament that is special to children. Second, the lessons learned from adult critical care. Third, understanding of how it is possible to intervene in developmental physiology and biology.

Diseases and Predicaments Special to Children

We are now able to intubate the trachea, and manage the infant and child airway for prolonged periods with pediatric tubes ranging from 1.5 to 6.0 mm. Outside early infancy two conditions have driven the need for such 'airway care' in critically illness: acute epiglottitis caused by *Haemophilus influenzae* type b and viral laryngotracheobronchitis, or croup. The development of heat-sensitive, plastic silicone tubes was a considerable advance on traditional approaches with either metal tracheostomy tubes or red-rubber orotracheal tubes. It meant that children could be managed safely with nasotracheal tubes that moulded to the shape of the airway with body temperature, rather than *visa versa*. Children did not have to receive neuromuscular blockade just because they were intubated, and, with careful handling, they could even be managed without the need for sedation.

After we had learnt these important lessons, we then discovered in the 1990s the influence on critical illness of good general pediatric health care. In my lifetime, acute epiglottitis has, in the main, disappeared from pediatric intensive care practice and that is because of the power of universal, infant primary immunization at 2-, 3- and 4-months of age [3, 4]. To a lesser extent, but equally dramatic, croup necessitating endotracheal intubation has also decreased. In this instance, it has been as a result of family doctors and general pediatricians treating croup early with short courses of steroids [5, 6].

We have also developed child-specific strategies for those needing neurological intensive care. This expertise was gained from the experience in the 1970s to 1990s of Reye's syndrome and post-resuscitation hypoxic-ischemic encephalopathy. Reye's syndrome came and went, but the condition did introduce pediatric critical care specialists to the complexities of neurological critical care [7], which has now had a beneficial knock-on effect on how we care for the severely head-injured [8]. At the time there was much debate about whether Reye's syndrome was related to influenza, occult or subacute forms of medium-chain acyl-CoA dehydrogenase deficiency, aspirin, or some combined interaction of all three factors. Interestingly, the greatest impact on pediatric intensive care was produced by a single public health intervention: the recommendation that aspirin should be avoided in children under 12-, and now more recently 16-years of age, resulted in disappearance of the condition. Post-resuscitation care of near-drowning victims introduced us to critical care neuroprotection. Although, in common with the adult experience, no effective drug therapies have been forthcoming in children [9, 10], it does seems likely that hypothermia may be of benefit in the post-asphyxiated newborn.

Last, we can now support even the most extremely preterm infant. The progress made from the 1940s through to the late 1990s was not without incident. We discovered the toxicity of oxygen and the now more recent problem of intensive care technology that can temporarily extend life beyond the extra-uterine limit of viability [11, 12]. That said, there have been positive impacts for our specialty: the knowledge of basic vegetative functions during development and the ability to manage homeostasis of patients as small as 300 g.

Lessons Learned from Adult Critical Care

The 'adult' approach to sepsis and shock came to fruition in pediatric intensive care, in the UK, during the meningococcal outbreak of the 1990s. A reduction in case fatality rate from meningococcal septicemia was associated with improved emergency health care, starting with early volume resuscitation and cardiorespiratory support [13, 14]. However, like our experience with *Haemophilus influenzae* type b, the major impact on pediatric intensive care has come with a public health initiative – meningococcal vaccine to all children and young people [15]. Like acute epiglotittis, the shocked patient with purpura fulminans is now a medical *curio* from the past. Other examples of cross-fertilization between adult and pediatric critical care include ventilatory treatment of acute lung injury and acute hypoxemic respiratory failure [16], and extracorporeal support for refractory cardiorespiratory failure [17, 18].

Treatments that Intervene in Developmental Physiology and Biology

In the 1970s, Flavio Coceani and Peter Olley discovered the role of prostaglandin E in the postnatal adaptation of the ductus arteriosus from a fetal- to an air-breathing circulation [19], and applied that knowledge clinically [20]. In so doing, they provided a new emergency therapy for certain cyanotic congenital malformations, and transformed the nature of infant cardiac surgery. No single intensive care therapy has had such an impact. A more modern example – although yet to stand the test of time – is, perhaps, the recent report of successful gene therapy for x-linked severe combined immunodeficiency [21]. This developmentally-directed therapy might prove to be a more effective strategy for restoring functional cellular and humoral immunity than conventional bone marrow transplantation, which as many intensivists know has a notorious track record in pediatric intensive care [22].

Taking all of these examples together – childhood infection, cross-fertilization from adult critical care medicine, and developmental biology – we can generate at least three hypotheses about the likely pattern of pediatric intensive care in 10 years time. First, in regard to infectious disease, we should expect that community-acquired infection would have a less prominent role with the development of new and wider ranging vaccines. Second, in regard to the broader field of critical care medicine, we should consider it likely that there will be greater convergence between adult, pediatric, and neonatal specialists in the practice of life-support and *reanimation*. Third, in regard to new intensive care therapies, we should be prepared for the most significant 'critical care' research to originate from outside our field and be later translated into new therapies.

Key Issues in the Delivery of Pediatric Intensive Care

If the above three predictions are in some way correct, then what will be the trend in pediatric and neonatal critical care 10 years from now? In order to answer this question we should consider the key issues in the delivery of pediatric intensive care in 2005. These are, the need for regionalization and the organizational consequences that follow, and the pattern of childhood critical illness.

Regionalization of Pediatric Intensive Care

In 1997, the UK Department of Health set about reviewing the national configuration of pediatric intensive care [1]. A multidisciplinary coordinating group was instrumental in shaping the future of the national service. Four types of hospital were defined and considered integral to meeting the profile of demand:

- District General hospitals (DGH) that admit children and are able to initiate pediatric intensive care;
- Lead Center hospitals that provide most of the pediatric intensive care that is needed in the area, as well as support the whole service for the area through the provision of advice and training;
- Major Acute General hospitals with large adult ICUs which already provide a considerable amount of pediatric intensive care in the older child; and
- Specialist hospitals that provide some pediatric intensive care in support for a defined specialty, e.g., cardiac, neurosurgical, and burns units.

Let us consider the child with severe head injury and acute subdural hematoma in order to illustrate the organizational operation of such a service. The annual incidence of head injury is between 100 and 300 per 100,000 population. It follows, therefore, that a population-based regionalization of pediatric neurosurgical and neurointensive care services is necessary because of the numbers of patients needed for a viable and sustainable clinical practice [1, 23]. However, one consequence of centralization for mixed suburban and rural regions, as opposed to those encompassing conurbations or metropolitan counties, is that the provision of an emergency practice has to contend with the problem of patient access, particularly if timeliness – surgical evacuation within 4 hours of injury – is a key requirement. In the UK region of East Anglia (a mixed urban and rural area) this time constraint for stabilization and transfer of the severely ill head-injured child translates into an operational range limited to DGH referrals up to ~45 minutes road distance from the lead center hospital [24].

If we consider the wider context of illness in children other requirements and patterns emerge. In the London Thames region of the UK the pediatric population is just above 3.1 million. In 1997, all children living in this area who met specific criteria for critical illness were included in a population-based audit [25, 26]. We found that there were over 6000 episodes of critical illness. Two-thirds of these episodes were managed on pediatric intensive care or cardiac units, and two-thirds of the patients were intubated. Throughout childhood the incidence of critical illness was 1.8/1000 pediatric population per year. The highest incidence, 13.6/1000/yr, was present in children under the age of 12 months.

Based on this analysis, the initial conclusions we can make about the current delivery of pediatric intensive care are as follows. First, given a relationship between volume and performance (i.e., higher equating with better) [27], then pediatric intensive care should be part of a population-based network. Second, an efficient national regional service necessitates adequate infrastructure to expedite equitable patient access [28]. Third, pediatric intensive care practitioners require significant training and expertise in the under 1-year-olds.

The Pattern of Childhood Critical Illness

The Paediatric Intensive Care Audit Network (PICANet) is a collaborative national (England and Wales) project funded by the UK Department of Health and by the Health Commission of Wales [29]. Its purpose is to audit pediatric intensive care activity and provide information on effective delivery of pediatric intensive care. For the one-year, March 2003 to February 2004, data are available from all 29 designated pediatric intensive care units (PICUs). In over 14,000 admissions, one-third was for support and monitoring following surgery. Half the admissions were unplanned emergencies, and of these 47% (3,092 children) came from a DGH or other acute facility, i.e., they needed interhospital transfer. The primary diagnostic groups, by age, are shown in Table 1. It is evident that pediatric intensive care is predominantly a specialty of surgery and cardiorespiratory illness in the under 5 year olds. If we go on to consider just those with a medical cause of acute respiratory failure, then the major etiologies are primary respiratory illness (52%), central nervous system insult (34%), and systemic disease such as sepsis (14%) [30]. Of those with a primary respiratory problem the major diagnoses include pneumonia in the immunodeficient and oncologic cases (25%), other forms of pneumonia (17%), acute bronchiolitis – usually due to respiratory syncytial virus (RSV) – 17%, and upper airway obstruction (17%).

Therefore, the next important conclusions about the current pattern of pediatric critical illness are as follows. First, pediatric intensive care has a significant function for children requiring complex surgery. Second, cardiorespiratory

Table 1. 2004 pediatric intensive care admissions in England and Wales by primary diagnostic group and age [29].

Diagnosis	Age (years)				Total (%)
	< 1	1 to 4	5 to 10	11 to 15	
Cardiac	2510	928	516	378	31.4%
Respiratory	1986	840	371	229	24.8%
Neurological	460	675	457	342	14.0%
GI	545	145	79	91	6.2%
Infection	232	237	96	80	4.7%
MS	50	96	134	258	3.9%
Oncology	53	147	113	108	3.0%
Other	721	388	239	301	11.9%
Total (n)	6557	3456	2005	1787	13805
Total (%)	47.5%	25%	14.5%	12.9%	

GI: gastrointestinal; MS: musculoskeletal.

failure in the under 5-year-olds appears to be the *sine qua non* of those needing pediatric intensive care. Third, out of the various illnesses producing respiratory failure, major infectious 'burdens' in pediatric intensive care are pneumonia in the immunodeficient, and acute bronchiolitis due to RSV.

Determining What will be Required for Infants and Children

Predicting the pediatric intensive care requirements for a future generation of specialists has risks. We may get everything horribly wrong. The only advantage is that many of the decision makers will no longer have any professional involvement in pediatric intensive care, and so be oblivious to the consequences of their (our) actions.

A Salutary Lesson of Mis-planning

In the early 1980s, the national hospital for children in the UK planned a 30-bedded unit for general pediatric intensive care. Health care planners had predicted that by the late 1990s the major problems necessitating intensive care in a national facility would be complex surgery, acquired immunodeficiency syndrome (AIDS), organ transplantation, and infection with multiresistant organisms. Half the bed-spaces were therefore planned as cubicles and many were built with barrier-isolation units. The new facility was opened in the mid-1990s. Within months it became obvious that the design was unworkable. The patients that were predicted to come never materialized. Sure, there were some cases with AIDS, multiresistant organisms, etc., but the major requirement for pediatric intensive care was for fast-track surgery. We quickly learnt that a cubicalized unit was not conducive to such management. The project over the next two years was therefore reconfiguring the space so that most of the cubicles could be dismantled – in effect redesigning an 'open' surgical unit.

Working With Children, 2004–2005

What are the current facts, figures and information about child health? Thursday December 30, 2004, Kofi Annan, the United Nations Secretary-General said of the Indian Ocean Tsunami "This is an unprecedented global catastrophe and it requires an unprecedented global response. Over the last few days it has registered deeply in the conscience of the World" [31]. The most pressing fact in 2005 worldwide child health is that child deaths from disaster, famine and infection remain considerable. We live in a complex world. At extremes we have countries with easy access to all potential resources and technologies, and those who have nothing. There are countries where basic food, water, immunization, and medical care are limited. Yet we have nation groups who are affluent, who have access to all modern resources and expect their children to have the full advantages of pediatric intensive care. How will a humane culture reconcile the inequalities?

By way of illustration of these inequalities between, and within nations, let us briefly consider death rates among under 5 year-old children. In September 2000, the United Nations set several millennium development goals, one of which was to reduce the 1990 death rates among the under 5 year-olds by two-thirds by 2015 – a fall from 93 to 31 in every 1000. Ninety countries are expected to meet this target, 53 of which are developing nations [32]. And, according to the UNICEF report *Progress for Children*, 98 countries are still falling far short of the 4.4% annual progress needed [33]. Table 2 shows mortality rates in under 5 year-old children for different regions in the world. In addition, summary data from individual member countries of the World Federation of Societies of Intensive and Critical Care Medicine (WFSICCM) are also included. In 2002, five of these countries had under 5 year-old mortality rate greater than 31 in every 1000 children: what is the answer - ventilators or vitamins? At the other end of the spectrum, all of the industrialized countries had a mortality rate below 10 in every 1000 children: is the answer really more ventilators?

If you were to walk around my unit on a typical winter's day you would find: a previously well 14-month-old child with pneumonia complicating influenza (current ventilated length of stay [vLOS] 5 days); an infant with RSV infection, and underlying pulmonary hypertension and trisomy 21 (current vLOS 15 days); another infant with RSV infection, and underlying ventricular septal defect (current vLOS 14 days); a 3-year-old child with an acute upper respiratory tract infection complicating an underlying airway anomoly (current vLOS 8 days); a 5-year-old child with chicken pox pneumonia and underlying severe cerebral palsy(current vLOS 12 days); and, a formerly preterm, 15-month-old child with post-hemorrhagic hydrocephalus and gross developmental delay who has recently undergone a twentieth cerebral-ventriculo-peritoneal (VP) shunt revision; etc. After a clinical round such as this example, you would be correct in wondering whether, with improvement in basic health, housing, nutrition and immunization, fewer and fewer individuals are consuming more and more of the pediatric intensive care resource. For example, long-stay pediatric intensive care patients (with length of stay > 12 days) account for 4.7% of the pediatric intensive care population, but use 36.1% of the days of care; they have less favorable outcomes, use more resources, and are more likely to require chronic care devices [34]. It also appears that in the developed world there is a recent trend for units to be occupied by more of such children [35]. If we look to the future then, we must ask ourselves "What form of pediatric intensive care will have the greatest effect on the largest number of children – where, when, how, why and to whom?"

Trends in Pediatric and Neonatal Critical Care

In this context, then, what are the likely trends over the next ten years? In regard to neonatal critical care, the rate of prematurity – year on year – remains unchanged at around 7%. There is no indication that numbers are diminishing so unless there are major developments in public health and obstetrics, such practice will continue in a manner similar to the present time [36]. We also know

Table 2. UNICEF under 5 year-old mortality figures (rates per 1000 children) [33]. The progress in reduction is measured as the average annual reduction rate. To achieve a two-thirds reduction between 1990 and 2015 requires a progress rate of 4.4% or higher.

	Under 5 mortality rate			Progress in reduction	
Region	1990	2002	2015 Target	1990-2002 Observed	2002-2015 Required
CEE/CIS, Baltic states	48	41	18	1.3	7.2
Latvia	20	21	7	-0.4	8.8
Romania	32	21	11	3.5	5.2
Macedonia	41	26	14	3.8	4.9
East Asia, Pacific	58	43	19	2.5	6.2
China	49	39	16	1.9	6.7
Indonesia	91	45	30	5.9	3.0
Singapore	8	4	3	5.8	3.0
Malaysia	21	8	7	8.0	1.0
Latin America, Caribbean	54	34	27	3.9	4.9
Venezuela	27	22	9	1.7	6.9
Panama	34	25	11	2.6	6.1
Argentina	28	19	9	3.2	5.5
Chile	19	12	6	3.8	5.0
Columbia	36	23	12	3.7	5.0
Mexico	46	29	15	3.8	4.9
Uruguay	24	15	8	3.9	4.8
Brazil	60	36	20	4.3	4.5
Ecuador	57	29	19	5.6	3.3
Middle East, North Africa	81	58	27	2.8	5.9
*Saudi Arabia	44	28	15	3.8	5.0
*United Arab Emirates	14	9	5	3.7	5.0
*Kuwait	16	10	5	3.9	4.9
South Asia	128	97	43	2.3	6.3
Pakistan	130	107	43	1.6	7.0
India	123	93	41	2.3	6.3
Sub-Saharan Africa	180	174	60	0.3	8.2
*South Africa	60	65	20	-0.7	9.1
Industrialized countries	10	7	3	3.0	5.8
Japan	6	5	2	1.5	7.0
United States	10	8	3	1.9	6.8
Canada	9	7	3	2.1	6.5
Switzerland	8	6	3	2.4	6.1
Finland	7	5	2	2.8	6.0
United Kingdom	10	7	3	3.0	5.8
Belgium	9	6	3	3.4	5.3
France	9	6	3	3.4	5.3
Ireland	9	6	3	3.4	5.3
Spain	9	6	3	3.4	5.3
Netherlands	8	5	3	3.9	4.7
Australia	10	6	3	4.3	4.6

Table 2. *Continued*

Region	Under 5 mortality rate			Progress in reduction	
	1990	2002	2015 Target	1990-2002 Observed	2002-2015 Required
Italy	10	6	3	4.3	4.6
Slovakia	15	9	5	4.3	4.5
Hungary	16	9	5	4.8	4.1
Austria	9	5	3	4.9	3.9
Germany	9	5	3	4.9	3.9
Slovenia	9	5	3	4.9	3.9
Israel	12	6	4	5.8	3.1
Sweden	6	3	2	5.8	3.1
Czech Republic	11	5	4	6.6	2.3
Norway	9	4	3	6.8	2.2
Portugal	15	6	5	8.6	0.5

Countries marked with "*" are those with pediatric intensive care units, but not members of the World Federation of Societies of Intensive and Critical Care Medicine.

that, in the developed world, formerly premature children are readmitted to the ICU more often during the same hospitalization, use more chronic technologies (e.g., ventilators, gastrostomy tubes, tracheostomy tubes, and parenteral nutrition), and have longer vLOS days [37]. Since we can expect continued improvements in neonatal care it is therefore likely that these individuals will have a significant impact on pediatric intensive care practice.

What are the other child health trends outside the perinatal period? In England and Wales the child population under 15-years-old is just over 11 million [36]. In 2002, there were 3,168 infant deaths under the age of 1-year [38] – equivalent to ~ 5.3/1000 live births. There were 187 sudden infant deaths (0.31/1000 live births), with the highest frequency in babies of mothers aged under 20-years at the time of birth – 0.97/1000 live births. In children aged 1– to 14-years there were 1,420 deaths – equivalent to 15/100,000 children. (The rate in 1– to 4-year olds is higher at 24/100,000). Table 3 summarizes the main causes of child mortality for 1998 to 2000 in children aged 1– to 15-years. Across the pediatric age-range cancer, accidents, and poisoning are the main causes of death. Of the cancers, leukemia is the most common in children.

If we think of the future, accidents and poisoning should be preventable with health education. In regard to accidents, just consider the following fact: a recent school survey of 10– to 15-year-olds in the UK identified that, during the previous year, around 40% of males had an accident that needed treatment by a doctor or at hospital [38]. The answer to this problem is not better or more health care!

Next, what are the chronic health conditions that might impact on pediatric intensive care? There are three major conditions that effect children – asthma, cerebral palsy, and diabetes. Up to 18% of 10– to 15-year-olds report having asthma [38]. However, with good primary medical care the need for pediatric intensive

Table 3. Main causes of child mortality 1998-2000 in England and Wales [35]

Causes	1 to 4 years Male	Female	5 to 15 years Male	Female
Infections	10%	9%	4%	6%
Cancers	15%	13%	24%	23%
CNS+S	13%	13%	15%	16%
Circulation	6%	8%	5%	5%
Respiratory	11%	9%	6%	8%
Congenital	13%	16%	6%	8%
Accident	16%	15%	27%	17%
Other	17%	16%	13%	16%
Total (n)	1,153	855	1,773	1,239

CNS+S: central nervous system and sense organs.

care should be avoided. In regard to cerebral palsy, 1 in every 400 babies born in the UK has cerebral palsy, i.e., 1,800 children every year. In total, in England and Wales (1998) there were 393,824 children under 16-years with disabilities (55,200 aged < 5-years). More than 100,000 were considered severely disabled and had at least two different sorts of significant impairment. These children require surgery (e.g., scoliosis, adductor tenotomy, Nissen's fundoplication, feeding gastrostomy, and VP shunt) and, because of their underlying condition, post-operative pediatric intensive care. Last, in the UK, there are 20,000 children with insulin-dependent diabetes mellitus. This condition is increasing in the northern hemisphere but in common with asthma, early diagnosis, and good primary and secondary medical care should avoid the need for pediatric intensive care.

In addition to these three conditions a new, acquired, life-impairing condition is emerging such that, if current trends continue, there will be an epidemic in 2015. In 2001 8.5% of 6-year-olds, and 15% of 15-year-olds met the criterion for obesity (body mass index > 30 kg/m^2). We are just beginning to see the ramifications of this epidemic in pediatric intensive care. For example, last month I looked after a 90 kg 12-year-old girl with cellulitis complicating intertrigo, and profound (and chronic) obstructive sleep apnea that came to medical attention only after hospital admission. This is new territory for pediatric intensive care – what maintenance fluids would you prescribe for a 90 kg 12-year-old, where the normal body weight should be half this amount?

In summary, the current trend in pediatric intensive care casemix suggests a future core practice devoted less to infectious disease. We will have to cope with seasonal variation and unexpected eventualities. But, by 2015 we would hope that vaccines for RSV infection in the under 1-year-olds should make this condition a thing of the past. Rather, core pediatric intensive care activity is increasingly committed to the current major killers and causes of chronic childhood disease. So in 10 years time this may mean a practice concentrated on support for oncology, accident, and surgical services, in their care of infants and children with underlying disease, susceptibility, and disability.

Conclusion

The history and current state of pediatric intensive care suggest that the trend in pediatric and neonatal critical care in 2015 will have the following core features.

1. A population-based network that includes adequate infrastructure to expedite patient access.
2. A workforce that has undergone significant training and expertise in the under 1-year-olds.
3. A caseload that is centered on children requiring oncologic, surgical and accident treatments.
4. A practice that, like the present, will contend with the extremes of life but from a new perspective. Late sequelae of extreme prematurity and obesity.

References

1. Paediatric Intensive Care: a “Framework for the future”. Department of Health, Health Services Directorate, UK. July 1997. At: http://www.dh.gov.uk/assetRoot/04/03/43/40/04034340.pdf Accessed July 2005
2. Downes JJ (1992) The historical evolution, current status, and prospective development of pediatric critical care. Crit Care Med 8:1–22
3. Garpenholt O, Hugossen S, Fredlund H, Bodin L, Olcen P (1999) Epiglottitis in Sweden before and after introduction of vaccination against Haemophilus influenzae type b. Pediatr Infect Dis 18:490–493
4. Midwinter KI, Hodgson D, Yardley M (1999) Paediatric epiglottitis: the influence of the Haemophilus influenzae type b vaccine, a ten-year review in the Sheffield region. Clin Otolaryngol 24:447–448
5. Cressman WR, Myer CM 3rd (1994) Diagnosis and management of croup and epiglottitis. Pediatr Clin North Am 41:265–276
6. Bjornson CL, Klassen TP, Wilhamson J, et al. (2004) A randomised trial of a single dose of oral dexamethasone for mild croup. N Engl J Med 351:1306–1313
7. Boutros A, Hoyt J, Menezes A, Bell W (1977) Management of Reye’s syndrome. A rational approach to a complex problem. Crit Care Med 5:234–238
8. Tasker RC (2000) Neurological critical care. Curr Opin Pediatr 12:222–226
9. Bohn DJ, Bigger WD, Smith CR, Conn AW, Barker GA (1986) Influence of hypothermia, barbiturate therapy, and intracranial pressure monitoring on morbidity and mortality after near-drowning. Crit Care Med 14:529–534
10. Biggart MJ, Bohn DJ (1990) Effect of hypothermia and cardiac arrest on outcome of near-drowning accidents in children. J Pediatr 117:179–183
11. Avery ME (1998) Pioneers and modern ideas: Neonatology. Pediatrics S1:270–271

12. Lorenz JM (2000) Survival of the extremely preterm infant in North America in the 1990s. Clin Perinatol 27:255–262
13. Booy R, Habibi P, Nadel S, et al (2001) Reduction in case fatality rate from meningococcal disease associated with improved healthcare delivery. Arch Dis Child 85:386–390
14. Pathan N, Faust SN, Levin M (2003) Pathophysiology of meningococcal meningitis and septicaemia. Arch Dis Child 88:601–607
15. Trotter CL, Andrews NJ, Kaczmarski EB, Miller E, Ramsay ME (2004) Effectiveness of meningococcal serogroup C conjugate vaccine 4 years after introduction. Lancet 364:365–367
16. Peters M, Tasker RC, Kiff K, Yates R, Hatch D (1998) Respiratory indices fail to predict outcome in acute hypoxemic respiratory failure in children. Intensive Care Med 24:699–705
17. UK Collaborative ECMO Trial Group (1996) UK collaborative randomised trial of neonatal extracorporeal membrane oxygenation. Lancet 348:75–82
18. Goldman A, Butt W, Kerr S, Tasker R, Macrae D (1997) ECMO for intractable cardiorespiratory failure due to meningococcal disease. Lancet 349:1397–1398
19. Coceani F, Olley PM (1973) The response of the ductus arteriosus to prostaglandins. Can J Physiol Pharmacol 51:220–225
20. Olley PM, Coceani F, Bodach E (1976) E-type prostaglandins: a new emergency therapy for certain cyanotic congenital heart malformations. Circulation 53:728–731
21. Gaspar HB, Parsley KL, Howe S, et al (2004) Gene therapy of x-linked severe combined immunodeficiency by use of a pseudotyped gammaretroviral vector. Lancet 364:2181–2187
22. Jacobe SJ, Hassan A, Veys P, Mok Q (2003) Outcome of children requiring admission to an intensive care unit after bone marrow transplantation. Crit Care Med 31:1299–1305
23. Shann F (1993) Australian view of paediatric intensive care in Britain. Lancet 342:68
24. Tasker RC, Gupta S, White DK (2004) Severe head injury in children: geographical range of an emergency neurosurgical practice. Emerg Med J 21:433–437
25. Steering Group for Pan Thames Study of Critically ill Children (1997) Should paediatric intensive care be centralised? Lancet 350:65
26. Maybloom B, Chapple J, Davidson LL (1999) The Use of Hospital Services in North and South Thames for the Care of Critically-ill Children: An Assessment of Need. Kensington & Chelsea and Westminster Health Authority, London
27. Tilford JM, Simpson PM, Green JW, Lensing S, Fiser DH (2000) Volume-outcome relationships in pediatric intensive care units. Pediatrics 106:289–294
28. Kanter RK (2002) Regional variation in child mortality at hospitals lacking a pediatric intensive care unit. Crit Care Med 30:94–99
29. Paediatric intensive care audit network. At: http://www.picanet.org.uk. Accessed July 2005
30. Tasker RC (2000) Gender differences and critical medical illness. Acta Paediatr 89:621–622
31. Bone J, Kennedy D (2004) The world digs deep. The Times, Friday December 31
32. White C (2004) Less than half the world is likely to meet target for cutting child deaths. BMJ 329:818
33. UNICEF (2004) Progress for Children. At: http://www.unicef.org/publications/index_23557.html. Accessed July 2005
34. Marcin JP, Slonin AD, Pollack MM, Ruttimann UE (2001) Long-stay patients in the pediatric intensive care unit. Crit Care Med 29:652–657
35. Briassoulis G, Filippou O, Natsi L, Mavrikiou M, Hatzis T (2004) Acute and chronic paediatric intensive care patients: current trends and perspectives on resource utilization. QJM 97:507–518
36. National Statistics (2000) Child Health Statistics. At: http://www.statistics.gov.uk/downloads/theme_health/Child_Health_Book_v4.pdf. Accessed July 2005

37. Slonin AD, Patel KM, Ruttimann UE, Pollack MM (2000) The impact of prematurity: a perspective of pediatric intensive care units. Crit Care Med 28:848–853
38. Horton C (2003) Working with children 2004–05. Society Guardian, London.

Diagnostic, Therapeutic and Information Technologies 10 Years from Now

The Patient Process as the Basis for the Design of an ICU

B. Regli and J. Takala

Introduction

What role does design play in the adult critical care environment? In the early 1990s, the Society of Critical Care Medicine (SCCM), the American Association of Critical Care Nurses (AACN), and the American Institute of Architects/Committee on Architecture for Healthcare (AIA/CAH) co-sponsored an Intensive Care Unit (ICU) design competition to focus awareness on the role of the critical care unit environment in promoting healing of the critically ill. The Swedish Medical Center of Englewood, Colorado, was honored with the first ICU Design Citation among 66 participants in 1992. Lessons learned in the process of conducting the competition were published by the SCCM in 1996, in a book titled *Critical Care Unit Design and Furnishing* [1]. Around the same time, the major American and European intensive care societies published statements concerning minimal requirements and optimal design [2–3].

Neither the SCCM nor the European Society of Intensive Care Medicine (ESICM) has published updated guidelines in the past decade. What has happened in the field of intensive care design in the meantime? What should we consider when designing the ICUs where we will treat our patients in the decades to come?

There is not exactly an abundance of recent technical literature on the topic of ICU design. Koay and Fock published "Planning and design of a surgical intensive care unit in a new regional hospital" in 1998 [4], and Hamilton published "Design for flexibility in critical care" in 1999 [5]. There were articles presenting the nursing perspective [6, 7] and investigating the effect of design on infection control [8–10]. More recently, the AIA published "Guidelines for Design and Construction of Hospital and Healthcare Facilities" [11]. A revised version of those guidelines is due out in 2006.

But the limited guidelines that exist for hospital construction and design are unlikely to address the changes that are sure to take place in healthcare delivery in years to come. While ICUs will certainly continue to exist over the next decades, the general hospital context around them will change substantially.

The importance of outpatient care will increase, and inpatient sectors will change from units with regular beds to step-down units, also referred to as intermediate care facilities. Progress in hospital construction will allow a more flexible ICU area. Flexibility will be an important principle, not only with regard to construction but even more so with respect to the mode of operation. Two critical resource factors – money and the availability of skilled personnel – will shape this operating mode.

There is no single approach to the task of designing the ICU of the future: the solutions depend on many factors within the hospital, in healthcare in general, as well as in society as a whole. Here, we look at how you can design your ICU using the different core processes of the ICU and the hospital, most importantly the patient care process, as the basis. We present our vision – one vision – of the ICU 10 years from now.

Basics/Approach

While the prerequisites for acute care of critically ill patients may seem rather obvious, ICU design is influenced by many factors that are not directly related to patient care within the ICU or even within the hospital. In order to assess the design features that are optimal for a specific ICU, it is useful to consider separately:

1) the environmental conditions outside the hospital that are likely to influence the ICU;
2) the environmental conditions within the hospital that are likely to influence the ICU;
3) the core processes within the ICU itself; and
4) the main support processes influencing the ICU.

Under what External Environmental Conditions does the Hospital operate?

- How many people live in the catchment area of the hospital, and how many ICU patients is it likely to produce? In order to assess the number of potential ICU patients, it is useful to separately assess the number of emergency patients (primarily dependent on the characteristics of the population and their expectations for care) and the number of patients requiring intensive care after elective surgery and other interventions (dependent on the available surgical and other interventional services among other factors).
- How is healthcare organized in the catchment area? What are the roles of private and public health care? Are there defined paths of patient flow for admissions and discharges?
- Do multiple hospitals with their own ICUs serve the same catchment area or compete in it?
- What is the hospital's mission? Is it expected to change?
- What is and what will be the strategy of the hospital in providing services and developing its role?
- What are the political plans of the government for healthcare and its financing?
- Is restructuring of healthcare planned or likely?
- What future scenarios can you envision in the next 5, 10, 15 years?

Under what Environmental Conditions within the Hospital does the ICU operate?

- What is the mission of the ICU?
- Are there different ICUs for specified tasks within the hospital?
- Which clinical specialties are available in the hospital? What is the actual patient mix for intensive care? Does the hospital have a special role, e.g., as a burn center or a trauma center?
- Are there serious problems with nosocomial infections in the hospital?
- What is the organizational structure of clinical services and how is intensive care organized within the hospital structure?
  - Is the ICU independent or part of another or several other services?
  - Are there other high dependency care units (i.e., other ICUs, intermediate-care or step-down units, post-anesthesia care units), and how are they organized?
- Is enough skilled staff available?
- To what extent is the capacity of the ICU utilized?

A major political issue that inevitably influences the design of the ICU and the utilization of its resources is the positioning of intensive care within the hospital structure. We strongly believe that concentrating ICU resources under one administration with an interdisciplinary intensive care concept offers many advantages, and that these should be considered in the design of future ICUs. For example:

- Resource allocation can be better controlled and efficiency facilitated
- Care and best practice models can be more systematically applied
- Optimizing the process of care is easier
- The continuous presence of ICU professionals can be better guaranteed
- There may be a fairer distribution of limited resources to patients who need it.

Our own experience at the University Hospital of Berne, where five ICUs (three surgical, two medical) from three different departments were merged into an independent department of intensive care medicine, supports this concept: the integration of the units resulted in increased admissions, reduced length of stay, and reduced ICU mortality, despite similar severity of illness (Table 1). Also, the number of patients discharged with a poor prognosis decreased.

To build interdisciplinary units you need a philosophy that encourages cross-specialty training and a broader skill mix. This may be more demanding and time-consuming than if you have staff members who are specialized in one discipline, but it will ultimately lead to more flexibility and foster interdisciplinary collaboration in the care of the critically ill patient.

Table 1. Patient data from 1998 to 2003. The merger of units started at the end of 1999, with full functional integration during 2000.

	1998	1999	2000	2001	2002	2003
# of patients	2,799	2,682	3,029	3,221	3,081	3,338
SAPS-2 (mean)	29.8	30.2	28.3	28.0	29.5	29.3
LOS ICU mean (days)	3.6	3.4	2.8	2.4	2.3	2.4
Age (mean)	60.1	59.9	60.8	59.6	60.0	59.5
Mortality (%)	8.2%	7.7%	6.5%	5.6%	6.0%	5.5%

LOS: lengh of stay

What are the Core Processes of the ICU?

The core processes of the ICU depend somewhat on the characteristics of the hospital and whether it is affiliated with a university. A pragmatic approach is to consider three main horizontal processes that are independent of the degree of specialization of the unit. All ICUs treat patients (patient care process) and provide teaching (education process; even in 'non-teaching' hospitals, education is still important for the ICU staff); if research belongs to the function, then it becomes the third main process. The relative weight of these processes may have consequences for the unit's design. In any case, over the short-term, the patient care process has the highest priority.

The core processes can be considered as:
- The patient care process
- The education process
- The research process

These processes are interrelated: each one influences the optimization of the others (Fig. 1). With a good education process, the risk of complications for patients can be reduced. Without the education process, the specialized knowledge and skills needed to care for patients will be limited. And without patients,

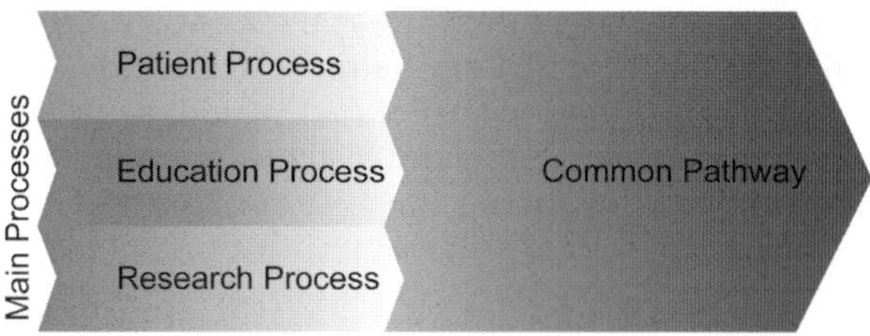

Fig. 1. The main processes – patient intensive care, education, and research – have a common pathway.

there are fewer options for teaching intensive care medicine. The same is true for research. The patients' diseases and problems form the basis for the questions asked, and research gives the answers needed for treating the patients. The three main processes may appear to exist in parallel, but ultimately they proceed in a common direction, and follow a common path.

The Support Processes

Support processes are essential for the main processes. Among those with greatest relevance for design are logistics, information technology, control, and administration. These processes should be adapted to the main processes, and not the reverse. The common aim of all of the processes should be steady improvement in organization and provision of intensive care medicine.

The Patient Process as the Central Task

It is important to recognize that an ICU is not a stand-alone organization. It is not an end in itself. The ICU is a central part of a complex horizontal patient process (Fig. 2).

Patient outcomes will depend not only on the expertise of the ICU team and the quality of the ICU facilities but also on the diagnostic tools available and the care provided in the emergency department, the operating room, and the units to which the patients are discharged. It is obvious that the physical paths should be short between the various departments involved. But it is not just the distance in meters that affects patient care; a safe and cost-efficient patient process is also dependent on the communication systems that link the various departments to the ICU.

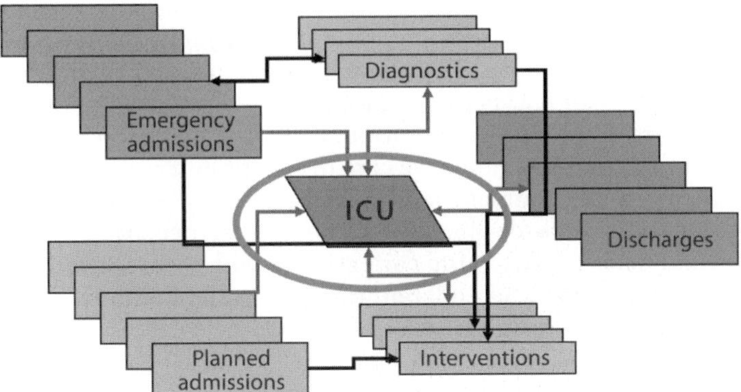

Fig. 2. The central position of the ICU in different patient processes and their interdependency. The function of several departments and services is typically influenced by the function and structure of the ICU. This should also be considered in the unit design.

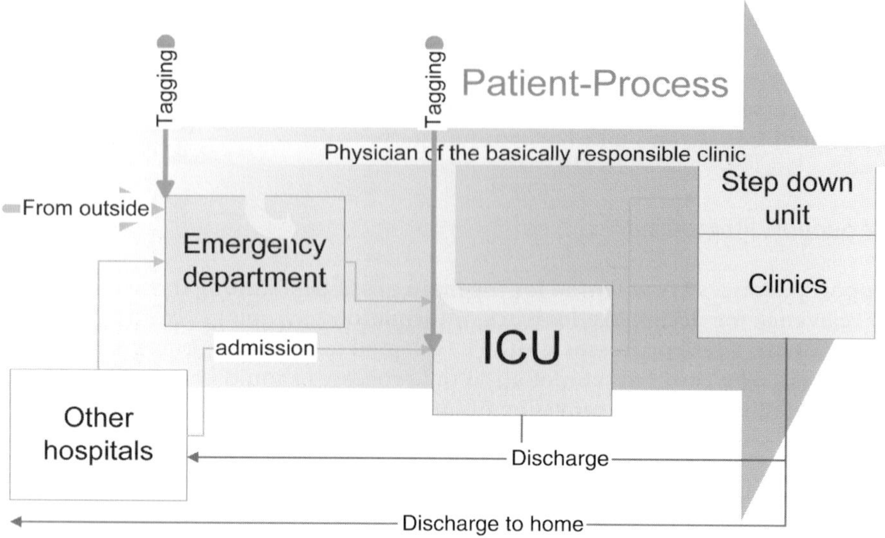

Fig. 3. The 'closed but integrative and communicating' model (from the ICU viewpoint). In a structured communication system, a physician accompanies the patient through the different departments.

The traditional division of ICU organizational models [12] into 'closed' (all decisions are the responsibility of the ICU staff) or 'open' (the primary physician is responsible for decisions concerning the intensive care, with or without an ICU physician in a more or less consultant role) should be obscure in the future. The future model should be seen as 'closed but integrative and communicating' (Fig. 3). The ICU team is involved in the care of patients from the moment they enter the hospital via the emergency department or are brought in by ambulance services, along with a physician from the unit that will receive the patient after the ICU stay. This physician accompanies the patient throughout the hospital stay. 'Tagging' is the term we use to describe the process of integrating another clinic in the responsibility for an ICU patient's care.

Tagging promotes interdisciplinary cooperation. Although it is necessary for the ICU physicians to be in charge of intensive care decisions and resources, the ICU should not be a closed environment, but rather a place where teams can work together. It should be possible for physicians from the partner specialties to be involved in important decisions affecting patients they will later receive from the ICU. Through communication and collaboration, the patient will profit (as will the economic interests of the hospital).

Process-Oriented Design

Planning and design can be facilitated using a structured system approach, which separately addresses the different levels of planning and the processes involved.

The Three-System Model [13]

Three separate levels of systems can be defined in planning, design, financing, and construction. The *primary system* consists of the walls of the building, the alignment of the different units within the building, and logistics between the ICU and the rest of the hospital. The *secondary system* refers to the layout of the unit and to functions inside the unit, including communications. The *tertiary system* consists of what is within a subunit (room), its layout, equipment, and furniture, i.e., the immediate patient treatment area and bedside design.

The primary system

The primary system determines the flexibility of the building. It is like the DNA for the development of a living thing. The primary system is a long-term investment.

The alignment of the units

To support the patient process in a general hospital, the ICU should be located in close proximity to:

- The emergency department
- The operating room
- Diagnostic facilities, such as computed tomography (CT) or magnetic resonance imaging (MRI)
- Other intervention facilities (cardiology laboratories, neurology stroke unit, angiology)
- Step-down facilities

These requirements depend on the specific characteristics of the hospital. More specialized hospitals (e.g., those without an emergency department) will have different priorities. For the alignment, there are three general concepts: horizontal, vertical, and mixed. Examples of these are shown in Figure 4.

Horizontal alignment locates all the important services next-door to the ICU on the same floor (A). Diagnostic modalities such as CT and MRI are gaining in importance, and transporting unstable patients is risky and resource-intensive. Whether portable diagnostic devices will be able to reduce transportation demands is currently not known. Also, close proximity to step-down facilities supports the continuum of care and helps to optimize resource utilization within the high-dependency care area.

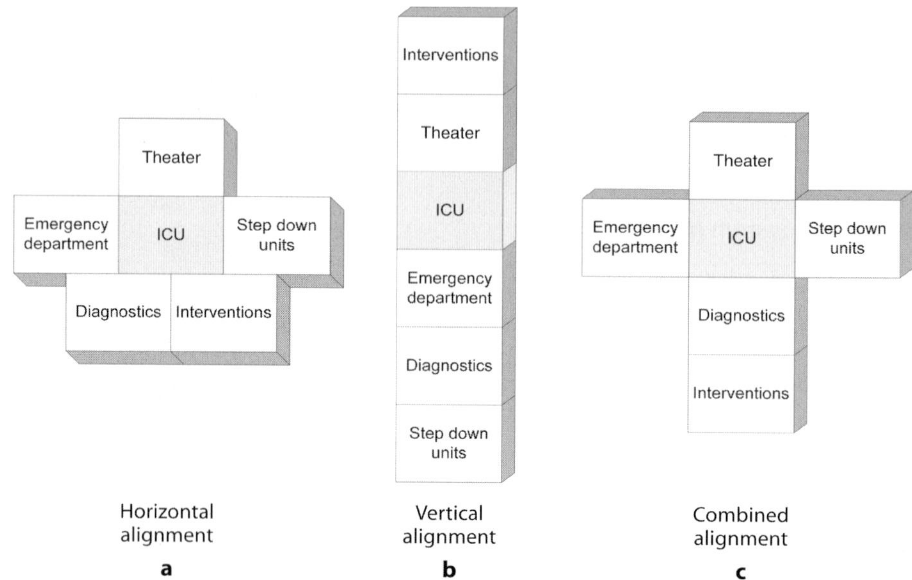

Fig. 4. Possible alignment of units close to the ICU. **a** is presented from above. **b** and **c** are viewed from the side.

Horizontal alignment also has drawbacks. Even a very compact ICU has fairly large dimensions, and distances to the neighboring units may become considerable. Arranging the unit to accommodate the different neighbors on all sides will require flexibility, and patient rooms will have no direct view to the outside.

If horizontal alignment is not feasible or desirable (your floor plan may not allow enough square meters, or access to too many services may be necessary), a more realistic alignment is vertical (B) or a combination of horizontal and vertical (C). In this case, wide lifts with dedicated capacity for ICU patient transport are necessary. These lifts should ideally lead to the center of the ICU. If the lifts are wide enough and there is enough capacity, distances are not very important. It is easier to examine and treat a patient in a wide lift than on a long corridor.

The patient lifts, the logistic imperative to connect units

A lift should be wide enough (approximately 2.15 x 3.20 m minimum) to enable transport of patients in complicated situations. Beds are becoming larger, and in the future some ICU equipment (monitoring, for instance) will be integrated into the patient's bed. Organ support systems consume space, and space is needed for the accompanying staff.

To have a redundant system, you should have two wide patient lifts in a tower-like building. For security reasons, the two lifts should not be in the same section of the building. If there is a fire, you must be able to evacuate patients from another area of the ICU floor.

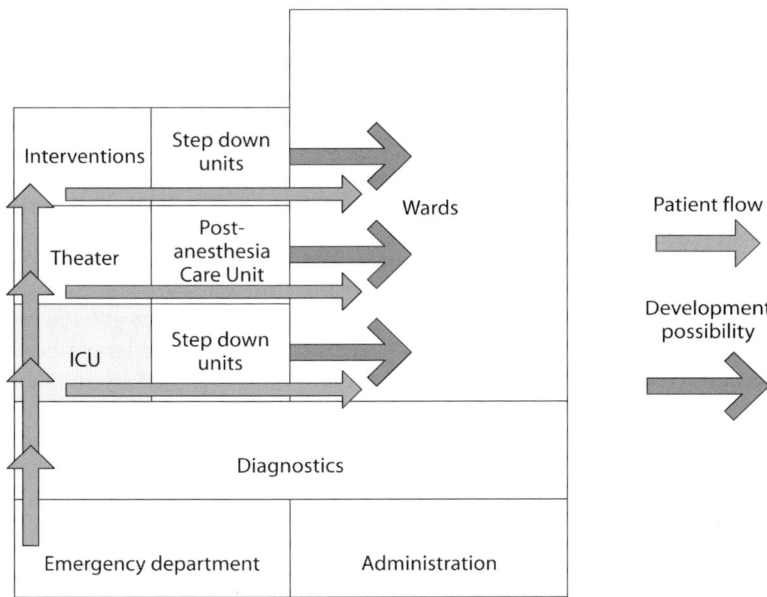

Fig. 5. Process-oriented alignment of units close to the ICU in a tower

Process-oriented alignment of units

If, as predicted, future hospitals will have more and more step-down beds instead of regular beds, then a tower will be the preferred primary system (Fig. 5).

In a changing healthcare environment you should have the flexibility to convert regular wards and patient rooms to high dependency care facilities.

The relationship between the ICU and the step-down unit

There are several reasons why hospitals have developed step-down units [14]:

- to facilitate earlier ICU discharge of stable patients who are thought to need more care than can be provided on general wards.
- to decrease the need for ICU readmission by providing more monitoring and nursing care than is available on hospital wards.
- to decrease patient mortality rates in hospitals that are experiencing marked pressure on the availability of beds in ICUs.
- to reduce the cost of treating patients who do not need the unique services of an ICU by providing care in areas with a lower nurse/patient ratio and less complex technology.

These step-down beds, providing care at a lower level than the ICU but a higher level than the general ward, can be organized in a quite different way. Principally there are two possibilities, with modifications:

- Step-down beds integrated in the ICU
  - based on cohorts or
  - based on flexible allocation of step-down patients throughout the ICU, with concomitant adjustment of personnel, monitoring, and care intensity
- Step-down beds outside the ICU
  - 24-hour post-anesthesia care unit
  - integrated in a surgical or medical clinical department

Each option has advantages and disadvantages. The aim should be to get the best quality of care at the lowest cost with the best possible outcome. Step-down beds located on the ward of a specialized department (e.g., cardiology) have the advantage of concentrating patients with very similar medical problems in one location. This reduces the breadth of knowledge and skills needed by the caregivers, and may enhance the treatment process for the majority of patients. But, as a result of the specialization, the care and treatment of patients with multiple or complex problems ('medical multiple trauma') is not optimal and may seriously interfere with the standard care process and result in wasting of resources. Locating step-down beds inside the ICU has the advantage of making it possible to change the level of care provided to patients without moving them from one place to another. The logistics for continual adjustment of care intensity and altering the staff/patient ratio may be easier to achieve. The entire staff will need a very broad knowledge of different medical specialties and will need skills covering a wide range of levels of care; thus, the staff will have to be much more flexible. Concentrating step-down patients in one area of the ICU has the advantage of easier planning and allocation of material and personnel within the ICU, while the lower intensity of care and severity of illness are predefined. At the same time, support from the normal ICU area will be readily available. Step-down bed cohorting may also facilitate training of less experienced staff, and may provide a temporary, less intensive working environment during periods of high work load in the normal intensive care area.

The secondary system

The secondary system is a medium-term investment. It is beyond the scope of this article to discuss all aspects of the secondary system. Therefore, we will concentrate on some key aspects that have a major potential impact on care processes.

The area requirements of a compact ICU

As intensive care medicine has developed into its own specialty, requirements for space have changed. Intensive care is now provided by trained intensivists and other professionals, who work exclusively in the perimeter of the ICU. Space is needed not only for treating patients, but also for education, research, and support processes, such as logistics, human resource management, informatics,

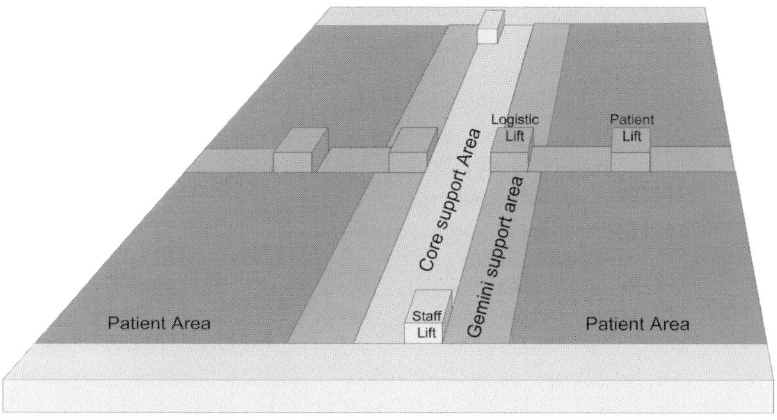

Fig. 6. Potential design of a compact ICU in a tower-like building. The dark gray area marks the patient rooms in subunits with a common communication center. The hatched area marks the twin (Gemini) support areas, each serving two subunits. The light gray area marks the core support area for all subunits (staff, main corridor, relatives, discussion facilities, secretary, research and education facilities).

control, and secretarial support. To meet all of these requirements, you will need about 100 square meters of floor space per bed.

The ICU of the future should be compact. The space allocated to patient care is dependent on the number of patient beds and on the treatment concept (the rate of high versus lower level of intensive care). The treatment area should contain a communication center (nursing station) serving a subunit of no more than 8–12 patients. Each subunit should have its own offices, toilets, storage rooms, sinks, lifts, waste disposal, etc. (Fig. 6).

The core support area contains kitchens and lounges for the staff and the relatives, the main corridors, storage rooms, meeting rooms (education, presentations, daily report), offices for staff and secretaries, an admissions point, clinical research facilities, staff lifts, and an area for the relatives to say their final goodbyes after a patient has died.

Nursing station

The 'nursing station' will look very different in the future. Although intensive care medicine organization as a whole will be more centralized, nursing and medical functions will be increasingly decentralized (Fig. 7). Centralized monitoring and observation will become less important as staff move closer to the patient's bed. However, central monitoring will not disappear completely, as it provides flexibility when there is a critical shortage of resources.

What was once a central monitoring and observation area will metamorphose into a communications area. In the communications area you will have the secretarial support staff, centralized telephone answering, personal computers, a fax machine, a tube station, and connection to the Picture Archiving and Com-

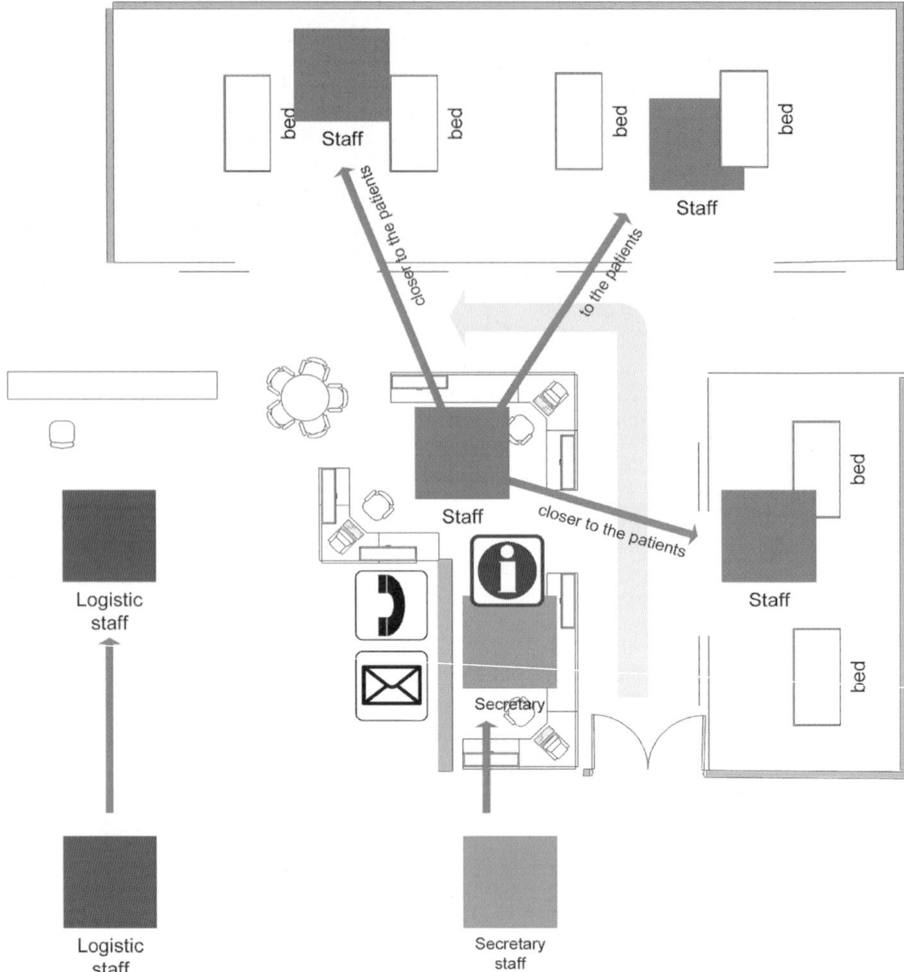

Fig. 7. In the nursing station of the future the medical and nursing staff are brought closer to the patients and the logistical and secretarial staff move closer to the front to relieve the medical and nursing staff.

munication System (PACS). The communication area will be one of the work sites for the numerous healthcare professionals who are involved in the treatment of the patients and support of the patients' relatives, and a point of information for the healthcare staff and relatives. Last but not least, it is a centralized area where informal communication can take place between staff members and the consulting specialties.

Wireless communications and personal hand-held communication terminals will be the norm; this is likely to reduce the administrative workload and enhance the link between administration and patient care process. The proximity

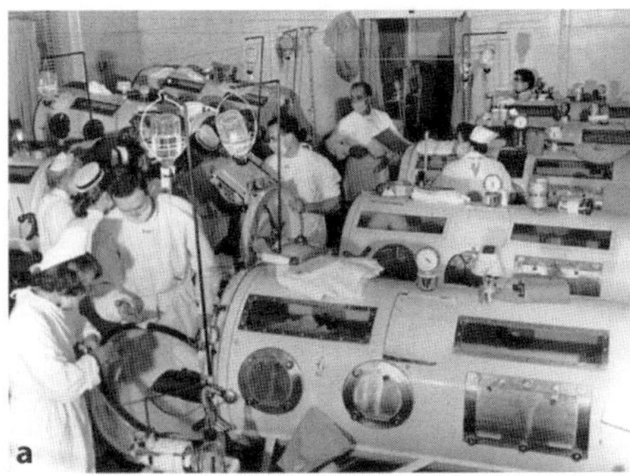

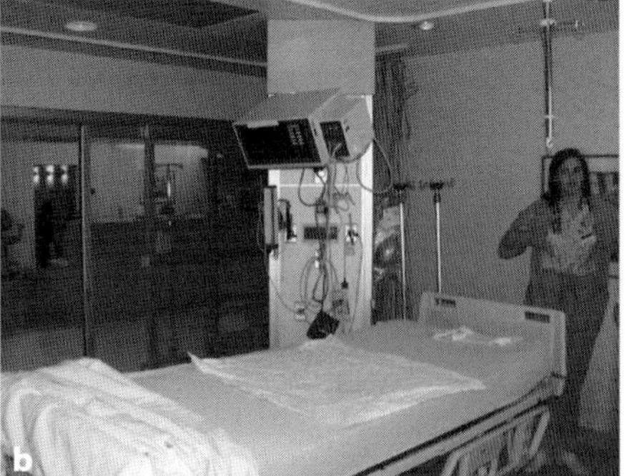

Fig. 8. a An ICU with an open design, showing multiple iron lungs during the polio epidemic in the Haynes Memorial Hospital in Boston, 1955 (Photo: AP Archive). **b** Swedish Medical Center, Englewood, Colorado, 1998 (Photo: B. Regli)

of the staff to the patients will remain essential; nevertheless, improved communication technology will facilitate flexible information exchange between different high-dependency areas, and may enhance the efficiency of resource utilization.

Patient rooms – open versus closed design

The configuration of many critical care units evolved from the recovery room model, which uses a so-called *open design* (Fig. 8a). The advantages of an open design include direct visualization of multiple patients, short distances between beds for the staff, and reduced needs for personnel and square meters. As part of a modular logistic concept, movable cupboards can offer a level of privacy between beds, and may be designed to provide protection from radiation.

Recently, there has been a trend toward a *closed design*, with smaller rooms for individual patients (Fig. 8b). The closed design has the advantage of shielding patients, who are awake and alert, from the constant activity in a high-level care environment (noise, light, traffic, interventions performed on patients in neighboring beds, relatives of patients in neighboring beds). In addition, the risk of hard-to-treat infections contributed to the trend toward a closed design.

How many beds should patient rooms contain?

It is likely that the room design of the future ICU will be a compromise. The unique situation and requirements of the hospital will determine the relationship between an open ward design and a closed design with individual rooms (Fig. 9). Flexibility should be the goal. The number of beds per room may vary widely and there are no solid arguments for any specific number. The authors' personal experience of many different room configurations and bed numbers between 1 and 8 per room suggests that 5 beds per room is a reasonable maximum number, providing that some degree of privacy between the beds can be

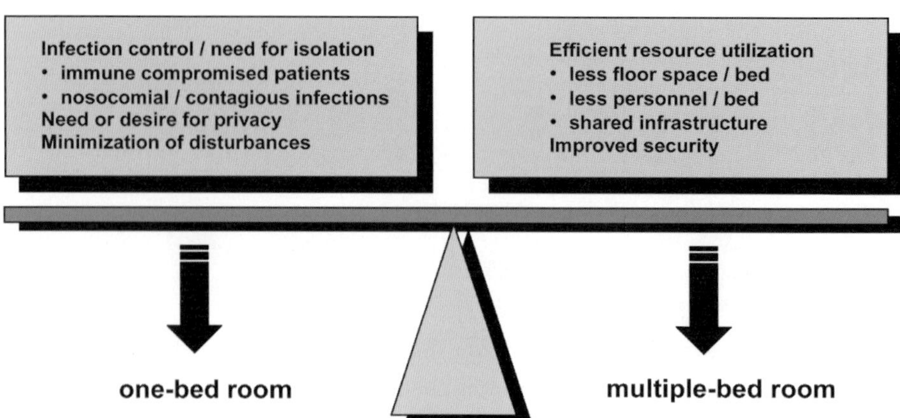

Fig. 9. Conditions influencing the choice of a one-bed or multiple-bed room

provided by mobile walls or cupboards. If the ICU treats a large number of postoperative patients with a very short ICU stay, even more patients per room may be reasonable.

The ICU of the future benefits from maximum flexibility in its secondary system. Mobile full- or partial-height walls (folding or sliding walls), other mobile dividers of floor space (e.g., cupboards or shelves), and sliding doors can be used to provide flexibility in the division of room space and the number of beds. The need to adapt rapidly and without major costs favors this approach in the secondary system, despite the sometimes higher initial investments needed.

Space around beds

Irrespective of the design you choose, you will need space around the bed. In 1965, the amount of space needed per patient in a multi-bed room was only 9 m^2. Thirty years later, in 1995, the ESICM recommended 20 m^2 per patient in a multi-bed room and 25 m^2 per patient in a private room [3], and the SCCM recommended even more space: 25 m^2 per patient in a multi-bed room and 28 m^2 per patient in a private room [2]. The increasing need for space has been in part related to the increasing number of devices used for patient care and diagnostics. On the other hand, modern technology has already enabled the size of many devices to decrease. Space needed per bed is unlikely to grow at the same pace as in past decades; if rooms are too large, distances increase and the advantages of compactness are lost.

Space is needed for:

- Interventions (e.g., insertion of catheters, minor surgery, tracheostomy, endoscopies)
- Organ support systems. Increases in the number of systems available or required to support organ failure (lung failure, renal failure, metabolic failure,

and liver failure) in the past few years have been accompanied by substantially increased requirements for space.
- Diagnostic tools. Many diagnostic tools are now brought to the patient's bedside (radiology, endoscopies, ultrasound examinations, metabolic measurements, scintigraphy). In the future, many current diagnostic technologies will develop into continuous monitoring technologies.
- Education and research.
  - New research tools, often prototypes, may not be integrated in the conventional monitoring or treatment application systems.
  - There should be sufficient space to conduct bedside teaching rounds.
- Contact isolation. If there is not enough space between the patient beds, it is very difficult to achieve contact isolation.
- Relatives. There is a growing trend toward allowing relatives to have access to the patient, sometimes almost continuously. These visitors need space.
- Supplies, such as often-used medications and dressings.

The need for space will continue to grow, as will the battle for financing that is associated with these increased needs.

Isolation requirements

One of the most challenging questions is how many patients will need to be isolated in the ICU of the future. Space is needed for both contact isolation, to prevent the transport of bacteria from one patient to another (most often difficult-to-treat nosocomial bacteria, such as methicillin-resistant *Staphylococcus aureus*), and aerosol isolation, for patients with very contagious infections like severe acute respiratory syndrome (SARS), which can infect other patients or the staff by contaminated drops in the air. Due to the negative atmospheric pressure needed for the aerosol isolation room and the separate logistics required for material delivery, disinfection and cleaning, and entrance/exit, these rooms will substantially reduce the flexibility of the ICU secondary system. Functional and financially sound technical solutions for flexibly converting sections of multiple-bed rooms to aerosol-isolation facilities is a clear challenge for the future ICU.

With a flexible secondary system that allows variation in room size, contact isolation of patients becomes much easier.

Where should staff members be when they are not at the bedside?

All core staff who work full-time in the ICU should have offices within the ICU perimeter. A dedicated area functioning as a workshop for education and training the staff should be integrated in the ICU to provide the nursing and medical staff with the opportunity for independent education in times of less activity. Real ICU equipment, simulation possibilities, and access to educational information should be provided. The workshop can be a multipurpose room; if it is also equipped as a patient room it can serve as a reserve.

Where should facilities for research staff and equipment be located?

Facilities for research staff should be located inside the ICU perimeter. The research staff will be better integrated in the ICU team, and clinical staff members engaged in research will benefit from better access and availability.

The logistic concept

Well-trained ICU personnel will remain an important commodity for the ICU. They should concentrate on their main special skills area and be relieved from logistical tasks, where possible. To do this, the logistic personnel should be brought to the front.

Material can be stored in modular units containing a predefined range of products ready for use. These can be delivered either to storage areas, directly to the patient care area, or both (Fig. 10). These modular units should be replenished by logistic personnel, and the consumption/supply controlled by a logistics software system. The modular supply concept can cover most bedside consumables, including medications.

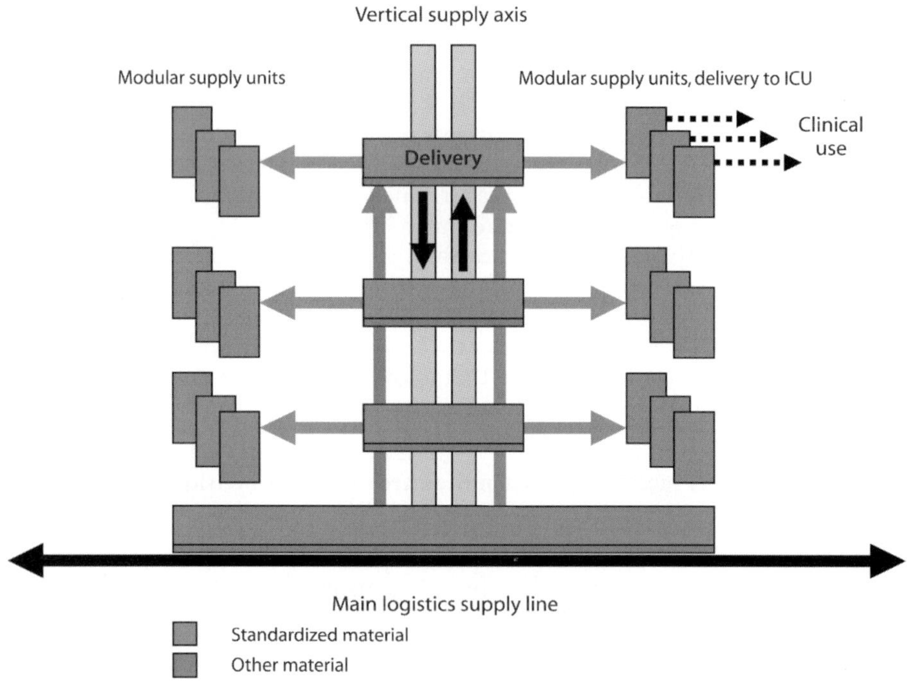

Fig. 10. The logistic process. Material is brought to a central storage area of the hospital. From there it is divided to the different departmental storage rooms or directly to the clinical units in modular units. The modular units are replenished by logistic personnel.

The tertiary system

For the future, flexibility is one of the key strategic issues. As discussed earlier, a flexible secondary system allows freedom to use different organization concepts. A lot of flexibility can be built into the design of the tertiary system as well. Flexibility can be considered either as 'adaptable flexibility', which allows a simple change in the current use, or 'convertible flexibility', which allows an inexpensive conversion to a new use [5]. In order to have 'adaptable flexibility' for a case-mix ranging from advanced intensive care to step-down patients, all patient beds need to be equipped with high-level monitoring. If the patient rooms are provided with maximum utilities capability (communication, medical gas supplies, electrical installations), but with different monitoring systems for high and lower levels of care intensity, there is a potential for convertible flexibility if the monitoring system can be changed or upgraded with an acceptable level of investment.

There are various options for installing the equipment for monitoring and treatment. Current approaches include a headwall, a ceiling service panel, and a column. With a headwall, it is not possible to have access to the patient from all sides. Ceiling service panels are extremely expensive. A power column/docking station may be the supply system of choice, providing the most flexibility.

A power column/docking station should be movable and should contain oxygen outlets, medical air outlets, vacuum outlets, electricity, and communications capabilities, including a local area network (LAN and W/LAN), a patient data management system (PDMS) interface, a telephone connection, and an alarm. It should be stable enough to also carry the monitoring system, a respirator, and the infusion pumps. The distances between the power column/docking stations should be adjustable. More power column/docking stations can be used to increase the number of beds in a room for patients who need a lower level of intensive care. If more space around a patient is needed, the distances between the power columns/docking stations can be widened. In the future, it will more than likely be possible to dock the ICU bed to this column, and some tools will be integrated into the ICU bed.

Conclusion

Intensive care professionals charged with designing ICUs of the future should begin by considering the environment in which the hospital operates. Evaluation of processes related to intensive care and within intensive care itself provides the key for successful design. Key points to keep in mind include:

- There are significant advantages to concentrating ICU resources under one administration, in a geographically compact area, with an interdisciplinary intensive care concept.
- Patient care, education, and research should be regarded as interrelated processes that follow a common path.
- A three-system model can help coordinate various aspects of planning, design, financing, and construction.

Considering it has been a decade since the major intensive care societies last published guidelines on the topic of ICU design, perhaps the time has come for them to revisit the issue. However, even if basic standards can be developed, the uncertainties in healthcare are likely to increase in the future. Thus flexibility will remain an essential goal at all levels of ICU design.

References

1. Harvey MA (1996) Critical Care Unit Design and Furnishing. Society of Critical Care Medicine, Anaheim
2. Guidelines/Practice Parameters Committee of the American College of Critical Care Medicine, Society of Critical Care Medicine (1995) Guidelines for intensive care unit design. Crit Care Med 23:582–588
3. Ferdinande P (1997) Recommendations on minimal requirements for Intensive Care Departments. Members of the Task Force of the European Society of Intensive Care Medicine. Intensive Care Med 23:226–232
4. Koay CK, Fock KM (1998) Planning and design of a surgical intensive care unit in a new regional hospital. Ann Acad Med Singapore 27:448–452
5. Hamilton DK (1999) Design for flexibility in Critical Care. New Horiz 7:205–217
6. Dyson M (1996) Modern critical care unit design. Nursing implications in modern critical care unit design: bed area ergonomics. Nurs Crit Care 1:194–197
7. Williams M (2001) Critical care unit design: A nursing perspective. Crit Care Nurs 24:35–42
8. Harvey MA (1998) Critical-care-unit bedside design and furnishing: impact on nosocomial infections. Infect Control Hosp Epidemiol 19:597–601
9. O'Connell NH, Humphreys H (2000) Intensive care unit design and environmental factors in the acquisition of infection. J Hosp Infect 45:255–262
10. Bartley J, Bjerke NB (2001) Infection control considerations in critical care unit design and construction: a systematic risk assessment. Crit Care Nurs Q 24:43–58
11. The American Institute of Architects (2001) Guidelines for Design and Construction of Hospital and Health Care Facilities: 2001 Edition (2001) The American Institute of Architects, Washington
12. Groeger JS, Guntupally KK, Strosberg MA, et al. (1992) Descriptive analysis of critical care units in the United States. Crit Care Med 20:846–863
13. Hettich Urs, Macchi Giorgio (1998) Nachdenken und umdenken - Über das dreiteilige Modell des Wettbewerbs INO Inselspital Bern. Special reprint from "Schweizer Ingenieur und Architekt", Nr. 13
14. Junker C, Zimmerman JE, Alzola C, Draper EA, Wagner DP (2002) A multicenter description of intermediate-care patients: comparison with ICU low-risk monitor patients. Chest 121:1253–1261

Information Technology

G. D. Martich, D. C. Van Pelt, and D. Lovasik

Introduction

The year is 2054; Tom Cruise plays a policeman in the Steven Spielberg movie, Minority Report. Detective Cruise works in the so-called 'pre-crime division' of the Washington DC police department. His job is to stop crimes before they happen. The premise of the story is that by using future-viewing technology, the police are able to arrest criminals, especially murderers, before they commit the crimes. In the opening scene of the movie, Detective Cruise manipulates data using advanced information technology and virtual reality gloves. These data then show him patterns of the murder before the crime actually happens. The 'pre-crime' policemen move in and apprehend the criminal before a drop of blood is spilled. In this scenario there is no victim, no blood, no death and the perpetrator is eliminated before the crime is committed.

The year is 2015; an intensivist uses advanced information technology to manipulate data without pen, paper or x-ray film, but with a mouse, monitors and wall-mounted voice recognition software. A clinical decision support system alerts the intensivist via her remote site virtual intensive care unit (ICU) that a pre-sepsis pattern exists in one of her patients. The intensivist has the patient's genomic and proteomic data immediately on-line via the monitor and prescribes the patient's personalized genetically engineered anti-microbial using voice recognition. Conversely, the intensivist can ask the computer to find all patients who have the same (or similar) clinical data. If she likes the matches, she can then look at their courses and outcomes and either repeat the therapies if the outcome was good or look for another path if it was not. In either of these scenarios, there is no infection, no distributive shock, no critical illness, no blood, no death and the microbe is eliminated before the disease becomes reality.

This has been a fun chapter to write since, like the movie Minority Report, it does not have to be reality-based to raise cultural, economic, technologic and real world questions. Postulating the look and feel of the ICU of the future may be as much fun and as exciting as the aforementioned scenario. On the other hand, the future could be as frightening as working with what we have now, except deleting care-givers because of the upcoming critical care physician and nursing shortages and the increased numbers of critically ill patients.

Physicians and the Evolution of Information Technology and ICUs

Before we consider where we are going with information technology in the ICU in the year 2015, we need to remember where we have come from both with information and intensive care technologies. In the mid 1800s in the US, a census was performed every ten years for one reason: It took ten years to count every American. In 1890, a physician, Dr. John Shaw Billings, working with Herman Hollerith, came up with a novel means of collecting census data in one-tenth the amount of time by using paper punch cards. Hollerith later started Tabulating Machines Corporation, which changed its name and became International Business Machines (IBM) Corporation in 1924. So, a physician had a part in starting IBM (Fig. 1).

Sixty years ago, the world's first digital computer, the electronic numerical integrator and computer (ENIAC), was built by the US Army to prepare for WWII. In reviewing the patent application for ENIAC, it is clear that much of what was desired in the mid 1900s for war preparations still applies to modern healthcare. "...With the advent of everyday use of elaborate calculations, speed has become paramount to such a high degree that there is no machine on the market today capable of satisfying the full demand of modern computational methods. The most advanced machines have greatly reduced the time required for arriving at solutions to problems, which might have required months or days by older procedures. This advance, however, is not adequate for many problems encountered in modern scientific work and the present invention is intended to reduce to seconds such lengthy computations..." [1]

The Army made ENIAC capable of processing two ten-digit multipliers in 2.6 milliseconds. The computer itself weighed 30 tons, had 19,000 vacuum tubes (bulbs) and hundreds of thousands of resistors and capacitors. ENIAC was

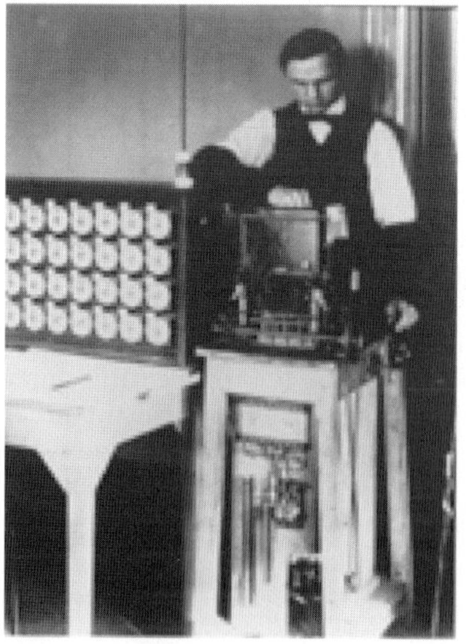

Fig. 1. The Hollerith Tabulating Machine which was developed using punch card technology to speed up the US census counting of Americans in 1880. Photo courtesy of IBM (http://www-03.ibm.com/ibm/history/history/decade_1890.html)

housed in a 20 x 50 foot room without air-conditioning and tended to by senior military officers day and night (Fig. 2). The officers replaced burned out computer vacuum tubes and removed insects that flew in through the windows of the building housing ENIAC. These insects frying on the hot vacuum tubes may have been the first instance of the term 'computer bug'.

Bill Gates dropped out of Harvard 30 years ago to write software for the MITS Altair personal computer for MITS' founder, Ed Roberts. MITS went out of business and Roberts pursued a childhood dream of becoming a doctor. Bill Gates developed a novel computer software program called disk operating system (DOS). Gates failed repeatedly to sell DOS to any computer company until his mother convinced the chairman of IBM to give her son's software programming a chance. Dr. Roberts is now a family physician in rural Georgia. Mr. Gates is now the richest man in the world.

Finally, just ten years ago, the widespread use of the internet came into being. We now have hundreds of thousands of websites a click away, almost instantly available for a multitude of educational, entertainment, and enterprise purposes. Who knows what the next ten years will bring for information technology?

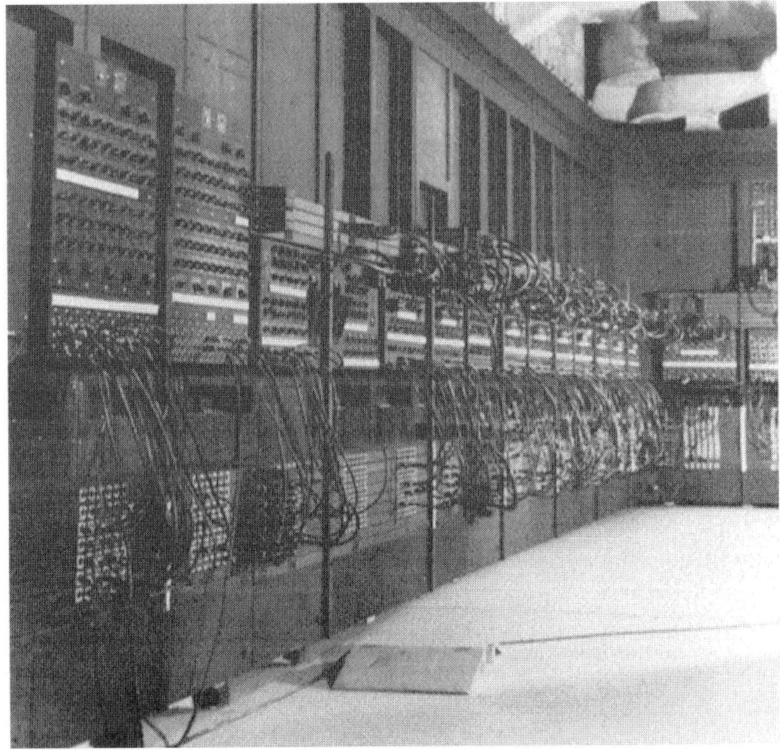

Fig. 2. The electronic numerical integrator and computer built by the US Army to prepare for World War II. The computer weighed 30 tons and took up a 20 x 50 foot room to run thousands of computations per second. (US Army Photo)

Will there be another disruptive technology like the Internet that changes the way people think and act? Or will healthcare and critical care in particular take advantage of the world wide web for the betterment of patient care, education and research in a fashion similar to other industries?

The development of the ICU has been along a parallel path. The first critical care unit opened in Copenhagen, Denmark in 1953 [2]. ICUs became the norm in large US hospitals by the late 1960s and nearly 70% of US hospitals had at least one critical care unit in a survey of hospitals published in 2000 [3]. Today, critical care beds comprise over 25% of the total licensed beds at the main campus of the University of Pittsburgh Medical Center.

Combining information technology and critical care has been a love-hate relationship with fits and starts. Because of the nature of the patients and caregivers, there is a need for extensive amounts of information in the ICU. These data need to be collected, reviewed and assimilated in order to appropriately care for the critically ill patient. But, while critical care clinicians value the biophysiologic monitors for blood pressure, heart rate, oximetry and continuous cardiac output, they are less enthusiastic about adopting information technology applications. By the early 1980s in the US, only a few large academic medical centers pursued electronic medical records (EMRs) and even fewer had any degree of penetration into the ICU. The early work of institutions such as the Regenstrief Institute in Indianapolis, Indiana; Duke University's TMR; and the HELP system at LDS hospital in Salt Lake City, Utah, pioneered the implementation of technology. In fairness to all of us in healthcare computers were quite expensive at the time of these installations. The IBM 7090 was a large computer, costing $20,000 per month to lease. Back then, staff were cheap, costing about 1/10th the amount of the computers. Times have changed, particularly in healthcare. Now, staff are more expensive. The people who use computers cost their companies tens to hundreds of times as much as the personal computer (PC) that they use. A powerful PC today costs $2,000–3,000 to purchase while the average non-physician employee of the University of Pittsburgh Medical Center costs the system approximately $45,000/year. How do we leverage the increased cost of personnel and decreased cost of information technology to improve the care provided to our critically ill patients?

The Need

In 1998, the Institute of Medicine (IOM), part of the National Academy of Sciences in the US, published a report on quality of health care in America. That report, "To Err Is Human", indicated that up to 98,000 Americans die each year from preventable medical mistakes they experience during hospitalizations [4].

Fig. 3. Screen print of vital sign flowsheet used in each of the ICUs at the University of Pittsburgh Medical Center. Calculations for infusion rates are performed by the computer system based on patient weight or body surface area. All data are "owned" by a clinician so that specific elements can be queried later for research or quality improvement efforts.

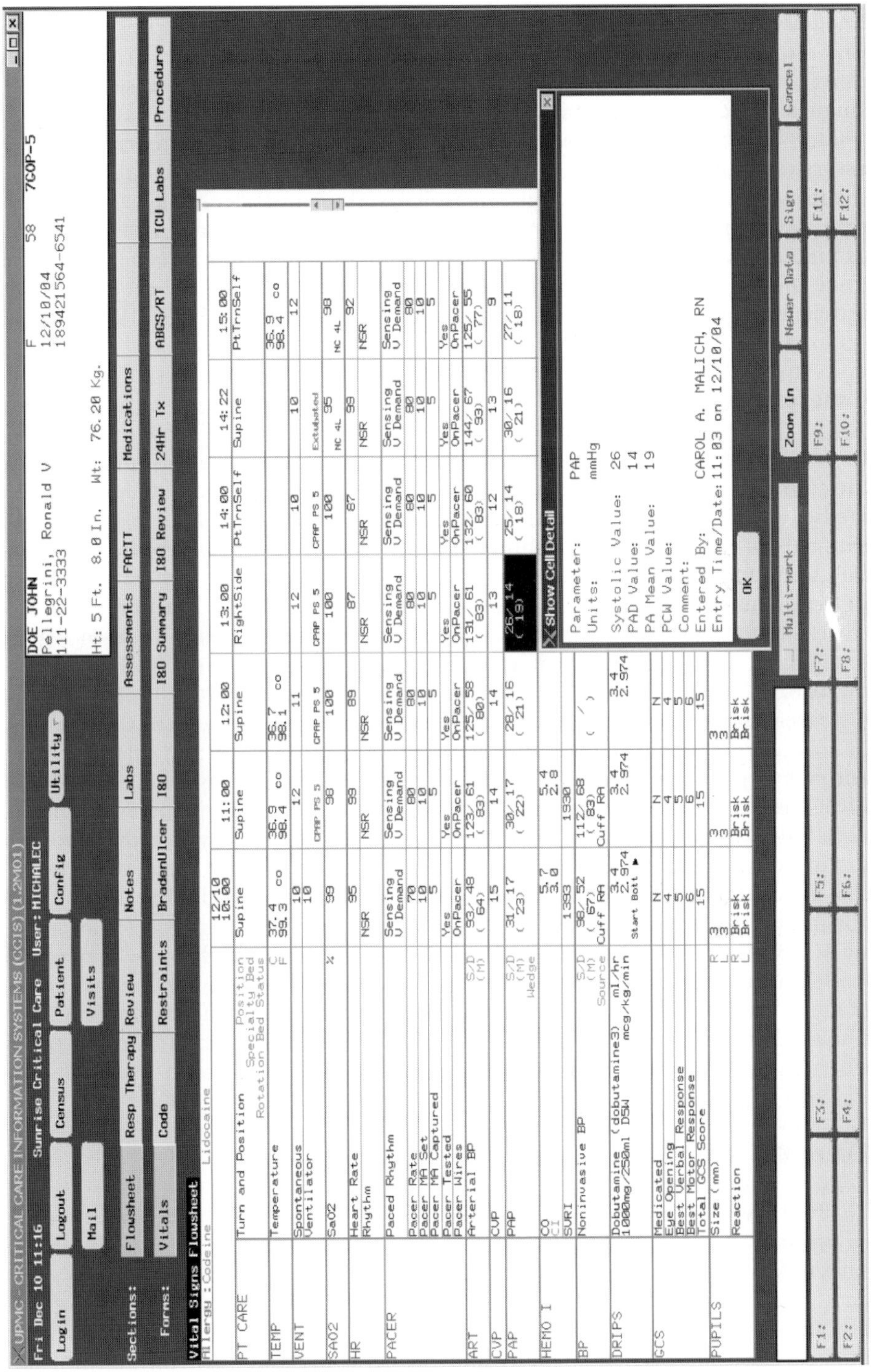

UPMC - CRITICAL CARE INFORMATION SYSTEMS (CCIS) (1.2M01)

Fri Dec 10 11:16 Sunrise Critical Care User: MICHALEC

Login | Logout | Census | Patient | Config | Utility
Mail | Visits

DOE JOHN F 58 7COP-5
Pellegrini, Ronald V 12/10/04
111-22-3333 189421564-6541
Ht: 5 Ft. 8.0 In. Wt: 76.20 Kg.

Sections: Flowsheet | Resp Therapy | Review | Notes | Labs | Assessments | FACTT | Medications

Forms: Vitals | Code | Restraints | BradenUlcer | I80 | I80 Summary | I80 Review | 24Hr Tx | ABGS/RT | ICU Labs | Procedure

Vital Signs Flowsheet

Allergy : Codeine Lidocaine

			12/10 10:00	11:00	12:00	13:00	14:00	14:22	15:00
PT CARE	Turn and Position	Position / Specialty Bed / Rotation Bed Status	Supine	Supine	Supine	RightSide	PtTrnSelf	Supine	PtTrnSelf
TEMP	Temperature	C / F	37.4 / 99.3 co	36.9 / 98.4 co	36.7 / 98.1 co				36.9 / 98.4 co
VENT	Spontaneous		10	12	11	12	10	10	12
	Ventilator		10	CPAP PS 5	CPAP PS 5	CPAP PS 5	CPAP PS 5	Extubated	
SAO2	SaO2	%	99	98	100	100	100	95 NC 4L	98 NC 4L
HR	Heart Rate		95	99	89	87	87	99	92
	Rhythm		NSR	NSR	NSR	NSR	NSR	NSR	NSR
PACER	Paced Rhythm		Sensing V Demand	Sensing V Demand	Sensing V Demand	Sensing V Demand	Sensing V Demand	Sensing V Demand	Sensing V Demand
	Pacer Rate		70	80	80	80	80	80	80
	Pacer MA Set		10	10	10	10	10	10	10
	Pacer MA Captured		5	5	5	5	5	5	5
	Pacer Tested		Yes	Yes	Yes	Yes	Yes	Yes	Yes
	Pacer Wires		OnPacer	OnPacer	OnPacer	OnPacer	OnPacer	OnPacer	OnPacer
ART	Arterial BP	S/D (M)	93/ 48 (64)	123/ 61 (83)	125/ 58 (80)	131/ 61 (83)	132/ 60 (83)	144/ 67 (93)	125/ 55 (77)
CVP	CVP		15	14	14	13	12	13	9
PAP	PAP	S/D (M) Wedge	31/ 17 (23)	30/ 17 (22)	28/ 16 (21)	26/ 14 (19)	25/ 14 (18)	30/ 16 (21)	27/ 11 (18)
HEMO I	CO		5.7	5.4					
	CI		3.0	2.8					
	SVRI		1393	1930					
BP	Noninvasive BP	S/D (M) Source	98/ 52 (67) Cuff RA	112/ 68 (83) Cuff RA	(/)				
DRIPS	Dobutamine (dobutamine3) 1000mg/250ml D5W	ml/hr mcg/kg/min	3.4 2.974 Start Bott ▶	3.4 2.974	3.4 2.974				
GCS	Medicated		N	N	N				
	Eye Opening		4	4	4				
	Best Verbal Response		5	5	5				
	Best Motor Response		6	6	6				
	Total GCS Score		15	15	15				
PUPILS	Size (mm)	R / L	3 / 3	3 / 3	3 / 3				
	Reaction	R / L	Brisk / Brisk	Brisk / Brisk	Brisk / Brisk				

Show Cell Detail

Parameter: PAP
Units: mmHg
Systolic Value: 26
PAD Value: 14
PA Mean Value: 19
PCW Value:
Comment:
Entered By: CAROL A. MALICH, RN
Entry Time/Date: 11:03 on 12/10/04

OK

Multi-mark | Zoon In | Newer Data | Sign | Cancel

F1: | F3: | F5: | F7: | F9: | F11:
F2: | F4: | F6: | F8: | F10: | F12:

The IOM report goes on to indicate that there are more deaths in hospitals each year from preventable medical mistakes than there are from motor vehicle accidents, breast cancer, or acquired immunodeficiency syndrome (AIDS). The single leading type of error is the medication error with estimates ranging from 4% to 20% of all hospitalized patients encountering medication errors. These errors result in excess costs of $2595 to $4685 per adverse drug event [5]. While the IOM report did not focus on care in ICUs, the report does suggest that critically ill patients are at a particularly high risk for adverse events. The ICU risk is as high as 17.7% for death or disability, and nearly 46% for any type of adverse event [6]. One of the oft-repeated recommendations from this IOM report is that information systems could reduce these mistakes considerably [7].

Unnecessary Variation

In 2003, Elizabeth McGlynn published a report indicating that compliance with the standard for quality of care for patients in the US based on evidence-based medicine (EBM) guidelines was approximately 55% [8]. This article opened our eyes to how extensive the variability of health care delivery, and hence opportunity for improvement, is in current practice. This was not the typical variability in treatment of disease that had been active fodder for public health researchers since the 1980s when many publications reported on the variability from region to region of the US on such disparate procedures as cesarean section, hysterectomy, cardiac catheterization and coronary artery bypass grafting [9–11]. Not only did researchers demonstrate variability among different regions of the country, but from urban to rural, female to male (where appropriate), and distinct racial and socio-economic differences. Yet another type of variability that is not unique to critical care medicine, but has been observed in the ICU, is intra-individual variability. The authors have observed that a critical care physician's responses to different problems varies based on the time of day, and not based on patients' clinical characteristics or ventilator setting. Unnecessary variability can be detrimental to patient care. How do we take advantage of the increasing affordability of information technology and ease the workload of our hospital personnel while improving the quality of patient care delivered? How do we change the art of medicine from a cottage industry mentality with individual variability as the standard of practice to a hardened precision-driven, highly-engineered process where the best therapies are consistently applied to every patient?

Current State

The ICU is where the pressures of a hospital converge. An ICU is also a data-rich environment where medical and information technologies converge. In health care, data are facts, such as heart rate, and observations, including clinical signs and family history. The sum of the data becomes information. Organizing and evaluating the information generates knowledge and provides the framework for medical decisions. When so many data elements must be turned into information and knowledge, errors occur because of sheer volume. A physician may be confronted with more than 200 variables during typical morning rounds [12]. Even an experienced physician is often not able to develop a systematic response to any problem involving more than seven variables [13]. Moreover, humans are limited in their ability to estimate the degree of relatedness between only two variables. This problem is most pronounced in the evaluation of the measurable effect of a therapeutic intervention. Computers and clinical information systems (CIS) are not consistently incorporated into patient monitoring, medication administration, ventilator or other life-support devices across ICUs the world over. Despite recognized problems of legibility, accessibility and their role in errors, handwritten records are still the strongholds of clinical record keeping. There is variable market penetration with CIS. When these systems are used, they provide critical care clinicians with timely physiologic data to help direct patient care. In addition, the computerized databases provide critical care clinicians with the ability to analyze care practices, improve patient safety, and evaluate quality and process improvement.

In 1991, we began using a CIS in the ICUs at the University of Pittsburgh Medical Center. Patient data, including demographics, biophysiologic data, ventilator settings and laboratory results, are collected from a number of sources and fed into an electronic vital sign flowsheet. This information is correlated with medication administration and medication infusion rates. Supportive information such as allergies, i.v. infusion ranges and calculations are configured into the system. The nurses record their narrative notes using either a drop-down menu or free text typing. In addition to collecting clinical data, the system also interfaces with the APACHE III database. The combination of the two databases provides a large medical data warehouse that can be queried for clinical, administrative, quality improvement and research objectives. There are also many opportunities for improvement: the current processors and monitors are large, bulky and outdated; their electrical cords and cables tether them and also create a safety hazard for tripping. Keyboards become contaminated if used without appropriate handwashing and our CIS support team replaces at least one mouse a day due to damage or misuse. There is a complex system of interfaces and servers that send data from laboratories, pharmacy, admit/transfer/discharge services that are each at risk from network problems including power outages and server crashes.

CIS are proven to enhance workflow and outcomes, and yet hospitals often face staff resistance when systems are installed. Even when a change is the best course of action, some groups of clinicians change slowly. The natural history of technology acceptance has been described as consisting of five groups: the innovators, early adopters, early majority, late majority and laggards. The innovators, or champions, pave the way for new technologies with early adopters following quickly behind. Most users fit in the early and late majority groups while the laggards, or nay-sayers, are resistant to change and new technology (Fig. 4) [15]. Two important factors for system acceptance are ease of use and speed. Hospital culture, physician and nursing champions, and personal relationships are key to the success of the CIS [16]. Hardware and software that succeed in one facility may not be effectively transferred to another facility. While the advan-

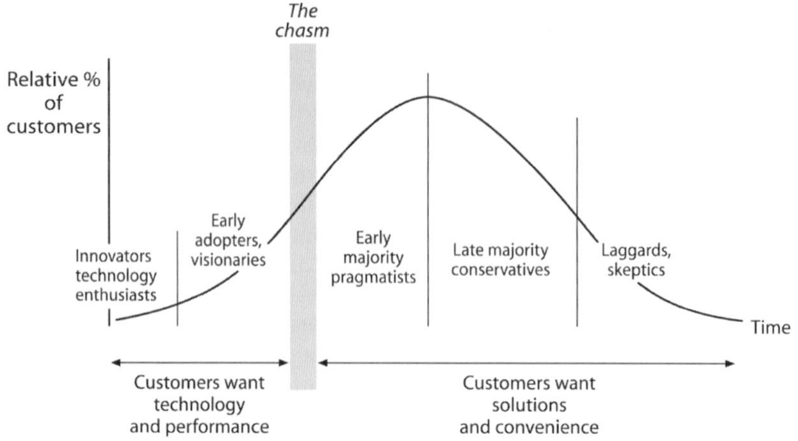

Fig. 4. The natural history of technology acceptance has been described as consisting of five groups: the innovators, early adopters, early majority, late majority and laggards. From [14] with permission

tages of the system include reducing transcription errors and quick accessibility, disadvantages such as the cost of installation and training along with concerns about patient confidentiality must also be considered.

Although many vendors offer software systems for critical care, very few ICUs are using paperless documentation. While these software systems have proven to be a huge advantage over the paper ICU systems, they are far from mature. Widespread adoption and evolution of these systems contribute to developing an appropriate level of maturity. Critical care information system implementation must mirror an adoption cycle similar to that of the automobile, (invented around 1890, reached 10% penetration in about 1908, and became 'mature' in the 1920s with 50% penetration). The key to widespread acceptance of the automobile was the assembly line – ICU information technology has yet to find its own 'assembly line', making its use commonplace in health care.

Pieces of the Future State 'Puzzle'

Picture Archiving and Communication System (PACS)

A PACS is a comprehensive computer system that is responsible for the electronic storage and distribution of medical images. The system is highly integrated with digital acquisition and display devices. The images are viewed within the hospital or via remote access for consultation. Facilities that use PACS reduce their use of film, film-processors and the associated costs. There has been constant growth in clinical implementation of PACS over the past few years as a means to reduce expenses and improve patient care, a trend that is expected to continue and increase. These systems can be web-based, much more affordable and provide diagnostic quality images from personal computers.

One of the unpredicted advantages of PACS has been the development of an international radiology staffing model. Teleradiology is used extensively in the US for both subspecialty consultations and overnight coverage of imaging services at selected US hospitals. Some US medical centers are investigating the potential to help provide staffing support from outside of the US. For example, a recent study documents how a staff radiologist in India interprets computed tomographic (CT) image cases that originated at a US university hospital. A radiologist using PACS in Bangalore, India viewed non-emergent CT scans obtained at Yale-New Haven Hospital. The radiologist was a former faculty member who maintained hospital privileges and an academic appointment at the parent institution. Following the radiologist review, the CT imaging reports were transcribed, then uploaded into Yale's radiology information system [17].

Quality Improvement

In the United States, the government is the largest purchaser of healthcare services. Recently, the US government announced that there would be pay-for-performance quality initiatives put into place for both inpatient and ambulatory care of patients [18].

In Germany, in conjunction with disease related groups (DRGs) as the sole method for inpatient reimbursement, healthcare authorities will require hospitals to publish quality benchmarks and also accumulate accreditation data after 2005. This can realistically only be captured by means of an electronic patient record.

In the UK, a recent government initiative has set up the Modernisation Agency for Critical Care to try and ensure standardization of protocols for transfers and the introduction of care bundles for stress ulcer prophylaxis and deep venous thrombosis (DVT) prophylaxis with hopes to address other issues such as the management of head-injured patients not requiring neurosurgery in district general hospitals. Now that over two-thirds of UK ICUs subscribe to the Intensive Care National Audit and Research Centre, it has been possible for ICUs to measure themselves on case-mix, adjusted outcome against other units. Each of these initiatives, including data collection and standardization requires the use of information technology by the ICUs.

Clinical Decision Support Systems

The goal of clinical decision support (CDS) systems is to supply the best recommendation under all circumstances. In its 2001 report, the IOM strongly recommends the use of sophisticated electronic CDS systems for radically improving safety and quality of care. Clinical information systems that generate CDS-driven electronic reminders and CDS-assisted computerized prescriber order entry (CPOE) have proven to both improve quality and cost effectiveness of care. Electronic reminders can significantly improve physicians' compliance with guidelines, reduce the rate of human errors and make physicians more responsive to specific clinical events [19].

CDS comes in three distinct varieties. Asynchronous CDS provides the clinician with information that requires the end-user to look for the data. Examples of this type of CDS include determining adjusted calcium based on the patient's albumin and calculating the anion gap based on the patient's electrolytes. This is a so-called 'pull' technology because the user needs to search for the values for it to be viewed. Synchronous CDS or 'push' technology requires the end-user to be at the computer terminal and an alert pops up into the user's view. Examples of synchronous CDS include a computer alert indicating that the dose of aminoglycoside antibiotic should be adjusted based on the patient's renal function and prompting the end user to note an elevated digoxin level while ordering the medication (Fig. 5). A tangible benefit of these types of CDS systems reported in the literature involves the review of all doctors' orders at a large US institution for drug interactions. The CDS alerts fired on approximately 400 of 15,000 orders, which resulted in changes daily. Most of these CDS-recommended changes were to avert potential adverse drug events [20].

The most complex and promising type of CDS is closed-loop CDS. This 'automatic' CDS implements detailed and explicit algorithms that adjust therapies

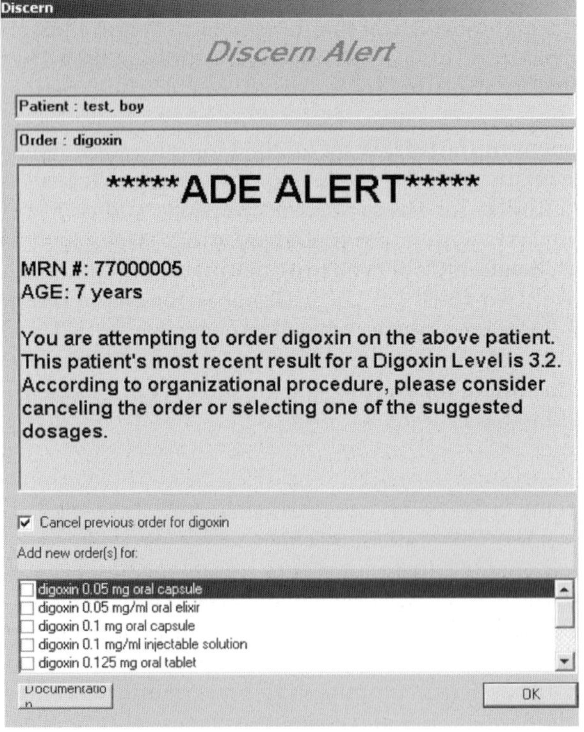

Fig. 5. An example of synchronous clinical decision support using 'push' technology. The physician attempts to prescribe digoxin for a patient with an elevated digoxin level. The system pushes a recommendation to the physician to either cancel the order or to select an alternative dose. The ultimate decision making is left to the physician.

without human intervention. To these authors' knowledge, there are only a few closed-loop CDS systems in critical care today; for example ventilators and isolettes. Although not labeled as one, every new ventilator is a closed-loop system [21]. In the past, we set tidal volume, respiratory rate, positive end-expiratory pressure (PEEP), and inspiratory time (I-time). Now pressure support ventilation changes the I-time with every breath without clinician intervention of any sort. Another, far simpler, closed-loop system used in most every neonatal ICU is the isolette. We place a baby in an isolette and connect him to a skin temperature probe, and the isolette automatically adjusts the heater output to keep the baby's temperature stable. The interesting caution about this latter system is that the providers must be sensitive to the closed-loop CDS to understand the child's physiology. A newborn in an isolette with a skin temperature of 37.4° in a system whose heater output has just fallen by 80% may be just as 'pre-septic' as the adult whose temperature has risen to 38.6° C.

Should closed-loop CDS be part of the information technology solution of the ICU of 2015? What kind of new closed-loop processes might work in critical care? Examples of possible closed-loop CDS alerts include changing the ventilator settings based on arterial blood gases or adjusting vasopressor infusions based on the biophysiologic data read out from the bedside monitor. Closed-loop CDS need impeccable inputs (ventilator flow rates) and/or default to 'off' when the input becomes questionable as when the skin temperature decreases in the neonate. Closed-loop CDS must be overridden when artifact is possible. Until we can clearly 'trust' that the blood gas was not a venous sampling erroneously put into the system as arterial or that the arterial line trace is valid, creating factitious hypotension or hypertension, we should continue to rely upon human interaction and reaction to all CDS alerts.

Multiparameter alerts are essential to improve the signal to noise ratio of accurate closed-loop alerts. Input signals must be interpreted in the appropriate context. Knowing that the patient's blood pressure has decreased is helpful as a single parameter. However, a concomitant increase in heart rate (i.e., physiologic response) or conversely a drop (i.e., vagal or medication response) will help separate the 'dampened' arterial line's factitious hypotension from a real hypotensive episode.

The movies, once again, have excellent examples of how to and how not to implement closed-loop CDS. "I'm afraid that I can't do that, Dave", was the eerie computer generated voice in Stanley Kubrick's film *2001: A Space Odyssey*. The computer had just performed a closed-loop decision support rule that locked the pilot outside of the spacecraft in deep space, sealing his fate. However, the original *Star Wars* film illustrated the value of overriding the CDS when Luke Skywalker is reminded to "use the Force" as he boards his spaceship to attack what is the only known weakness of the Death Star. The rebel attack on the Death Star is completely guided by computer systems. An early sequence of this ending finds the lead rebel using his computer-guided system to launch the crucial missile at the right time – and he misses. The final sequence has Luke flying into the same spot under the computer-guided control of R2–D2. He again hears the admonition to "use the Force" and he finishes the job shooting by hand. Luke's shot hits the mark and blows up the Death Star. The rebels are saved. The message in this scenario is that Luke needed R2–D2 behind him, adjusting power, etc. with a closed-loop efficiency to locate his target. His line of attack depended on the computer-guided weapons destroying the Death Star's perimeter weapons. But the success of the mission required Luke to administer hands-on control at a crucial point in the battle. Closed-loop CDS in the ICU must be the same as the above scenario. Let the CDS get us as far as they can. The role of the clinician in 2015 will be to understand when to override the CDS and shoot by hand.

Voice Recognition

Within and outside of healthcare, voice recognition technology is currently being used to automate services such as customer support and document transcription. Radiology departments have dramatically reduced overhead by using voice recognition and decreasing transcription costs [22]. The current 95% accuracy rate is acceptable in this field where modular content, the presence of a visual reference (i.e., the patient film), and the predominant physician 'audience' can overcome transcription errors. However, before this technology can be adopted in critical care, the accuracy rate must be closer to 100%. Using current systems, a typical 250 word progress note would have 12 syntax errors that could translate into medical errors. In critical care, patient complexity and variability make modular content more difficult to implement. Moreover, the physician's dictation is the 'snap shot' of a patient's condition at one point in time for which there is no other reference. An inaccurate report of antibiotic start date or wound size could result in poor decision-making, which goes unrecognized. However, as accuracy improves, voice recognition in combination with wireless technology, will become an important way of automating documentation.

Handheld Computing

Handheld computers are widely used in business and medicine alike. They are affordable reference and organization devices that can store several textbooks' worth of information in addition to appointments, memos, and contacts. Today they are used for point of care reference, medical calculations and patient tracking [23]. A $150 Personal Data Assistant (PDA) with 16-megabytes of memory can store up to 5 textbooks; such as Harrison's Manual of Medicine, Griffith's 5 Minute Clinical Consult, Washington Manual, and Epocrates Rx. With the use of a memory card, storage capacity can be increased more than 10 fold. Their functionality is restricted due to their small screen, limited battery power, and security issues. Ultimately, this technology will be integrated with hospital records through wireless connections. Secure access of records from any location by the mobile clinician will improve the provider reaction time to patient problems.

Virtual ICUs

The internet has rapidly become a part of daily life for many homes and businesses. It is likewise becoming more commonplace in the daily practice of medicine. Recent applications show that it has the power to ameliorate important problems facing critical care today; namely communication failures and manpower shortages. Creative web-based programs have been used to improve communication between families and providers and also reduce medical errors [24, 25]. The most comprehensive system to date, *e*ICU®, has the potential to be a working solution for manpower shortages. This model provides around-the-clock, centralized intensivist care to multiple ICUs. In an observational study applying this system to two open ICUs, reductions were demonstrated in ICU length of stay and average case cost [26]. The VISICU system implements an assortment of decision support tools in order to integrate disparate sources of patient information at a remote location. In 2015, patient-centered software applications with CDS, video conferencing, telemedicine monitors, and radiographic image displays along with a team of physicians will provide the kind of process consistency we have come to expect from airline cockpit crews. When supervising trainees this centralized patient information will allow more time for teaching by reducing efforts spent tracking down patient information.

Simulation Training

The military and aviation industries are decades ahead of medicine in understanding how simulation training can help overcome the inefficiencies of apprentice training. In these high-risk, time pressure environments where inefficiency is lethal, teamwork can save lives.

With this in mind, they have pioneered simulation training in order to reduce errors by identifying and preventing problems in communication and decision-making [27]. Such training is at odds with traditional Advanced Cardiac Life Support (ACLS) courses where a clinician is tested on his personal ability to save a mannequin from a megacode scenario without assistance. Recently, however the creative application of information technology to mannequin training has been used to train hospital teams for 'code blue' events [28]. Hypothetical scenarios capture the complexity of real life crises and teach pattern recognition for both common and uncommon situations. A computerized, talking mannequin has life-like physiology including breath sounds, heart tones, palpable pulses, chest wall movement, and even a difficult airway. Vital signs can be monitored with standard electrocardiogram (EKG), pulse-oximetry and blood pressure devices. With this technology, the consequences of team decisions are played out in real time and a detailed electronic record of events provides immediate feedback. In this way, errors of omission and commission can be critiqued from a team perspective without putting lives in jeopardy. Ten years from now full scale human simulator training will be a valued adjunct to medical training and continuing education. It will provide a safe environment for clinicians to develop and maintain proficiency with critical team actions, rare medical cases, and risky procedures.

Passwords and Automatic Identification

A common unintended consequence of ICU information technology is the use of ad hoc applications that parse the patient record into disparate systems. A clinician suspecting ventilator-associated pneumonia might have to use three passwords at three different workstations to locate the patient's temperature, bronchoalveolar lavage culture, and chest x-ray results. Beyond inconvenience, poorly integrated information technology prevents the recognition of important patient trends. The Clinical Context Object Workgroup (CCOW) of the HL7 committee designed a programming standard that can alleviate such workflow problems. By applying a 'context management' architecture it allows the clinician to access multiple patient applications at a single computer terminal with a single password [29]. Programming tools called mapping agents enhance the interaction between computer applications allowing information to be synchronized with respect to individual patient results at designated time points. Eventually, CCOW will improve clinician pattern recognition through graphical summaries, which incorporate data from multiple applications.

Automatic identification is used in commercial industry for inventory control and its application in medicine can dramatically reduce medication errors and equipment waste. One example already in use, Bar-Code Medication Administration (BCMA), is an effective means of reducing adverse medication events. A handheld infrared device is used to crosscheck medication bar codes with patient and nurse identification badges to ensure that medications are delivered as ordered. Important sources of error can be eliminated using BCMA to support nursing decisions and automate the typical handwritten medication administration record.

Radiofrequency identification (RFID) is a more sophisticated form of this wireless technology. It uses a tiny computer chip, or tag, to store unique product information and overcomes many bar-code limitations. For example, bar-code stickers require a direct line of sight to be read, cannot be modified, and can be impossible to read if they are wet, wrinkled, or torn. Originally developed in the 1970s, RFID has been used in a wide range of industries including pistachio suppliers, easy-pass toll booths and retail stores [30]. In the ICU of the future, this technology will do more than reduce adverse medication events. It will electronically track hospital supplies, reducing time wasted on hunting for a 20 cm dialysis catheter or rapid infusion i.v. tubing. Additionally, read-write tags will give providers the ability to store information at the bedside. Central lines can be programmed with the date of insertion, and patient identification tags can store past medical history. In addition to inventory control, RFID technology will soon enable hospitals to track patients and staff. Currently, cost is a barrier to widespread use. Today, at 25 cents per tag, an 800-bed hospital would have to spend several thousand dollars per day on RFID [31]. However, the recent announcement that the largest department store chain in the US, Walmart, is to use RFID on every one of its products will put these costs more in line with that of bar-code stickers.

Context Awareness

An integrated CIS makes data available at the patient bedside by interfacing with patient monitoring devices and the cumulative data that are provided will support clinical decision making, assist in patient management, support outcome measurement and facilitate research. However, health care providers will find themselves spending time on the computer to access this information. Just as automated teller machines (ATMs) have decreased bank-customer interactions and on-line reservations have impacted the travel agencies, CIS places the ownership for accessing the patient data back to the clinician. While working toward a goal of a paperless system through the EMR, CPOE, world wide web (www) access and e-mail communication has clear benefits, managing all these means of electronic communication also expends time and energy. Measurable end user benefit must be clearly demonstrated before clinicians will invest the time and money required to adopt information technology-induced work flow changes into everyday practice.

In our future ICU, the technology will be wireless, the monitors will have large, flat screens. The data will flow without interruption or disturbances. Graphical displays with large letters, numbers and symbols will be easy to read. This is an important point since the average age of a US nurse is 47 years [32]. A single log-in, perhaps by voice recognition or RFID, would access all of the clinical systems and the data would interface to provide information in bundles. As the user approaches the system, it will recognize their particular role (intensivist, nephrologist, nurse, etc.), how long it had been since the last interaction, report what has transpired while they were away and offer suggestions for patient management based on user specific CDS.

Today, experienced clinicians rely on the data to provide critical information, then use their expertise and pattern recognition to identify patient problems as well as the appropriate actions. With increased utilization of protocols and EBM, the system can be programmed to assist in identifying gaps in care, alerting busy clinicians to rapidly changing patient status and perhaps suggest changes in therapy based on programmed conditions.

Acuity Systems and Outcome

The search for an organized and standardized report using clinical data for patient care and quality assurance led to the development of APACHE (Acute Physiology and Chronic Health Evaluation) in 1981. APACHE and APACHE II, introduced in 1985, are severity of illness systems that combine existing clinical knowledge with computer-based statistical search techniques. The next iteration, APACHE III, included a prognostic estimate for mortality and length of stay that created some controversy with concerns that it could become a self-fulfill-ing prophecy. There are other acuity scoring systems as well, but none have ever suggested that a particular patient's mortality is 100% based on the system. In the US, ICU admission at the end of life is commonplace. What is the value and role of any acuity mortality prediction models for ICU care? We speculate that the use of acuity scoring systems to ration care is unlikely to be widely adopted until the probabilistic calculation of death is 100% by the system. Furthermore, we conclude that the most important technical deficiency is the lack of automated information technology to provide outcome predictions to decision makers. This barrier pales in comparison, however, to the cultural and policy acceptance toward rationing care at the end of life [33].

Security and Confidentiality

All of the advantages of sharing information via CIS can be wiped out with one high profile example of inappropriate sharing or access to electronic patient records. Not exclusive to physicians or other clinicians, the concern over widespread distribution of confidential medical information has been mentioned numerous times by the lay press with a multitude of celebrity cases. The physicians who begin with skepticism over adoption of CIS can rightly point to the lack of data security stewards scrutinizing access to every piece of a person's record.

Some health care computer security measures including firewalls and password-aging processes were first implemented in other industries such as banking and credit card companies. Others are unique to health care. In the US, the Health Insurance Portability and Accountability Act (HIPAA) was designed to protect patient confidentiality. Private patient information is visible on the monitor screen, necessitating a lock-out period to protect patient confidentiality. Non-secure email consultations among physicians or between a physician and a patient may be violated through a breach in security. Wireless technology creates additional security concerns. The threat of hackers, viruses, even terrorism has clinicians, administrators and information technology engineers working together to protect private patient information. Security measures in the future will require unique identifiers, such as fingerprint matching, retinal scans, voice recognition or RFID.

Stability and Downtime Preparedness

Contingency plans must be in place for either planned or unplanned downtime. In the US, HIPAA requires that responsible entities have established policies and procedures for responding to an emergency or other occurrence that may damage confidential health information. At a minimum, a data back-up plan to maintain exact, retrievable copies of the electronic protected health information is required. Disaster recovery must be in place to restore any lost data caused by human, technical or natural events. If the system is in an emergency mode operation, the security of the record must be maintained while operating during the emergency. Procedures must be in place to test and revise contingency plans, usually through drills and updates. The relative criticality of the applications and data must be evaluated since different components of the system must be prioritized and the information recovery-time identified. These security procedures mirror other hospital drills (internal and/or external drills) and should be performed routinely.

Conclusion

With this emphasis on technology, one could ask if information technology is inappropriately displacing the art of medicine. It is clear that the technology helps us collect the data, but medicine and nursing remains a unique contract with the patient. With care expanding horizontally across specialties, even geographically, there is an ever-increasing potential to be a contributor to patient care. There is currently a shortage of qualified intensivists and critical care nurses in the US and around the world. Since clinicians provide the compassion and care that technology cannot, they are irreplaceable at the bedside. CIS reduce paperwork to allow the health care providers to be with the patient. Clinicians must manage and adapt to technological, economic, social, and regulatory forces that are redefining our approach to health care delivery. In order to meet the growing need for improved data communication between various providers in the healthcare domain, it is necessary to overcome barriers of software heterogeneity and lack of broadly accepted standards.

In the information technology-laden ICU of 2015, innumerable patient variables will be seen more as an asset than a distraction. A wide array of integrated, secure tools will transform data into dynamic, context specific information that focuses clinician cognition on appropriate patient management strategies. Without even logging on to a computer, clinician attention will be guided by immediate information displays that appear as the bedside is approached. An integrated graphical summary of vital signs and test results as well as relevant consult notes, and online decision support will keep cognition on the task at hand. As the treatment plan comes into focus, voice recognition technology will simultaneously document morning rounds and relay pharmacy orders. Immediate feedback will warn of potential errors and suggest evidence-based approaches. When the physician leaves the bedside, mobile wireless and Internet devices will immediately apprise him/her of important clinical changes or trends whether he/she is in the hospital, at home, or in transit. In this way the robust, integrated information technology systems of the future will inspire clinician confidence by capturing the scope of complexity that is modern ICU patient care.

Acknowledgements

We thank Dr. James C. Fackler of Cerner Corporation and Dr. Martin Doerfler of VISICU for their thoughtful comments of earlier versions of this manuscript.

References

1. Eckert JP, Mauchly JW (1964) Electronic Numerical Integrator and Computer. United States, Patent No: 2,577,141
2. Berthelsen PG, Cronqvist M (2003) The first intensive care unit in the world: Copenhagen 1953. Acta Anaesthesiol Scand 47:1190–1195
3. Halpern NA, Pastores SM, Greenstein RJ (2004) Critical care medicine in the United States 1985–2000: an analysis of bed numbers, use, and costs. Crit Care Med 32:1254–1259
4. Kohn LT, Corrigan JM, Molla S (1999) To Err Is Human: Building a Safer Health System (1999) Committee on Quality of Health Care in America, The Institute of Medicine, National Academy Press, Washington
5. Bates DW, Spell N, Cullen DJ, et al (1997) The costs of adverse drug events in hospitalized patients. Adverse Drug Events Prevention Study Group. JAMA 277:307–311
6. Andrews LB, Stocking C, Krizek T, et al (1997) An alternative strategy for studying adverse events in medical care. Lancet 349:309–313
7. Bates DW, Gawande AA (2003) Improving safety with information technology. N Engl J Med 348:2526–2534
8. McGlynn EA, Asch SM, Adams J, et al (2003) The quality of health care delivered to adults in the United States. N Engl J Med 348:2635–2645
9. Bernstein SJ, McGlynn EA, Siu AL, et al (1993) The appropriateness of hysterectomy. A comparison of care in seven health plans. Health Maintenance Organization Quality of Care Consortium. JAMA 269:2398–2402
10. Winslow CM, Kosecoff JB, Chassin M, Kanouse DE, Brook RH (1988) The appropriateness of performing coronary artery bypass surgery. JAMA 260:505–509
11. Leape LL, Hilborne LH, Park RE, et al (1993) The appropriateness of use of coronary artery bypass graft surgery in New York State. JAMA 269:753–760
12. Morris A (1998) Algorithm-based decision-making. In: Tobin JA (ed) Principles and Practice of Intensive Care Monitoring. McGraw-Hill, New York, pp 1355–1381
13. Miller G (1956) The magical number seven, plus of minus two: Some limits to our capacity for processing information. Psychol Rev 63:81–97
14. Norman DA (1998). The Invisible Computer: Why Good Products Can Fail, The Personal Computer Is So Complex, And Information Appliances Are The Solution. MIT Press, Cambridge
15. Moore GA (1999) Crossing the Chasm. Harper Business, New York
16. Clemmer TP, Spuhler VJ, Berwick DM, Nolan TW (1998) Cooperation: the foundation of improvement. Ann Intern Med 128:1004–1009
17. Kalyanpur A, Neklesa VP, Pham DT, Forman HP, Stein ST, Brink JA (2004) Implementation of an international teleradiology staffing model. Radiology 232:415–419
18. Martich GD, Waldmann CS, Imhoff M (2004) Clinical informatics in critical care. J Intensive Care Med 19:154–163
19. Kucher N, Koo S, Quiroz R, et al (2005) Electronic alerts to prevent venous thromboembolism among hospitalized patients. N Engl J Med 352:969–977
20. Sharpe VA, Faden AI (1998) Medical harm: Historical, Conceptual, and Ethical Dimensions of Iatrogenic Illness. Cambridge University Press, Cambridge
21. Sailors MR, East TD (2000) Computerized management of mechanical ventilation. In: Grenvik A, Ayres SM, Holbrook PR, Shoemaker WC (eds) Textbook of Critical Care, 4th edn. WB Saunders, Philadelphia, pp 1329–1355
22. Mehta A, McLoud TC (2003) Voice recognition. J Thorac Imaging 18:178–182
23. Fischer S, Stewart TE, Mehta S, Wax R, Lapinsky SE (2003) Handheld computing in medicine. J Am Med Inform Assoc 10:139–149
24. Braner DA, Lai S, Hodo R, et al (2004) Interactive Web sites for families and physicians of pediatric intensive care unit patients: a preliminary report. Pediatr Crit Care Med 5:434–439

25. Major K, Shabot MM, Cunneen S (2002) Wireless clinical alerts and patient outcomes in the surgical intensive care unit. Am Surg 68:1057–1060
26. Breslow MJ, Rosenfeld BA, Doerfler M, et al (2004) Effect of a multiple-site intensive care unit telemedicine program on clinical and economic outcomes: an alternative paradigm for intensivist staffing. Crit Care Med 32:31–38
27. Helmreich RL (2000) On error management: lessons from aviation. BMJ 320:781–785
28. DeVita MA, Schaefer J, Lutz J, Dongilli T, Wang H (2004) Improving medical crisis team performance. Crit Care Med 32:S61–S65
29. Seliger R (2000) Overview of HL&'s CCOW Standard. At: http://www.hl7.org/special/Committees/ccow_sigvi.htm. Accessed July, 2005
30. RFID Journal At: http://www.rfidjournal.com/article/articleview/207. Accessed July, 2005
31. Becker C (2004) A new game of leapfrog? RFID is rapidly changing the product-tracking process. Some say the technology–once costs drop–could displace bar-coding. Mod Healthc 34:38, 40
32. Buerhaus PI, Staiger DO, Auerbach DI (2000) Implications of an aging registered nurse workforce. JAMA 283:2948–2954
33. Barnato AE, Angus DC (2004) Value and role of intensive care unit outcome prediction models in end-of-life decision making. Crit Care Clin 20:345–viii

Diagnostic Technologies to Assess Tissue Perfusion and Cardiorespiratory Performance

M. R. Pinsky

Introduction

Fundamental to the management of critically ill patients is the on-going assessment of both cardiorespiratory status and the adequacy of tissue perfusion. However, the management of the critically ill is also context specific. What measures one makes in the operating room, where tight titration of support in the face of surgical trauma is the rule, to field and Emergency Department settings where invasive monitoring is impractical and steady state conditions rarely present, limit the generalizability of statements about specific devices and their utility. Furthermore, no monitoring device will improve outcome unless coupled to a treatment, which, itself, improves outcome. The next five years should witness a closer synchrony between monitoring techniques and goals in terms of patient-centered outcomes. Within the context, some truths have sustained clinical scrutiny and speak to consistent treatment logic that should progress more over the next five years, although they will probably not develop into mature applications.

Tissue hypoperfusion, or circulatory shock, induces a profound sympathetic response that aims to restore central arterial pressure to sustain cerebral and coronary blood flow. The body does this at the expense first of the skin, non-active muscles and renal ultrafiltration, followed closely by splanchnic vasoconstriction [1]. Fundamentally, therefore, a blood pressure within the normal range and the presence of mentation in a patient do not insure cardiovascular sufficiency. Regrettably, the opposite is true. In previously healthy trauma patients, mentation and mean arterial pressures in excess of 90 mmHg often exist within the context of profound hypoperfusion and ischemic injury to the gut mucosa and renal medulla. Such states are often referred to as compensated shock, to describe this masquerade. Furthermore, delayed resuscitation even if it restores regional blood flow, may not prevent organ injury or rapidly restore organ function. The increased morbidity and mortality from delayed or inadequate resuscitation efforts have been documented in the trauma literature [2].

Finally, monitoring and resuscitation are also context specific. Differing groups of patients reflect differing needs and can be assessed well to differing degrees. One must apply differing filters to the review of the literature and the application of technologies in assessing tissue perfusion and monitoring techniques based on a variety of criteria. However, here we shall discuss several new

and exciting developments that should become commonplace within the next five years. These advances can be broadly placed in the following categories:
1) continuous non-invasive or minimally invasive measures of tissue wellness;
2) assessments of cardiopulmonary reserve and responsiveness to therapies; and, finally
3) protocolized care to minimize medical errors, practice variation and apply best practices across broad groups of patients independent of the training of the bedside healthcare provider, sophistication of the intensive care unit (ICU) and patient population differences.

Within the framework monitoring of tissue perfusion and tissue wellness will become increasingly integrated into treatment protocols, defining not only who is ill but also the end-points of therapy.

Assessment of Tissue Wellness

A reasonable therapeutic goal is to restore blood flow to tissues so as to reverse tissue hypoperfusion, progressive ischemic cellular injury and their associated organ dysfunction. Preventing sustained tissue hypoperfusion is usually associated with a far better outcome than treatment strategies that allow tissue hypoperfusion to persist to the point of inducing organ injury or if the resuscitation is inadequate so that tissue perfusion is not fully restored to a level that will result in no perfusion deficit. However, tissue perfusion is a relative concept. Tissues need only as much blood flow as required to meet their metabolic demands. Although one can make the distinction between flow and oxygen delivery, under most conditions these two variables are coupled. Assessment of tissue wellness usually revolves around estimates of the adequacy of aerobic metabolism and the associated performance of the tissue being monitored. Measures of tissue or venous PCO_2 are often used to assess blood flow because CO_2 production is remarkably constant for all organs, except the kidney, as blood flow decreases up until the point that oxygen extraction cannot sustain oxidative phosphorylation [3]. Numerous probes have been developed and studied to assess oxygen sufficiency, regional blood flow for Doppler or CO_2 flux, and mitochondrial energy state.

Oxygen Sufficiency

Of all the measures of regional perfusion, oxygen measures are the least accurate because they rely on too many unproven assumptions. On a global level, one can measure mixed venous oxygen saturation (SvO_2). Assuming arterial oxygen saturation (SaO_2) is > 92% then SvO_2 will be a function of the oxygen carrying capacity, the mean weighted flow to all organs and metabolic demand. Over a short time interval, hemoglobin and hemoglobin oxygen binding affinity usually do not change, and if metabolic demand is controlled, then one can use SvO_2 as a measure of global oxygen delivery (DO_2) sufficiency. Under normal conditions

SvO_2 stays around 72%. However, if it becomes ≤ 70% then circulatory stress is occurring and, if SvO_2 becomes < 65%, some areas of tissue ischemia probably exist [4]. However, an SvO_2 > 72% does not insure that all tissues have adequate blood flow because shunt flow may artificially increase end-capillary PO_2 in hyperperfused regions masking tissue ischemia. In fact, this is often the argument given for why organ dysfunction is seen in septic patients when their SvO_2 is > 72%, cardiac output elevated, but hyperlactatemia is present. Although other reasonable explanations for these findings can be given, including mitochondria block, decreased lactate clearance and failure of lactate dehydrogenase to convert lactate to pyruvate [5], clear documentation of microcirculatory derangements in septic patients has also been described [6]. Decreases in SvO_2 have also been used to identify those ventilatory-dependent subjects who will fail to wean from mechanical ventilatory support, as weaning successes did not display a decrease in SvO_2 during their spontaneous breathing trials [7].

Recently, interest in using central venous SO_2 ($ScvO_2$) as an alternative to SvO_2 has been proposed, because $ScvO_2$ can be measured from a central venous catheter, is similar though not identical to SvO_2 and eliminates the need for pulmonary arterial catheterization to measure SvO_2 [8, 9]. A resuscitation protocol based on $ScvO_2$ as a surrogate of SvO_2 resulted in better outcome from septic shock in patients treated in an emergency department than similar patients treated without the aid of $ScvO_2$ or SvO_2 guided therapy [10]. Thus, measures of compensated shock, even if measured using degraded measures, such as $ScvO_2$, may still improve outcome if coupled to an aggressive treatment protocol. Although this approach has been endorsed by the SCCM and ESICM Surviving Sepsis campaign for the treatment of patients with septic shock [11], the published protocol [10] did not treat acutely ill in-patients within an ICU, but subjects presenting to an emergency department whose entire protocolized treatment was done there. Furthermore, care once in the ICU was not controlled and this emergency department protocol used very large red blood cell transfusions independent of fluid resuscitation, which could have independently altered outcome. Furthermore, using threshold values of $ScvO_2$ to drive these protocols is problematic, since the relation between $ScvO_2$ and SvO_2 may vary markedly in shock states and during therapy [12]. However, this study clearly documented that using measures of oxygen extraction stress as a marker of compensated shock identified patients whose outcome improved if resuscitation persisted further to resolve this presumed deficiency.

Although regional measures of tissue PO_2 are possible, including splanchnic oxygen consumption [13], in-dwelling oxygen-sensitive electrode catheters placed into tissues [14] and non-invasive measures of tissue PO_2 [15], the clinical utility of these devices has not been shown and their use has been limited to a few research centers. When muscle PO_2 levels are measured during experimental hemorrhagic shock and resuscitation, the trends appear to reflect ischemia and its recovery. Thus, measures of oxygen sufficiency exist and on a global level have proven useful to drive therapy in one clinical trial. Still, the sensitivity of global measures of oxygen sufficiency is poor, whereas regional measures of tissue PO_2 have not been used to drive treatment protocols. Finally, in subjects with prolonged cardiovascular insufficiency, as may occur in patients with severe sepsis and septic shock, the potential exists that mitochondrial dysfunction may develop owing to impaired mitochondrial protein synthesis needed to drive oxidative phosphorylation [16]. Under these conditions, otherwise adequate tissue PO_2 levels (i.e., > 10 mmHg) may still be associated with impaired energy metabolism. However, under these circumstances of metabolic block, both oxygen consumption and CO_2 production will be limited. To date, no studies have reported decreased CO_2 production as part of high output circulatory shock.

Regional Blood Flow

Regional blood flow is heterogeneous both among organs and within organs, and regional blood flow distribution may vary over time in response to changes in sympathetic tone and treatments [17]. However, under most circumstances, regional blood flow is proportional to regional metabolic demand. Since regional metabolic demand reflects oxidative phosphorylation, CO_2 production is also proportional to regional blood flow. Thus, tissue PCO_2 remains remarkably constant across tissues as metabolic rate varies as long as blood flow can co-vary with metabolic rate. Since total PCO_2 is also dependent on tissue CO_2 stores, measures of a specific threshold value for tissue PCO_2 are less informative than are measures of the differences between tissue PCO_2 and arterial PCO_2. This so-called regional PCO_2 gap can be used to measure regional blood flow in the gut, if measured by gastric tonometry [18], the mouth, if measured by sublingual PCO_2 [19] in muscle and subcutaneous tissues, if measured by indwelling PCO_2 electrodes [20], and in the bladder musoca using surface electrodes [21]. Gutierrez et al. used an elevated gastric PCO_2 gap equivalent to identify compensated shock in critically ill subjects following an initial resuscitation [22]. Others have shown that gastric tonometry can identify occult circulatory failure during weaning [23]. Subjects who fail to wean from mechanical ventilatory support also develop an elevated gastric PCO_2 gap, consistent with gastric vasoconstriction during the stress of weaning [7]. Interestingly, when PCO_2 measures are coupled with pH measures, one has the unique opportunity to access the emergency of regional tissue metabolic acidosis, as the point wherein tissue pH decreases more rapidly than can be explained by the associated increase in PCO_2 based on the Henderson-Hasselbalch equation. Potentially coupled pH-PCO_2 measures will be used in the future to identify critical DO_2 states and the onset of metabolic acidosis. Thus, measures of regional blood flow exist and may be more robust than measures of oxygen sufficiency. However, their primary limitation at the present is the difficulty in acquiring reliable measures of PCO_2 and its change over time.

Regional gastric mucosal blood flow can also be measured by local laser Doppler techniques; although this technique is useful for research purposes, it has not been used to document results of resuscitation or drive resuscitation protocols in humans. Presumably, this lack of study is due to the invasive nature of the technique and its instability over time. Finally echo-imaging techniques allow for the assessment of renal cortical blood flow and myocardial blood flow. Similarly, trans-cranial Doppler measures are used to assess cerebral blood flow. Along this same line, echo-derived estimates have been reported for numerous regional vascular beds. However, although such echo-derived measures of regional blood flow can be used to describe large vessel blood flow, their ability to assess actual tissue blood flow or effective blood flow is limited.

Cellular Energy Status

Cellular energy production through metabolism of three-carbon units within the tricarboxylic acid cycle to produce CO_2 and reduced cytochromes needed to feed mitochondrial oxidative phosphorylation for the production of ATP and consumption of oxygen reflects the basic means by which cells, organ and whole animals survive and adapt to the environment. Although anaerobic metabolism of glucose to pyruvate and then lactate can generate some ATP, this strategy is grossly inefficient and unable to sustain cellular metabolism at any but the most quiescent level. Accordingly, numerous techniques have been studied that aim to assess mitochondrial redox state. With increased hypoxic stress, oxidative phosphorylation is impaired with increased intracellular reduced cytochrome a/a3 and NADH levels. Since adequate oxygen flux from capillaries to mitochondria represents the final pathway of oxygen transport to the cells, measures of reduced cytochrome a/a3 and NADH levels represent a direct evaluation of the effectiveness of resuscitation to sustain cellular function [24]. Although circulatory shock states have been demonstrated to induce impaired intracellular oxidative phosphorylation, and resuscitation has been shown to improve these measures, they have not been used in clinical trials. The reasons for this are multiple, not the least of which is the reality that such measures are, by necessity, highly localized and marked regional differences in tissue oxygen sufficiency often exists in both health and disease. Potentially, measuring these parameters non-invasively over a spectrum of tissues and sites within tissues may give a clearer picture of tissue wellness. The second major weakness of these approaches is the lack of a calibrated threshold below which injury occurs and above which tissue energy production is adequate. In essence, absolute levels of any oxidative phosphorylation factor or co-factor are less important than the rate of ATP turnover. Levels of these agents are analogous to the number of wheels on a car, not the rate at which the car is moving. Furthermore, increased reduced cytochrome and cofactor levels, using this same analogy, reflect the state of inflation of those tyres, not their potential rate of turn given an adequate substrate.

Assessment of Cardiorespiratory Reserve and Responsiveness to Therapy

Hypoxemia

Hypoxemia, defined as an $SaO_2 < 92\%$, usually corresponds to an arterial PO_2 of approximately 65 mmHg. As arterial PO_2 decreases below this value SaO_2 rapidly decreases owing to the shape of the hemoglobin oxygen dissociation curve. Although chronic hypoxemia can be tolerated remarkably well, acute arterial desaturation usually causes end-organ dysfunction. Although one may accurately measure SaO_2 during arterial blood gas analysis, this approach has been largely superseded by the indirect measure of SaO_2 using pulse oximetry to derive pulse oximetry saturation (SpO_2). Pulse oximeters determine SO_2 by measuring the light absorption of arterial blood at two specific wavelengths, 660 nm (red) and 940 nm (infrared). While pulse oximetry is accurate in reflecting one-point measurements of SaO_2, it does not reliably predict changes in SaO_2 [25]. Moreover, the accuracy of pulse oximeters deteriorates when SaO_2 falls to 80% or less. Still, since the lungs and the body do not store sufficient oxygen reserves to meet metabolic demands, changes in arterial oxygenation may be seen in changes in SpO_2. Importantly, titration of positive-end expiratory pressure (PEEP) and inspired oxygen fraction (FiO_2) in patients with acute lung injury (ALI) is usually done to achieve a $SpO_2 < 90\%$ [26].

Subjects with acute exacerbations of chronic obstructive lung disease often have arterial desaturation. The etiology of this desaturation is often complex and includes ventilation/perfusion (V/Q) mismatching, increased metabolic demand and intrapulmonary shunting [27]. Importantly, exercise, by increasing both cardiac output and pulmonary arterial pressure tends to minimize V/Q mismatch while not affecting shunt. Since exercise also increases oxygen consumption, SvO_2 usually decreases as well. Since V/Q mismatch is amenable to small increases in FiO_2 and is not influenced greatly by low SvO_2 values, patients with predominately V/Q mismatch will improve their SpO_2 with sitting up, whereas those patients with primarily fixed intrapulmonary shunts will demonstrate a decrease in SpO_2. The advantage of this simple test is that the treatments for V/Q mismatch and shunt are different, thus allowing a simple non-invasive measure to both make a diagnosis and define therapy. Such provocative uses of non-invasive SpO_2 monitoring represent the new frontier of this technique, which has gone underutilized for too long.

Preload-responsiveness

Over the past few years it has become increasingly evident that static measure of left ventricular (LV) volumes or indirect estimates of LV preload, such as pulmonary artery occlusion pressure (PAOP) and right atrial pressure, do not reflect actual LV end-diastolic volume or predict the subsequent change in LV stroke volume in response to volume loading [28]. However, other provocative monitoring techniques have been documented to be very sensitive and robust parameters of preload-responsiveness.

Volume challenge: The traditional method of assessing preload-responsiveness in a hemodynamically unstable patient is to rapidly give a relatively small intravascular bolus of volume and observe the subsequent hemodynamic response in terms of blood pressure, pulse, cardiac output and related measures [11]. Volume challenges, if given in too large a volume, carry the risk of inducing acute volume overload with its associated right ventricular (RV) failure (acute cor pulmonale) or LV overload (pulmonary edema). Importantly, several surrogate methods of creating reversible or transient volume challenges include passive leg raising and using ventilatory maneuvers.

Passive leg raising: Passive leg raising transiently increases venous return [29]. In one study, subjects who demonstrate a sustained increase in mean cardiac output or arterial pressure 30 seconds after the legs were raised were found to be preload responsive [30]. The advantage of this approach is that it can be used in patients who are breathing spontaneously, on mechanical ventilation or partial ventilatory assist, and it can be used even in the setting of atrial fibrillation. One limitation of this technique is that the volume mobilized by leg raising is also dependent on total blood volume and could be small in severely hypovolemic patients.

Central venous pressure (CVP) and inferior vena caval (IVC) diameter changes during spontaneous ventilation: Since the primary determinant of preload-responsiveness is RV performance, tests that specifically assess RV performance are inherently attractive. During spontaneous inspiration, the pressure gradient for venous return increases and intrathoracic pressure becomes more negative. CVP will decrease in preload-responsive patients [31] because the right ventricle can accommodate the increased inflow without over-distending. Similarly, IVC diameter measured in its intrahepatic position will collapse if CVP is < 10 mm Hg [32]. Unfortunately, the changes in CVP are quite small and may be within the error of measurement of most ICUs. Similarly, measures of IVC diameter require an expert bedside echocardiographer to visualize the intra-hepatic IVC.

Changes in LV output during positive-pressure ventilation: During positive-pressure ventilation, changes in LV output reflect combined RV-LV performance. Positive-pressure inspiration transiently decreases venous return, causing LV filling to vary in a cyclic fashion as well. If the RV–LV system is preload-responsive, then these small cyclic changes must also alter LV stroke volume. Since the greater the increase in tidal volume, the greater the transient decrease in venous return and subsequently greater decrease in LV output [33], one can program a ventilator to deliver a series of increasing tidal volumes and assess the degree of stroke volume decrease as a measure of preload-responsiveness [34]. During fixed tidal volume positive-pressure ventilation cyclic variations in systolic pressure [35], pulse pressure [36], LV stroke volume [37] or aortic flow [38] quantify preload-responsiveness. Several monitoring devices are available to measure these pressure and flow variations, although none have been studied prospectively as a guide to treatment. Importantly, since measures of systolic pressure, pulse pressure, aortic flow, and descending aortic flow and flow velocity all have different relations to the dynamic change in LV end-diastolic volume to stroke volume relation for the same subject, the threshold values for each parameter predicting preload-responsiveness must be different between parameters and may demonstrate different degrees of robustness in their clinical utility [39].

Dobutamine challenge: Assuming that some preload-reserve is present but limited by impaired cardiac contractility, then one may increase inotropic state as a challenge and observe its effect of regional oxygenation. Using this test, Creteur et al. [40] demonstrated that occult splanchnic ischemia could be unmasked in approximately 30% of critically ill patients who were otherwise considered stable.

Use of Protocolis Driven by Physiological End-Points to Standardize Resuscitation

The application of evidence-based guidelines to clinical practice has gained increased acceptance in recent years. Using a rigorous and open method of grading the scientific evidence and then placing it within the framework on known physiology and local practice patterns can produce remarkable treatment algorithms that, though not perfect, even at their inception, are still better than the nearly random behavior of the present practice of medicine. There are obvious potential advantages of introducing decision-making that is rational and based on evidence. Clinical care can be simplified by the use of treatment algorithms that may facilitate cooperation between different healthcare professionals. This approach may also reduce costs for healthcare purchasers [41]. Unfortunately, standardization of care by the use of guidelines and protocols may not necessarily be a success. There are no certainties in clinical care and individual patients may have needs that fall outside standard guidelines. The rigid application of protocols cannot replace clinical judgment. Furthermore, practice guidelines imposed from outside and without clear rational or perceived benefit may not be accepted by the practicing physicians. However, by merging bedside monitoring technologies with clinical information technology that can assess tissue wellness to run decision-support systems, real-time support and monitoring can be accomplished, and in a cost-effective fashion.

For example, fluid optimization as an endpoint of resuscitation has been shown to reduce length of hospital stay and important complications in patients undergoing a variety of major surgical procedures [42]. This is usually achieved with an esophageal Doppler monitor to evaluate changes in flow in response to fluid challenges [43–45]. Markers of tissue perfusion have also been used as endpoints for resuscitation. These include SvO_2, $ScvO_2$, lactate, base excess and gut mucosal pH using gastric tonometry. The use of these endpoints is attractive, because ensuring optimal blood flow to the vital organs is the ultimate aim of hemodynamic resuscitation. Those patients who spontaneously achieve target hemodynamics fall into a low mortality group and those who are non-achievers despite treatment have a high mortality. These differences must be due to the underlying fitness of patients [46]. Protocolized care plans should use best evidence, aim to reverse those processes known to increase morbidity and mortality, and at the same time be simple enough to be applied across care centers.

Another such protocol that lends itself to this approach is referred to as Functional Hemodynamic Monitoring, because it asks of the monitoring information what treatments should be given, not what is the diagnosis [47]. One needs to first know that a patient is unstable with tissues at risk or existing in an ischemic state. Once this has been identified, then how to treat the patient can be greatly simplified. Fundamentally there are only three questions asked of the cardiovascular system regarding response to resuscitation efforts during shock. First, will blood flow to the body increase (or decrease) if the patient's intravascular volume is increased (or decreased), and if so, by how much? Second, is any decreased in arterial pressure due to loss of vascular tone or merely due to inadequate blood flow? And third, is the heart capable of maintaining an effective blood flow with an acceptable perfusion pressure without going into failure? If taken in this order, one can develop a logical treatment algorithm. If the patient is hemodynamically unstable and preload-responsive, then treatment must include immediate volume expansion as part of its overall plan. However, if the patient is also hypotensive and has reduced vasomotor tone, then even if cardiac output were to increase with volume expansion, arterial pressure may not increase in parallel. Thus, vital organ blood flow may remain compromised despite increasing cardiac output. Since the goal of resuscitation is to restore tissue perfusion, knowing that perfusion pressure will decrease despite an increasing cardiac output, defines that the physician should also start a vasopressor agent in tandem with the initial fluid resuscitation so that both pressure and flow increase. If the patient is not preload-responsive but has reduced vasomotor tone, then a vasopressor alone is indicated, since fluid resuscitation will not improve organ perfusion and may precipitate RV or LV overload. In the patient with circulatory shock who is neither preload-responsive or displaying reduced vasomotor tone, the problem is the heart and both diagnostic and therapeutic actions must be taken to address these specific problems (e.g., echocardiography, dobutamine). The exact cause of cardiac compromise is not addressed by this approach. For example massive pulmonary embolism (acute cor pulmonale), acute hemorrhagic tamponade and massive myocardial infarction would all fall into this category but would have markedly different treatments. However, since the diagnostic development can rapidly default to this group within minutes of initiating the algorithm, appropriate diagnostic approaches could then be used in a highly focused fashion. Although this simplified algorithm has not been used in clinical trials, it has the advantage of being easy to defend on physiological grounds, as well as being simple and easy to apply at the bedside across patient subgroups.

Acknowledgement

The work was supported in part by NIH grants HL67181–02A1 and HL07820–06

References

1. Schlichtig R, Kramer D, Pinsky MR (1991) Flow redistribution during progressive hemorrhage is a determinant of critical O_2 delivery. J Appl Physiol 70:169–178
2. Ivatury RR, Sugerman H (2000) In quest of optimal resuscitation: tissue specific, on to the microcirculation. Crit Care Med 28:3102–3103

3. Schlichtig R, Kramer DJ, Boston JR, Pinsky MR (1991) Renal 0_2 consumption is supply-dependent at all levels of renal 0_2 delivery during progressive hemorrhage. J Appl Physiol 70:1957–1962
4. Robin ED (1980) Of men and mitochondria: coping with hypoxic dysoxia. The 1980 J. Burns Amberson Lecture. Am Rev Respir Dis 122:517–531
5. Pinsky MR (2004) Goals of resuscitation in circulatory shock. Contrib Nephrol 144:31–43
6. Ince C, Sinaasappel M (1999) Microcirculatory oxygenation and shunting in sepsis and shock. Crit Care Med 27:1369–1377
7. Jabran A, Mathru M, Dries D, Tobin MJ (1998) Continuous recordings of mixed venous oxygen saturation during weaning from mechanical ventilation and the ramifications thereof. Am J Respir Crit Care Med 158:1763–1769
8. Scheinman MM, Brown MA, Rapaport E (1969) Critical assessment of use of central venous oxygen saturation as a mirror of mixed venous oxygen in severely ill cardiac patients. Circulation 40:165–172
9. Rady MY, Rivers EP, Martin GB, Smithline H, Appelton T, Nowak RM (1992) Continuous central venous oximetry and shock index in the emergency department: use in the evaluation of clinical shock. Am J Emerg Med 10:538–543
10. Rivers E, Nguyen B, Havstad S, et al (2001) Early goal-directed therapy in the treatment of severe sepsis and septic shock. N Engl J Med 345:1368–1377
11. Dellinger RP, Carlet JM, Masur H, et al (2004) Surviving Sepsis Campaign Guidelines for management of severe sepsis and septic shock. Crit Care Med 32:858–873
12. Reinhart K, Kuhn HJ, Hartog C, et al (2004) Continuous central venous and pulmonary artery oxygen saturation monitoring in the critically ill. Intensive Care Med 30:1572–1578
13. Creteur J, De Backer D, Vincent JL (1999) Does gastric tonometry monitor splanchnic perfusion? Crit Care Med 27:2480–2484
14. Boekstegers P, Weidenhofer S, Kapsner T, Werdan K (1994) Skeletal muscle partial pressure of oxygen in patients with sepsis. Crit Care Med 22:640–650
15. McKinley BA, Marvin RG, Cocanour CS, Moore FA (2000) Tissue hemoglobin O_2 saturation during resuscitation of traumatic shock monitored using near infrared spectrometry. J Trauma 48:637–642
16. Singer M, De Santis V, Vitale D, Jeffcoate W (2004) Multiorgan failure is an adaptive, endocrine-mediated, metabolic response to overwhelming systemic inflammation. Lancet 364:545–548
17. Eckert R, Randall D, Burggren W, French K (2002) Circulation. In: Randall D, Burggren W, French K (eds) Eckert Animal Physiology. Mechanisms and Adaptations, 5th ed. WH Freeman & Co, New York pp 473–523
18. Tang W, Weil MH, Sun S, Noc M, Gazmuri RJ, Bisera J (1994) Gastric intramural PCO_2 as a monitor of perfusion failure during hemorrhagic and anaphylactic shock. J Appl Physiol 76:572–577
19. Nakagawa Y, Weil MH, Tang W, et al (1998) Sublingual capnometry for diagnosis and quantification of circulatory shock. Am J Respir Crit Care Med 157:1838–1843
20. Sims C SP, Menconi M, Matsuda A, Pettit J, Puyana JC (2000) Skeletal muscle acidosis correlates with the severity of blood volume loss during shock and resuscitation. J Trauma Injury Infect Crit Care 49:1167–1173
21. Clavijo-Alvarez JA, Sims CA, Menconi M, Shim I, Ochoa C, Puyana JC (2004) Bladder mucosa pH and PCO_2 as a minimally invasive monitor of hemorrhagic shock and resuscitation. J Trauma 57:1199–1210
22. Gutierrez G, Palizas F, Doglio G, et al (1992) Gastric intramucosal pH as a therapeutic index of tissue oxygenation in critically ill patients. Lancet 339:195–199

23. Mohsenifar Z, Hay A, Hay J, Lewis MI, Koerner SK (1993) Gastric intramural pH as a predictor of success or failure in weaning patients from mechanical ventilation. Ann Intern Med 119:794–798
24. Chance B, Cohen P, Jobsis F (1962) Intracellular oxidation-reduction state in vivo. Science 137:499–508
25. Van de Louw A, Cracco C, Cerf C, et al (2001) Accuracy of pulse oximetry in the intensive care unit. Intensive Care Med 27:1606–1613
26. The Acute Respiratory Distress Syndrome Network (2000) Ventilation with lower tidal volumes as compared with traditional tidal volumes for acute lung injury and the acute respiratory distress syndrome. N Engl J Med 342:1301–1308
27. Calzia E, Radermacher P (2003) Alveolar ventilation and pulmonary blood flow: the V_A/Q concept. Intensive Care Med 29:1229–1232
28. Kumar A, Anel R, Bunnell E, et al (2004) Pulmonary artery occlusion pressure and central venous pressure fail to predict ventricular filling volume, cardiac performance, or the response to volume infusion in normal subjects. Crit Care Med 32:691–699
29. Thomas M, Shillingford J (1965) The circulatory response to a standard postural change in ischaemic heart disease. Br Heart J 27:17–27
30. Boulain T, Achard JM, Teboul JL, Richard C, Perrotin D, Ginies G (2002) Changes in blood pressure induced by passive leg raising predict response to fluid loading in critically ill patients. Chest 121:1245–1252
31. Magder SA, Georgiadis G, Tuck C (1992) Respiratory variations in right atrial pressure predict response to fluid challenge. J Crit Care 7:76–85
32. Kircher BJ, Himelman RB, Schiller NB (1990) Noninvasive estimation of right atrial pressure from the inspiratory collapse of the inferior vena cava. Am J Cardiol 66:493–496
33. Reuter DA, Bayerlein J, Goepfert MS, et al (2003) Influence of tidal volume on left ventricular stroke volume variation measured by pulse contour analysis in mechanically ventilated patients. Intensive Care Med 29:476–480
34. Perel A (1997) Analogue values from invasive hemodynamic monitoring. In: Pinsky MR (ed) Applied Cardiovascular Physiology. Springer-Verlag, Berlin, pp 129–140
35. Perel A (1998) Assessing fluid responsiveness by the systolic pressure variation in mechanically ventilated patients. Systolic pressure variation as a guide to fluid therapy in patients with sepsis-induced hypotension. Anesthesiology 89:1309–1310
36. Michard F, Boussat S, Chemla D, et al (2000) Relation between respiratory changes in arterial pulse pressure and fluid responsiveness in septic patients with acute circulatory failure. Am J Respir Crit Care Med 162:134–138
37. Slama M, Masson H, Teboul JL, et al (2002) Respiratory variations of aortic VTI: a new index of hypovolemia and fluid responsiveness. Am J Physiol Heart Circ Physiol 283: H1729–H1733
38. Feissel M, Michard F, Mangin I, Ruyer O, Faller JP, Teboul JL (2001) Respiratory changes in aortic blood velocity as an indicator of fluid responsiveness in ventilated patients with septic shock. Chest 119: 867–873
39. Pinsky MR (2004) Using ventilation-induced aortic pressure and flow variation to diagnose preload responsiveness. Intensive Care Med 30:1008–1010
40. Creteur J, De Backer D, Vincent JL (1999) A dobutamine test can disclose hepatosplanchnic hypoperfusion in septic patients. Am J Respir Crit Care Med 160:839–845
41. McKee M, Clarke A (1995) Guidelines, enthusiasms, uncertainty and the limits to purchasing. BMJ 310:101–104
42. Fenwick E, Wilson J, Sculpher M, Claxton K (2002) Pre-operative optimisation employing dopexamine or adrenaline for patients undergoing major elective surgery: a cost-effectiveness analysis. Intensive Care Med 28:599–608
43. Mythen MG, Webb AR (1995) Perioperative plasma volume expansion reduces the incidence of gut mucosal hypoperfusion during cardiac surgery. Arch Surg 130:423–429

44. Venn R, Steele A, Richardson P, Poloniecki J, Grounds M, Newman P (2002) Randomised controlled trial to investigate influence of the fluid challenge on duration of hospital stay and perioperative morbidity in patients with hip fractures. Br J Anaesth 88:65–71
45. McKendry M, McGloin H, Saberi D, Caudwell L, Brady AR, Singer M (2004) Randomised controlled trial assessing the impact of a nurse delivered, flow monitored protocol for optimisation of circulatory status after cardiac surgery. BMJ 329:438–443
46. Yu M, Levy M, Smith P, Takiguchi S, Miyasaki A, Myers S (1993) Effect of maximizing oxygen delivery on morbidity and mortality rates in critically ill patients: a prospective randomized controlled trial. Crit Care Med 21:830–838
47. Pinsky MR (2002) Functional hemodynamic monitoring: Applied physiology at the bedside. In: Vincent JL (ed) Yearbook of Emergency and Intensive Care Medicine. Springer-Verlag, Berlin pp 537–552

Microcirculatory Distress in Critically Ill Patients: Meaning and Future

C. Ince

Introduction

This chapter reflects thoughts about the manner in which new inroads into the diagnosis, monitoring and treatment of sepsis and septic shock may be resolved in the future. It is a view from a physiologist interested in the circulatory aspects of critical illness. It is based more on growing insights into the pathophysiology of sepsis rather than on clinical perspectives about things to come. Whatever the perspective, however, it is clear that the major challenge ahead is the adequate prevention, diagnosis and treatment of sepsis and shock. These conditions will dominate intensive care medicine for the foreseeable future [1]. Systemic variables can be adequately monitored and to a large extent, unless the disease is too severe, corrected. The current challenge now and for the foreseeable future is to monitor and correct regional, microcirculatory, cellular and even sub-cellular (e.g., mitochondrial) distress not being sensed by monitoring systemic hemodynamic variables.

Understanding the pathophysiology of sepsis and being able to monitor the physiological processes directly related to outcome will be realized in the foreseeable future. Being mainly focused on cardiovascular function in critical illness, the view presented in this chapter is primarily centered around the notion that achievement of adequate tissue oxygenation and perfusion is a prime target in the care of the critically ill. Only a functioning (micro)circulation can ensure adequate tissue oxygenation and transport of other nutrients and therapeutic agents in support of cell and organ function. The pathophysiology of sepsis, however, is a complex and dynamic process. It is changing all the time, and in a manner dependent on a host of mostly unknown factors. Several advancements will need to be achieved before comprehensive evaluation, monitoring and guiding of therapy are routine.

Current monitoring techniques are mainly based on systemic variables and have been shown to provide incomplete information about the severity of disease and have not provided affective resuscitation end-points. New monitoring technologies that measure more relevant physiological parameters will need to be introduced. Since systemic variables have been shown to provide inadequate information about the severity of disease and outcome [2], it is clear that new monitoring approaches will concern assessment of microcirculatory and cellular function at the bed-side. These technologies will need to be embedded in a comprehensive integrative model of the disease. Such an approach will allow clinicians to guide therapy in an integrative way with well defined end-points based on a clear understanding of the mechanisms driving the disease.

Central to this line of thought is that the essential end-points are parameters, which can be directly targeted by a therapeutic intervention and are not dependent on downstream variables, such as lactate concentration or strong ion difference. Sensitive non-invasive monitoring techniques based on optical spectroscopy are expected to play an important role in the development of this approach. Clinical trials aimed at implementing such techniques and demonstrating that end-points derived from these techniques improve outcome will need to be undertaken [3]. In this chapter, I present such a model, describing the progression of sepsis to severe sepsis and discuss techniques, which are currently being used or are under development. These techniques, together with this model, may contribute to improved diagnosis and treatment for sepsis and shock in the future.

Microcirculatory and Mitochondrial Distress Syndrome: A New View of Sepsis

The major challenge in the critically ill is the treatment of distributive shock [4]. Resuscitated sepsis, characterized by persistent regional and microcirculatory dysfunction and mitochondrial dysfunction, carries a poor prognosis [2, 5–9]. Systemic variables are unable to detect microcirculatory and cellular dysfunction effectively due to shunting and heterogeneity, leaving the clinician without suitable end-points for treatment [8].

The clinical relevance of the microcirculation in sepsis was underscored recently by the excellent study of Sakr et al. [2]. These investigators measured systemic hemodynamic parameters and systemic oxygen transport over time. These investigators also made measurements over time of the sublingual microcirculation, using orthogonal polarization spectral (OPS) imaging. They then analyzed the sensitivity and specificity of the various parameters measured on day one in predicting outcome. They found that neither systemic hemodynamic or oxygen transport variables were able to predict outcome. Derangements in the sublingual microcirculation were the most sensitive and specific predictor of mortality. Besides showing the predictive value of monitoring the microcirculation, this study also showed that conventional resuscitation strategies are capable of improving and correcting microcirculatory failure. When these strategies are ineffective, the prognosis is bad. This study underscores the importance of recruiting and restoring the microcirculation.

The complicated multi-factorial syndrome called sepsis needs a new description and analysis with associated monitoring techniques, if new therapies and resuscitation procedures are to be affective in treating microcirculatory and cellular disorder in such critically ill patients. Thus, we use the term Microcirculatory and Mitochondrial Distress Syndrome (MMDS), because it emphasizes the pathophysiologic compartments where the disease takes place [12]. This syndrome is poorly reflected by systemic hemodynamic variables, which can explain why those parameters provide poor resuscitation end-points. Until now, because of the lack of adequate technology, it was not possible to determining the adequacy of resuscitation by examining the tissue and cellular levels. With the development and improvement of new non-invasive techniques, we are discovering the real role that components of the microcirculation and mitochondria play in diseases. Furthermore new therapies are going to be directed to this level.

In our model of MMDS, factors different from the initial insult contribute to and modulate the pathophysiology and outcome of the disease. These factors include the patient's genotype, the patient's co-morbid conditions, the therapy being applied, and the duration that the condition has persisted (Fig. 1). From a physiological point of view, a patient who is receiving vasopressors in high doses in the presence of diminished circulatory volume, is different from a patient who has been well resuscitated with fluids. The functional behavior of the microcirculation and mitochondria depends on the duration of the septic process and the effects of the drugs that are being administered (Fig. 1).

This view leads to the conclusion that therapy being applied forms a defining component either in the positive or negative sense to the MMDS of resuscitated sepsis and should therefore be regarded as an input parameter (Fig.1). A good example in this respect is the use of corticosteroids for the treatment of sepsis. Besides treating adrenal insufficiency, corticosteroids inhibit expression of inducible nitric oxide (NO) synthase (iNOS), the enzyme thought to be responsible for excessive production of NO and unresponsive hypotension in patients with sepsis [14]. Furthermore, iNOS is expressed in some areas of organs and not in others, resulting in a pathological distribution of regional blood flow [16, 17]. Fig.2 shows how fluid resuscitation can be ineffective for resuscitating the microcirculation in one area of an organ (in this example, the intestinal mucosa where iNOS is expressed) and not in another (the intestinal serosal where iNOS is not expressed). In this figure, microcirculatory oxygen pressures were measured simultaneously in the intestinal serosa and mucosa, using the palladium (Pd) porphyrin phosphorescence technique, in a porcine model of sepsis [18, 19].

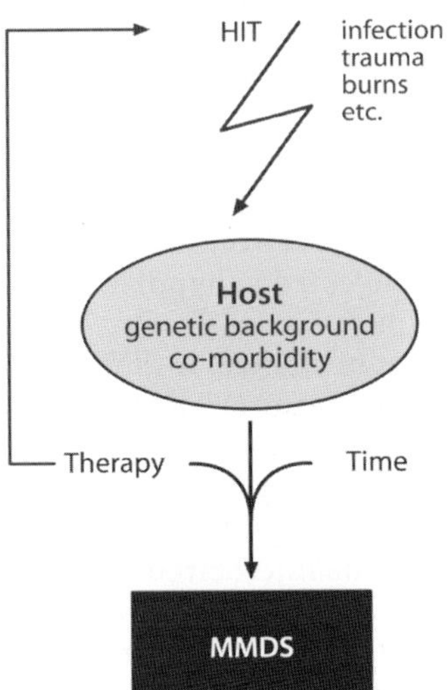

Fig. 1. Microcirculatory and mitochondrial dysfunction syndrome (MMDS) depends on the stimulus (HIT), specific host factors, time, and therapy.

Fluid resuscitation alone resuscitates the mucosa but not the serosa. In the presence of an iNOS inhibitor, however, which inhibits hyperdynamic flow to the iNOS expressing mucosa and restores autoregulation [20], both compartments are resuscitated and gastric CO_2 production corrected. It seems that iNOS is going to be a main target in the treatment of sepsis [15]. Thus, the presence or absence of corticosteroids in the treatment regime of septic patients directly affects autoregulation and blood flow distribution and needs to be taken into account as a defining element in the pathophysiology of MMDS. Of course, other less beneficial affects of corticosteroids also will contribute to the nature of MMDS, underscoring the need to include therapy as an independent input variable in classifying subtypes of MMDS. In this way MMDS can be categorized into subclasses when defining its pathology. For example, MMDS occurs as subtypes with and without steroids. Further subclasses of MMDS could depend upon the use of blood transfusion, the type of asanguinous intravenous fluid being utilized, and the degree to which vasopressors or vasodilators are used. As techniques and insights are put into clinical practice, different approaches and treatments will apply. Thus, we will be able to characterize genetic factors, NO production level, and the type of infection at the time of admission to the hospital. Therapy will be tailored to the individual patient. Some MMDS patients may benefit from the early use of corticosteroids, whereas others might benefit from the administration of NO donors or scavengers of reactive oxygen species.

The use of vasopressors versus vasodilators has a direct effect on the functioning of the cardiovascular system. Vasocontrictors increase arterial blood pressure and even systemic oxygen transport but fail to alleviate microcirculatory distress [13]. Boerma and co-workers found that administration of the vasopressinanalog, terlipressin, to a patient with catecholamine-resistant septic shock, ameliorated profound hypotension and oliguria, but also markedly impaired the sublingual microcirculation as observed by OPS imaging [22]. In contrast, the administration of vasodilators (after ensuring that circulating volume is adequate) ameliorates microcirculatory distress in patients with sepsis [23, 25]. In many forms of shock, microcirculatory flow in the sublingual region correlates very well with data obtained using gastric tonometry. Thus, the sublingual area seems to be a suitable place to evaluate organ perfusion in acutely ill patients. If the inhibition of the sublingual microcirculation observed by Boerme and colleagues during the infusion of vasopressin is a surrogate for what is happening in the splanchnic area, then one should realize that while arterial blood pressure is maintained, other organs are subjected to hypoxia that if not corrected will lead to the development of organ failure. Guzman et al., using a canine model of endotoxin shock, tested the patterns of change of sublingual and intestinal mucosal circulation [24]. They showed that restoration of systemic parameters can be accompanied by persistent tissue hypercarbia when a vasopressor is used to normalize systemic hemodynamic variables. The type of vasodilators and or vasopressors used in a given septic patient will thus define the (patho)physiological state of oxygen transport through the microcirculation.

Time also can be considered as a key input parameter defining the severity of MMDS (Fig.1). Although the terminology of early and late sepsis has been used in the literature, the true impact of time as a pathogenic factor was convincingly demonstrated by Rivers and colleagues [26]. They showed that titrating resuscitation to a systemic parameter, such as central venous oxygen saturation ($ScvO_2$), was beneficial in early sepsis, whereas previous studies of the same strategy applied later in the septic process generated contrary findings. The true challenge for the future will be to determine the effects of time on the persistence of MMDS. But, more insight is needed into the nature MMDS and its impact on microcirculatory blood flow as well as regional tissue oxygen handling by the mitochondria.

Light at the End of the Tunnel

Optical spectroscopy has contributed in a major way to gaining insight into sensing oxygen transport pathways to the tissue cells in health and disease. Optical spectroscopy makes use of the oxygen-dependent properties of native molecules, such as hemoglobin (Hb) in red blood cells and cytochrome oxidase and reduced nicotinamide adenine dinucleotide (NADH) in mitochondria. Optical methods also can take advantage of extrinsic diagnostic dyes, such as Pd-porphyrin [27]. The great advantage of optical spectroscopy is that it is non-invasive and can provide detailed information about oxygen transport pathways at the microcirculatory and cellular levels. Optical spectroscopy also has made important impacts on the clinical monitoring of the circulation. Examples include pulse oximetry, near infrared spectroscopy (NIRS) and reflectance spectrophotometry [27]. In animal models, more advanced techniques, not applicable in humans, can be used to investigate dysfunction of oxygen transport pathways from lung to mitochondria during disease. Such techniques applied to models of critical illness are providing clues about which parameters need to be monitored and corrected in the clinical settings. Based on such insights, clinical techniques will need to be developed to provide this needed information at the bedside. It is expected that, based on such measurements, the severity of disease and the response to therapy can then be judged in a more comprehensive way.

Quenching of Pd-porphyrin phosphorescence for measurement of microcirculatory PO_2 has provided important insights into the behavior of oxygen transport pathways between and within organ systems in experimental animal models of shock, sepsis and resuscitation. Originally developed by Wilson and co-workers [28] and further perfected by us, this technique relies on the infusion of albumin-bound Pd-porphyrin in experimental animals. The technique allows measurements of microvascular PO_2 (μPO_2) *in vivo* [29–31]. We developed and validated a fiber optic phosphorimeter that permits measurements of μPO_2 on organ surfaces in clinically relevant large animal models of human acute diseases (e.g., Fig. 2, [18]). In an intravital study, we were able to demonstrate that it is possible to use the fiber to selectively measure capillary and venular PO_2 [32]. Comparison of this signal to venous PO_2 then allows measurement of the presence and severity of microcirculatory shunting, which is present when μPO_2 is less than venous PO_2 [8, 18]. We further developed a multi-fiber device, which made it possible to follow the time course of μPO_2 simultaneously in different organs, such as the heart, kidney and gut (e.g., Fig. 2, [33]). Investigations we have carried out over

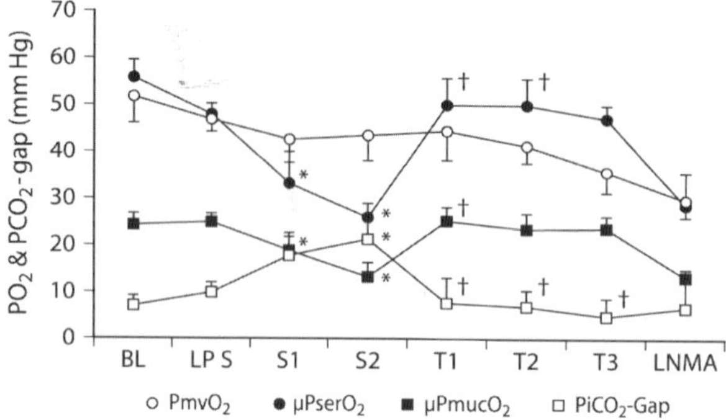

Fig 2. Microvascular oxygenation (μPO_2) and intestinal PCO_2-gap in pigs at baseline, after endotoxin infusion and a shock phase (shock), 3 hours of resuscitation (t1, t2, t3) with 0.5 $mg{\cdot}kg^{-1}{\cdot}min^{-1}$ of the selective iNOS inhibitor 1400W. At the end of the experiment all animals received the non-selective NOS inhibitor L-NAME. Microvascular PO_2 of the ileal serosa ($\mu PserO_2$). Microvascular PO_2 of the ileal mucosa ($\mu PmucO_2$) and calculated difference between $PaCO_2$ and $PiCO_2$ measured by tonometry ($PiCO_2$-gap) (see [19])

the years have identified redistribution of oxygen transport among organ systems and within organ systems, and documented that shunting within the microcirculation is a major response of the circulation to sepsis, shock and resuscitation [8, 34]. For translating such insights into the clinic, we use NIRS (deep penetration) with reflectance spectrophotometry (superficial monitoring) to monitor oxygen transport in the sublingual microcirculation [35]. These observations in combination with the findings of Sakr et al. [2], concerning the predictive value of monitoring the sublingual microcirculation, support the view that this form of monitoring will become routine in intensive care medicine in the future. Sublingual capnography also may be integrated into this form of monitoring [36].

Prior to an understanding of what happens in models of critically illness, however, we will first have to understand what happens in resuscitation procedures when there has been no insult. In other words, we need to know the normal physiological reaction to the procedures employed during critical illness in the absence of inflammation, ischemia or shock. It is striking how little information is available about oxygen transport pathways under such conditions, let alone during critical illness. What is particularly lacking is an understanding of the interactions among the systemic circulation, regional circulations, the microcirculation, and cellular oxygen transport pathways. The reason for this lack of information has been the unavailability of suitable techniques and the lack of investigations in clinically relevant large animal models. In a recent study in a clinically relevant porcine model of acute normovolemic hemodilution (ANH), we investigated the response of the circulation to hemodilution. We investigated the relationships among cerebral and intestinal microcirculatory oxygen transport parameters as well as the redistribution of the oxygen transport pathways within an organ system. We studied the relationship between mucosal and serosal μPO_2 in the intestines. Our results showed that ANH caused a redistribution of oxygen transport away from the intestines and toward the brain. Within the gut, there was microcirculatory shunting of serosal μPO_2 in favor of the mucosal microcirculatory PO_2 [34, 37]. These results suggest that there is a tendency to favor more vital organs, and parts of organs when oxygen transport becomes impaired.

From the above and the literature, it is clear that redistribution and shunting of the microcirculation are prominent responses of the circulation to distress. A disadvantage of the Pd-porphyrin technique for detecting these effects is its limited penetration depth from the organ surface (about 500 μM; [18]). Multi-fiber phosphorimeter measurements have shown that different microcirculatory compartments in different organ systems have different rest values for microcirculatory PO_2. For example, in the intestines under normal conditions, the mucosal microcirculatory PO_2 is less than the serosal microcirculatory PO_2 (Fig. 2). Also, the epicardial microcirculatory PO_2 is much higher than the intestinal microcirculatory PO_2 because of the large amounts of oxygen that are consumed by the myocardium [33]. Being able to measure microcirculatory PO_2 distribution in depth and increasing the penetration depth of the phosphorescence signal would therefore be an important advancement of the technique. It would provide valuable information about the normal and pathological redistribution of microcirculatory oxygen transport as well as its response to therapy. Two-photon excitation is a technique whereby this goal can be achieved. We recently showed that this technique can be applied to Pd-porphyrin phosphorescence and validated its use [31]. An example of the possibilities of this technique is shown in Fig. 3. In this figure, we show how non-invasive and controlled measurement of the kidney microcirculatory PO_2 as a function of penetration can be achieved [31]. This example not only shows a new method to study the distribution of oxygen transport pathways in organs in more detail, but also illustrates the heterogeneous nature of resting oxygen tensions in organs, with kidney cortex microcirculatory PO_2 being much higher than the inner layers of the kidney. Fig. 4 shows how the distribution of microcirculatory PO_2 in the rat kidney cortex is affected by sepsis (T. Johannes, unpublished observations). The cortex of the kidney is more severely affected by sepsis because oxygen is shunted to the advantage of

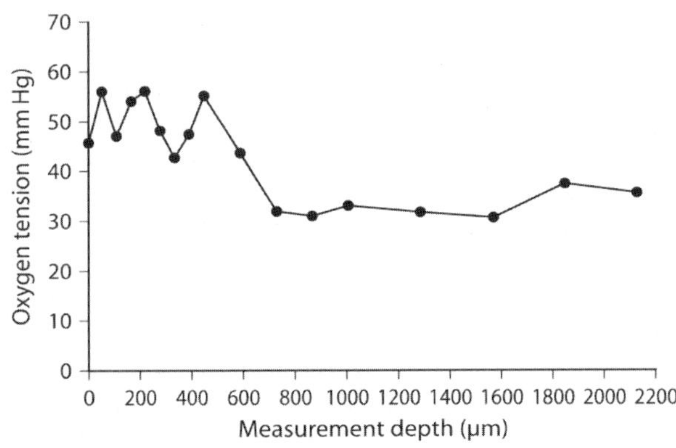

Fig. 3. An example of longitudinal oxygen scanning through the kidney cortex measured by two-photon excitation of Pd porphyrin. The figure shows the PO_2 as a function of measurement depth, measured from the outer surface of the kidney. From [31] with permission

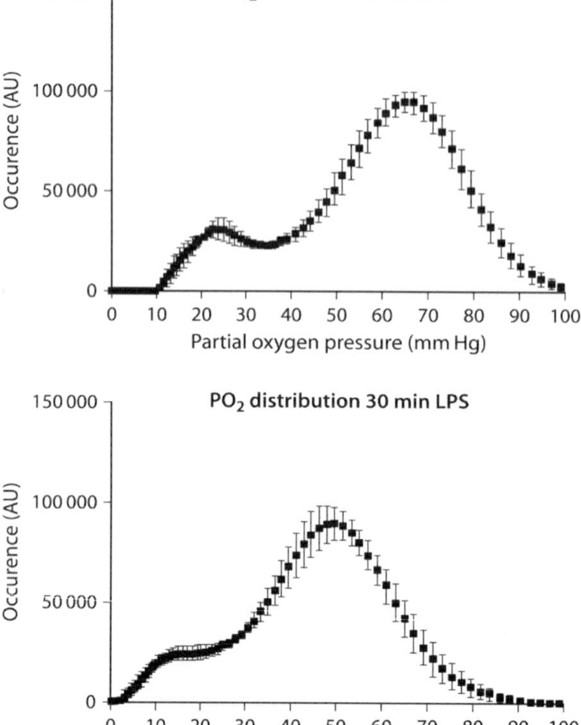

Fig. 4. The distribution of renal cortex microvascular PO_2 measured by Pd porphyrin phosphorescence before and after infusion of 0.1mg/kg endotoxin iv into a rat.

the deeper layers of the kidney. It is anticipated that more such investigations will provide the needed insights into the nature of microcirculatory and cellular distress during critical illness in the intensive care of the future.

Sidestream Dark Field Imaging

In the ICU of the future, insight from the pathophysiology of microcirculatory and cellular dysfunction will provide the basis for evaluation the state and severity of MMDS. Applying these insights to the care of the critically ill patient will thus require routine clinical monitoring of microcirculatory and cellular function at the bedside. The importance of doing so has been highlighted in recent years by the application of OPS imaging to the monitoring of the sublingual microcirculation in sepsis [2, 5, 22, 25]. OPS imaging is a pioneering technology, because it allows clinicians to assess the microcirculation at the bedside [38–41]. The technique has, however, a number of shortcomings. The major drawback of OPS imaging is relatively poor image quality, making it difficult to observe the granular nature of flowing red blood cells and to identify leukocyte kinet-

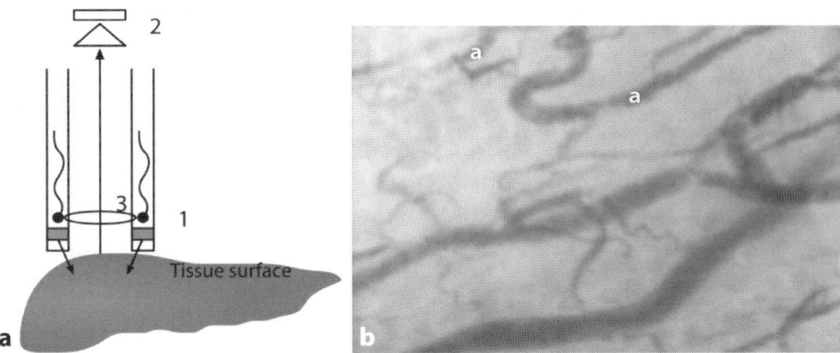

Fig. 5. SDF (Sidestream Dark Field) imaging, an improved technique to observe the microcirculation. a) shows 1, indicating the position of the green light-emitting diodes, 2, the CCD camera capturing the images; and 3, the magnifying lens. b) shows an example of sublingual microcirculation with improved image quality capillary and arteriolar (a) detection visible. From [42] with permission

ics. Also the relatively poor image quality of OPS imaging has hampered the development of image processing software able to automatically analyze the images. Currently such analysis is mainly done by hand, and is a very cumbersome procedure.

To improve microcirculatory imaging technology, we developed a new optical modality, which we have called Sidestream Dark Field (SDF) imaging [42]. This technology provides better image quality of the microcirculation and capillaries. Because of the improved image quality, automatic image analysis software has been successfully developed. SDF imaging uses a light guide to image the microcirculation. The light guide is surrounded at the tip by green light-emitting diodes whose emitting light is optically separated from the inner imaging pathway. Green light is absorbed by the Hb of the red blood cells. By this separation, light is pumped straight into the tissue and no tissue surface reflections can interfere with the reflected image of the underlying microcirculation. This complete separation of emission and reflected light provides much better imaging and can be regarded as an ultimate form of dark field microscopy. It is expected that a combination of SDF imaging with other spectroscopic modalities will give more integrative knowledge about the functional state of the microcirculation and tissue cells at the bedside.

Treating MMDS: Towards an Integrative Monitoring of Cellular, Microcirculatory and Systemic Variables

The basic challenge for the future is to develop a good model of the disease by which the various monitoring variables including microcirculatory and cellular variables are assessed at the bedside. The most difficult aspect of this endeavor will be to take into account the heterogeneous nature of the (micro)circulation. Ultimately being able to sense mitochondrial energy state in a reliable way will further add to the arsenal of techniques able to monitor the nature and severity of MMDS. Much more detail will be collected and add input into comprehensive model of the circulation. It is expected that new, more integrative drugs will be developed targeting microcirculatory dysfunction. Such an integrative model of disease, monitoring and therapy will provide the much needed information about the impact of shock and resuscitation on the progress of disease and provide end-points which can be targeted more precisely than before.

References

1. Angus DC, Linde-Zwirble WT, Lidicker J, Clermont G, Carcillo J, Pinsky MR (2001) Epidemiology of severe sepsis in the United States: analysis of incidence, outcome and associated costs of care. Crit Care Med 29:1303–1310
2. Sakr Y, Dubois MJ, De Backer D, Creteur J, Vincent JL (2004) Persistent microcirculatory alterations are associated with organ failure and death in patients with septic shock. Crit Care Med 32:1825–1831
3. Sibbald B (2004) Shockingly complex: the difficult road to introducing new ideas to critical care. Crit Care 8:419–422
4. Vincent JL (2001) Hemodynamic support in septic shock Intensive Care Med 27:S80–S92
5. De Backer D, Creteur J, Preiser JC, Dubois MJ, Vincent JL (2002) Microvascular blood flow is altered in patients with sepsis. Am J Respir Crit Care Med 166:98–104
6. Kaplan LJ, Kellum J (2004) Initial pH, base deficit, lactate, anion gap, strong ion difference, and strong ion gap predict outcome from major vascular injury. Crit Care Med 32:1120 –1124
7. Brealey D, Brand M, Hargreaves I, et al (2002) Association between mitochondrial dysfunction and severity and outcome of septic shock. The Lancet 360:219–223
8. Ince C, Sinaappel M (1999) Microcirculatory oxygenation and shunting in sepsis and shock. Crit Care Med 27:1369–1377
9. Spronk PE, Zandstra DF, Ince C (2004) Bench-to-bedside review: sepsis is a disease of the microcirculation. Crit Care 8:462–468
10. Joly HR, Weil MH (1969) Temperature of the great toe as an indication of the severity of shock. Circulation 39:131–138
11. Fink MP (1997) Cytopathic hypoxia in sepsis. Acta Anaesthesiol Scand (suppl 110):87–95
12. Spronk PE, Kanoore-Edul VS, Ince C (2004) Microcirculatory and mitochondrial distress syndrome (MMDS) a new look at sepsis In: Pinsky M, Payen D (eds) Functional Hemodynamic Monitoring. SpringerVerlag, Heidelberg, pp 47–67
13. LeDoux D, Astiz ME, Carpati CM, Rackow EC (2000) Effects of perfusion pressure on tissue perfusion in septic shock. Crit Care Med 28:2729–2732
14. Duma D, Silva-Santos JE, Assreuy J (2004) Inhibition of glucocorticoid receptor binding by nitric oxide in endotoxemic rats. Crit Care Med 32:2304 –2310
15. Hollenberg SM, Broussard M, Osman J, Parillo JE (2000) Increased microvascular reactivity and improved mortality in septic mice lacking inducible nitric oxide synthase. Circ Res 86:774–779
16. Revelly JP, Ayuse T, Brienza N, Fessler HE, Robotham JL (1996) Endotoxic shock alters distribution of blood flow within the intestinal wall. Crit Care Med 24:1345–1351
17. Morin M J, Unno N, Hodin RA, Fink MP (1998) Differential experession of inducible nitric oxide synthase messenger RNA along the longitudinal and crypt-villus axes of the intestine in endotoxemic rats. Crit Care Med 26:1258–1264
18. Sinaasappel M, van Iterson M, Ince C (1999) Microvascular oxygen pressure measurements in the intestine during hemorrhagic shock and resuscitation. J Physiol (Lond) 514:245–253

19. Siegemund M, van Bommel J, Schwarte LA, Emons M, Ince C (2001) Selective blockade of iNOS by 1400W, but not by LNMA, is beneficial to intestinal oxygenation after endotoxaemia. Intensive Care Med 27:S180 (abst)
20. Avontuur JA, Bruining HA, Ince C (1997) Nitric oxide causes dysfunction of coronary autoregulation in endotoxemic rats. Cardiovasc Res 35:368–376
21. Raat NJ, Verhoeven AJ, Mik EG, et al (2005) The effect of storage time of human red cells on intestinal microcirculatory oxygenation in a rat isovolemic exchange model. Crit Care Med 33:39–45
22. Boerma EC, van der Voort PHJ, Ince C (2005) Sublingual microcirculatory flow is impaired by the vasopressin-analogue terlipressin in a patient with catecholamine-resistant septic shock. Acta Anaesth Scand (in press)
23. Buwalda M, Ince C (2002) Opening the microcirculation. ... can vasodilators be useful in sepsis? Intensive Care Med 28:1208–1217
24. Guzman JA, Dikin MS, Kruse JA (2005) Lingual, splanchnic, and systemic hemodynamic and carbon dioxide tension changes during endotoxic shock and resuscitation. J Appl Physiol 98:108–113
25. Spronk PE, Ince C, Gardien MJ, et al (2002) Nitroglycerin promotes microvascular recruitment in septic shock after intravascular volume resuscitation. The Lancet 360:1395–1396
26. Rivers E, Nguyen B, Havstad S, et al (2001) Early goal-directed therapy in the treatment of severe sepsis and septic shock. N Engl J Med 345:1368–1377
27. Siegemund M, van Bommel J, Ince C (1999) Assessment of regional tissue oxygenation. Intensive Care Med 25:1044–1060
28. Wilson DF, Pastuszko A, DiGiacomo JE, et al (1991) Effect of hyperventilation on oxygenation of the brain cortex of newborn piglets. J Appl Physiol 70:2691–2696
29. Sinaasappel M, Ince C (1996) Calibration of Pd-porphyrin phosphorescence for oxygen concentration measurements in vivo. J Appl Physiol 81:2297–2303
30. Mik B, Donkersloot K, Raat NJH, Ince C (2002) Exciatation pulse deconvolution in phosphorescence lifetime analysis for O2 measurements in vivo. Photochem Photobiol 76:12–21
31. Mik EG, Van Leeuwen TG, Raat NJ, Ince C (2004) Quantitative determination of localized tissue oxygen concentration in vivo by two-photon excitation phosphorescence lifetime measurements. J Appl Physiol 97:1962–1969
32. Sinaasappel M, Donkersloot K, van Bommel J, Ince C (1999) PO2 measurements in the rat intestinal microcirculation Am J Physiol 276:G1515–G1520
33. Zuurbier CJ, van Iterson M, Ince C (1999) Functional heterogeneity of oxygen supply consumption ratio in the heart. Cardiovasc Res 44:488–497
34. Schwarte LA, Fournell A, van Bommel J, Ince C (2005) Redistribution of intestinal microcirculatory oxygenation during acute hemodilution in pigs. J Appl Physiol. 98:1070–1075
35. Atasever B, van der VeenA, Goedhart P, de Mo B, Ince C (2005) Sublingual NIRS and reflectance spectrophotometry: new methods to monitor sublingual oxygen availability. Crit Care 8:A542 (abst)
36. Weil MH, Nakagawa Y, Tang W, et al (1999) Sublingual capnometry: a new noninvasive measurement for diagnosis and quantitation of severity of circulatory shock. Crit Care Med 27:1225–1229
37. van Bommel J, Trouwborst A, Schwarte L, Siegemund M, Ince C, Henny ChP (2002) Intestinal and cerebral oxygenation during severe isovolemic hemodilution and subsequent hyperoxic ventilation in a pig model. Anesthesiology 97:660–670
38. Mathura KR, Alic L, Ince C (2001) Initial clinical experience with OPS imaging. In: Vincent JL (ed) Yearbook of Intensive Care and Emergency Medicine. Springer-Verlag, Heidelberg, pp 233–244
39. Mathura KR, Vollebrecht KC, Boer K, de Graaf JC, Ubbink DT, Ince C (2001) Comparison of OPS imaging to intravital capillarosopy of nail fold microcirculation. J Appl Physiol 91:74–78

40. Mathura KR, Bouma GJ, Ince C (2001) Abnormal microcirculation in brain tumours during surgery. Lancet 358:1698–1699
41. Pennings F, Bouma GJ, Ince C (2004) Direct observation of the human cerebral microcirculation during aneurysm surgery reveals increased arteriolar contractility. Stroke 35:1284–1288
42. Ince C (2005) Sidestream Dark Field (SDF) imaging: an improved technique to observe sublingual microcirculation. Crit Care 8:A477 (abst)

Managing Infection: From Agar Plate to Genome Scan

J. Cohen

Introduction

Sepsis is the systemic injurious response to infection [1]. There is wide agreement that sepsis is currently one of the most common, and most challenging conditions encountered on the intensive care unit (ICU) and it is implausible to believe that it will not continue to be a problem for the foreseeable future. The management of the septic patient – and in particular, a patient who develops septic shock – is complex and multi-faceted [2]. In this chapter I will focus specifically on the diagnosis and management of the infection *per se*, while acknowledging that this forms only one part of the treatment plan.

The epidemiology of infection on the ICU has been discussed extensively elsewhere [3–5]. Suffice it to say here that the organisms most frequently identified are common enteric bacteria (*Escherichia coli*, *Klebsiella*, *Citrobacter*), non-fermenting Gram-negative bacteria such as *Pseudomonas* and *Acinetobacter* species, and Gram-positive bacteria, in particular staphylococci. The commonest sites of infection in septic patients are the respiratory tract, the abdomen, bacteremias, and skin and soft tissue infections. It is interesting to reflect that despite these clinical syndromes being common and well-recognized, until recently there has been no agreement on epidemiological definitions of infections at these sites that could be used for comparative purposes in clinical trials in septic patients. Given the widely acknowledged difficulties there are in defining, for instance, exactly what is meant by ventilator-associated pneumonia (VAP), this is a surprising oversight. Recently, the International Sepsis Forum convened an Expert Panel to agree a set of working definitions that could be used for these purposes [6].

An important question that needs to be asked – and answered – is why is it necessary to try and diagnose the infection at all? After all, if the clinical syndrome is sepsis (septic shock) surely it is *this* that needs to be recognized promptly? In the ICU of the future, what will be gained by trying to identify the infection: will this be simply academic curiosity? I think there are at least three good reasons why the answer is clear: we will certainly want to be able to diagnose the infection, and indeed, to do it considerably more quickly than we can at the moment. Let me briefly set these out:

a) Establishing the diagnosis. There is no need to rehearse the arguments that establishing a precise diagnosis is likely to lead to quicker, safer, and more appropriate care for the patient. For instance, there is already an abundance of evidence that shows that treating patients with the correct antibiotic (that is, an antibiotic active against the organisms shown to be the cause of the infection) is more likely to lead to a better outcome [7, 8].

b) Dealing with antimicrobial resistance. The problems posed by the spread of antibiotic resistance and the diminishing number of effective antimicrobial agents are unlikely to go away. It is unclear how much longer we will be able to use an empirical antibiotic regimen with sufficient confidence that there is a reasonable chance that it will be active against the infecting pathogen. Furthermore, widespread use of broad-spectrum antibiotics tends to drive resistance. It would be greatly to the advantage of the individual patient – and the wider community – if we were able to identify the susceptibility pattern of the pathogen at a very early stage, hence allowing much more specific antimicrobial therapy.

c) Deploying targeted therapy. The biomedical research community is continuing an active program aimed at developing adjunctive agents for the treatment of sepsis and septic shock (reviewed in [9]). The first of these agents – drotrecogin alfa (activated) – has already entered clinical practice. In many cases, these drugs are targeted at specific microbial components (for instance, the lipopolysaccharide [endotoxin] of Gram-negative bacteria), or at host pathways that are predominantly activated by a particular type of organism, or an organism that bears a particular virulence determinant. Hence, proper use of these drugs, should they be shown to be clinically active, would depend on rapid early identification of the organism (or some component of the organism) in order to ensure that the drug is used appropriately. Indeed, it could be argued that these drugs cannot be properly tested unless the correct patients can be quickly identified.

Given that I believe that microbiological diagnosis (in the widest sense) will still be important for the foreseeable future, let me now turn to a consideration of what developments we might expect over the next 10–15 years. I will first consider the question of diagnosis, that is, identification of the organism or of microbial components, and then consider the monitoring of antimicrobial therapy. My purpose is to focus on those developments that relate to the organism itself. It should be acknowledged that there is a considerable literature concerned with the identification of non-specific markers of infection, such as procalcitonin or C-reactive protein (CRP) [10]. Some of these molecules may indeed help, in a categorical sense, in the diagnosis of the presence or absence of infection but a full discussion of their role is beyond the scope of this paper.

Developments in Rapid Diagnosis

Microbiological diagnosis has two main components: detection of microorganisms in clinical specimens, and antimicrobial susceptibility testing. I will consider each in turn.

Detecting Microorganisms

The first, and clinically most useful aspect of this, is the direct detection of microorganisms in clinical specimens. Various methods can be used (Table 1). Some very simple methods can be rapid and effective. Direct microscopy by Gram stain or the use of fluorescent antibody testing works well in many situations. Simple antigen detection, and of course, conventional culture will probably continue. Traditional microbiological culture-based methods have the great disadvantage of requiring at least several hours of incubation; often full diagnosis requires 12–18 hours. We are most interested here in new molecular or immunological approaches to diagnosis that may greatly reduce this delay (Table 2).

Table 1. Methods for the detection of microorganisms in clinical specimens

Method	Comments/Examples
Microscopic observation: direct staining	Gram; Ziehl-Neelsen (Mycobacteria); Fluorescent antibody (Legionella)
Antigen detection	*Neisseria meningitidis; Streptococcus pneumoniae*
Conventional culture	Available for most organisms, but usually many hours delay
Molecular assays	See Table 2

Table 2. Molecular and immunological methods that are available, or in development, for microbial detection

Method	Comment/Examples
Ribosomal RNA probes	Available commercially for *N. gonorrhoeae* and *C. trachomatis*, and others
ELISA	Galactomannan for Aspergillus
DNA amplification methods	Include PCR, ligase chain reaction, real time PCR.
Microarray	'Labchips', either used for rapid genome screening or for complex multiple biochemical assays
Fluorescent in-situ hybridization (FISH)	Developed for group B streptococci
Adenylate kinase biomass	Highly sensitive method for detecting bacterial
B cell sensor	Engineered B cells use bioluminescence to detect pathogens bound to cell surface antibodies

The possibility of using molecular probes or sequence-based diagnosis in microbiology was appreciated at an early stage, and enthusiastically embraced. Considerable effort has been expended in developing the various approaches (listed in Table 2) to make them clinically applicable, but it has become apparent that there are a number of significant problems with these methods. The first limitation relates to the ability to obtain 'clean' DNA for analysis. In the early studies, this was obtained from a single colony of the organism. Although this still has some value (see below) it of course vitiates the whole purpose of molecular methods (the speed of diagnosis) since it is first necessary to isolate the organism using conventional methods. It would be much more useful if the target DNA could be obtained directly from the clinical specimen (e.g., from blood culture) but this has proved technically challenging. The second difficulty is the fact that, like antigen testing, molecular methods do not distinguish between dead and alive bacteria. Polymerase chain reaction (PCR) techniques will detect that part of the organism's DNA that is the target sequence, and of course, it may still be present even if the bacterium has been killed. Indeed, it is not just that detecting the DNA from a dead organism might produce a 'false positive'; the extreme sensitivity of DNA amplification techniques means that very few viable organisms can be sufficient to lead to a positive test. This means that in many clinical sites it can be impossible to distinguish between a few, colonizing organisms and a large number of potentially pathogenic organisms using PCR-based methods. Finally, there is the real risk of laboratory contamination, again a consequence of the extreme sensitivity of the methods.

Despite these difficulties there are some encouraging and exciting developments using a variety of DNA-based approaches. The most attractive methods (from the standpoint of clinical utility) are those that can be used directly on clinical specimens. For example, Golden et al. have described a real-time fluorescent PCR assay for the rapid detection of group B streptococci in neonatal blood samples [11], and Artz et al. reported the use of FISH (fluorescent in-situ hybridization) directly on vaginal specimens to detect carriage of group B streptococci in pregnant women [12]. One step further away is a method in which a matrix of rRNA probes, chosen to select for the most commonly isolated blood culture isolates, is used to screen aliquots of blood that have been incubating in conventional isolator bottles. Although this introduces a delay while the organisms grow in the bottles, it cuts out the slow process of identification [13].

Not all rapid detection systems depend on DNA amplification. Perhaps of particular interest to intensivists is an enzyme-linked immunosorbent assay (ELISA) that has been used to detect intravascular catheter-related sepsis due to coagulase-negative staphylococci [14]. The assay measures IgG responses to an exocellular antigen, lipid S, which is produced by the bacteria. Other similar approaches, already in clinical use, include assays for galactomannan or D-glucan, designed to identify fungal infections. In the main though, antibody-detection systems such as these have proved less effective, in part because of the time needed to generate a sufficient signal and in part because of the difficulties in separating infection from colonization.

Others have begun to explore completely innovative approaches. Investigators at the Defence Science and Technology Laboratory at Porton Down, UK, wanted a method that simply provided an exquisitely sensitive tool to detect bacterial biomass. Their initial concept was that assuming the sample came from a normally sterile site, this would be *a priori* evidence of bacterial contamination. (The initial drive for this work was the need to have early warning of potential biological warfare agents). The method they have developed uses bioluminescence to detect the enzyme adenylate kinase, and by introducing a number of amplification steps they can distinguish the presence of fewer than 100 bacterial cells in a 5 minute semi-automated assay (Murphy M., Federation of Infection Societies meeting, Manchester, UK, 2004). By modifying the procedure they can introduce some specificity so that they can look specifically for methicillin-resistant *Staphylococcus aureus* (MRSA), for instance.

An extraordinarily ingenious method was reported recently by Rider et al. [15]. B lymphocyte cell lines were engineered to express cytosolic aequorin, a calcium-sensitive bioluminescent protein, and also to express membrane bound antibodies specific for pathogens of interest. Cross linking of the antibodies by even small numbers of the appropriate pathogen elevated intracellular calcium levels within seconds causing the aequorin to emit light. The system was used first for *Yersinia pestis*, the plague agent, and was shown to detect as few as 50 colony forming units (cfu) in a total assay time of less than 3 minutes. More prosaically, the assay could detect 500 cfu/g of the foodborne pathogen *Escherichia coli* 0157:H7 in contaminated lettuce in just 5 minutes, including sample preparation. Clearly this method has enormous potential for the rapid detection of pathogens in clinical samples.

Thus far, I have considered methods that are intended either to simply measure bacterial biomass, or to give a general indication of the bacterial genus, and sometimes species. In a conventional microbiology laboratory, this would be analogous to reporting that a urine sample contained a significant growth of coliform bacteria, for instance. The next stage would be to identify it specifically as an *E. coli*, with relevant antimicrobial sensitivity patterns. Both these steps take time. Identifying an isolate to species level is usually achieved by a combination of serological and biochemical methods that can sometimes require a further overnight incubation. Modern molecular methods can speed this up, for instance by using gene probes to demonstrate that a strain of staphylococcus is *S. epidermidis* rather than *S. aureus* [16]. More excitingly, and very much the way forward, is more precise determination of particular virulence characteristics. A good example is the use of PCR to detect the Panton-Valentine leukocidin gene in isolates of *S. aureus* [17]. This is of considerable clinical interest, since these strains have lately been associated with a particularly severe form of pneumonia in children [18]. The linear development of this approach is the gene chip, in which microbial DNA is scanned to produce a gene profile that could include information on not just the species identification, but virulence determinants and antimicrobial susceptibility [19].

Susceptibility Testing

For reasons noted above, there would be considerable clinical benefit to having rapid information about the sensitivity pattern of a particular isolate. This is not just because of the opportunity this would provide to choose more specific antimicrobial therapy, but also because it would give early warning of potential cross-infection problems (e.g., isolation of an MRSA).

One of the earliest uses of molecular probes in this context was the identification of the gene encoding isoniazid resistance in *M. tuberculosis*, a development that revolutionized the management of tuberculosis by obviating the need for a further period of prolonged incubation. Of more immediate interest to the intensive care physician is the use of gene probes (and other related approaches) for the rapid detection of MRSA. As an example of this, Warren et al. have described a method in which real-time PCR is used directly on a nasal swab and the DNA product is then detected using a fluorogenic probe [20]. A more sophisticated (and perhaps less practical approach at present) is described by Rolain et al. [21] in which they used real-time PCR to quantitate the DNA copies of either 16S RNA or *rpoB* genes that are present over time in experiments in which various antibiotics are added to the culture medium. The idea of this 'universal antibiotic susceptibility test' is simply that the more susceptible the organism the less DNA will be detected. It would seem more likely that more robust methods for detecting biomass (perhaps such as the adenylate kinase method described above) would be better than PCR in this case.

Developments in Monitoring Therapy

Once we have started a patient on antimicrobial therapy, be it empirical or directed against a known pathogen, how do we monitor the patient to ensure that they are responding satisfactorily (Table 3)? On many occasions simple clinical signs are adequate and it is perfectly obvious that the patient is improving. If in addition the blood cultures become negative and levels of procalcitonin are falling, we have more than enough evidence of success. But not infrequently on the ICU the picture is less clear: we have not been able to isolate an organism, or the patient remains unstable, or interpretation of biochemical markers is confounded by other pathology. Another scenario is the patient with a deep seated, or complicated infection, perhaps in the setting of an inadequate immune response as a result of immunosuppressive therapy, or a case in which we are dealing with an organism with marginal sensitivity to the only available antimicrobial agent. In these instances we need to ensure that the antimicrobial therapy is 'fine-tuned' to have maximum efficacy. At present, the only real tool we have to do this is measurement of antimicrobial drug levels. Although we understand the principles of pharmacokinetics and pharmacodynamics and how these may influence tissue levels of a drug, there is a relative paucity of data showing how we should interpret drug levels in the complex and dynamic setting of the critically ill patient. Indeed, studies have shown that in this patient group, nomogram-based dosing regimens can result in substantial under-dosage [22].

Table 3. Methods for monitoring the response to anti-infective therapy

Method	Comment
Clinical response	Vital signs
Eradication of the organism	Follow up cultures, where possible
Non-specific markers	Changes in C-reactive protein, procalcitonin etc
Antimicrobial drug levels	As indicated (usually for toxicity)

Historically, the serum bactericidal assay (or serum bactericidal test, or titer, SBT) was developed as the ideal way to assess the appropriateness of antibiotic therapy [23]. It is one of the few *ex vivo* tests performed in the clinical laboratory that reflects the interaction of the isolated pathogen, the antimicrobial agent and the patient, and at least theoretically, it should be able to take account of the problems inherent in interpreting antibiotic drug levels in ICU patients. However, most investigators regard the SBT as imprecise and time consuming, and because quality control schemes found it to be poorly reproducible it has generally fallen into disuse. Recently we have developed a novel approach to measuring bactericidal activity in blood, based on the concept of time-to-positivity (TPOS) [24]. This uses the same basic principle as the traditional SBT assay, but assumes that most microbiology laboratories use one of the modern continuous blood culture assay systems. These continuously monitor the bottle for growth, and signal as soon as there is a 'positive' that crosses a pre-determined threshold. We have shown that TPOS can be used as a surrogate for total bactericidal activity. Hence, if a patient is being treated adequately then the net antimicrobial activity in the blood will be high. If a specimen of that patient's blood, taken at a time when antimicrobial activity should be maximal, is inoculated with a test organism then the TPOS will be long: the effective therapy will substantially delay the bacteria 'growing out' in the culture. Conversely, if antimicrobial activity is subtherapeutic then TPOS will be short – the bacteria will quickly grow and the threshold for signaling will be crossed. When we carried out a pilot clinical study to test the potential clinical utility of this method we were surprised to find very substantial variations in TPOS in patients who were ostensibly all being adequately treated. For instance, in 20 patients receiving vancomycin for deep-seated staphylococcal infections, there was an 8-fold range in the TPOS. If these preliminary findings are borne out in more extensive studies, then it will be clearly be interesting to ask whether there is any correlation between TPOS and clinical outcome.

Monitoring the adequacy of antimicrobial therapy is potentially one of the areas that will see the most noticeable changes over the next 10–15 years. The various assays of bacterial biomass, described above, can probably be adapted reasonably easily to allow quick and easy quantitation of the microbial burden.

Alternatively, non-specific markers such as procalcitonin or its descendants, or even perhaps image-based approaches (scans that detect inflammation in a semi-quantitative fashion are already available) will be developed. The challenge will be to carry out the clinical trials that will show whether these more complex approaches are worthwhile in terms of hard clinical endpoints.

Microbiological Diagnosis will be Redundant in 2015 – Discuss

It is sometimes possible to detect an interesting tension between clinicians who believe the safest and easiest way to approach the treatment of the septic patient is to deploy broad spectrum antibiotics at an early stage (empiricists), and those (sometimes characterized as academic purists) who argue that the patient is best served by making a specific etiological diagnosis and prescribing carefully tailored therapy. Although this is obviously rather a caricature, it does nevertheless highlight an important question: will knowing more about the infection actually help the patient? At the beginning of this paper I argued that the answer was "yes". Let us now explore this in a little more detail. What specific changes in medical science and practice are likely over the next 10–15 years that might alter our view? First, what are the arguments that we will not need to worry about microbiological diagnosis in the future?

- New non-antimicrobial anti-infective drugs will become available that will supersede antibiotics. The hope is it will be possible to develop safe and cheap new molecular entities, probably small peptides or monoclonal antibodies, which will block virulence pathways or stimulate host defenses and so limit infection. One of the great attractions of such drugs would be that they would not drive antibiotic resistance. It is likely that there will be some successes in this field, but improbable that they will be of broad enough spectrum of activity, or sufficiently active, that antibiotics would not be needed as well.
- We will have better knowledge of host targets and so will be able to intervene in pathological processes, irrespective of the causative organism. The argument against this is much the same as that just stated. In addition though, it relies on the mistaken assumption that the inflammatory and injurious pathways that occur in the septic patient are independent of the causative organism, i.e., that there is some kind of final common pathway. This is only partly true at best: indeed, as we have learnt more about the mechanisms by which bacteria interact with the host it has become apparent that Gram positive and Gram negative bacteria, for instance, most certainly do activate explicit and differing pathways [25].
- Better early diagnosis and/or more effective prophylaxis will mean that sepsis will almost disappear. This is not so easy to dismiss. Indeed, it is likely that there will be significant advances in these areas. For instance, so-called 'lab chips' which allow rapid assay of multiple parameters using robotic mechanisms with frequent read outs and then employ bioinformatics to generate predictive outcomes are already well advanced in development. Better identification of high-risk patients is likely to help in the targeting of prophylactic

measures, which in turn will reduce the incidence of sepsis. But it seems unlikely that these measures will completely prevent the condition occurring. In contrast, what are the reasons that might suggest that we will need to continue to make a microbiological diagnosis?

- Bacteria – and resistance to antibacterial agents – are not going to disappear. Clearly bacteria themselves are going to continue to cause disease, and there is no evidence that the problems associated with antibacterial resistance are diminishing. The only practical way of achieving this would require an enormous cultural shift in the way that we as a society use antibiotics. Despite the extremely well-argued case of many professional bodies, that is most unlikely to occur. It is true of course that in the limited environment of ICUs there has been some interest in strategies such as short course therapy [26] or antibiotic cycling [27], but unfortunately these are likely to have only minimal impact on the problem as a whole.
- Bacteria, rather than the host are likely to be the safest point of intervention. The potential hazards of manipulating the host immune response have been apparent since the early days, and are most graphically illustrated by the increased incidence of tuberculosis that has occurred with some anti-tumor necrosis factor (TNF) antagonists [28]. It is true that these problems arose in the context of prolonged therapy, and that in the septic patient this is likely to be less of an issue, since the intervention is much more likely to be short-lived. However, drugs that target fundamental host cell process such as signal transduction pathways that are certainly involved in the pathogenesis of sepsis but are also key to many other processes, do run the risk of serious adverse events. Hence, therapeutic strategies aimed at the bacteria (even if the strategies are not conventional antimicrobial agents) are likely to be safer and much more attractive.
- There is no evidence of a great increase in new antimicrobial drugs. The dearth of novel antimicrobial compounds has been widely commented on [29, 30]; it would be unwise to think that we can rely in the future upon new, ultra-broad spectrum agents that will not fall victim to bacterial resistance mechanisms. It is more likely that we will need to use the antibiotics we already have, but deploy them with great care having regard to the particular type of infection and local patterns of antibiotic resistance.

Conclusion

It is hard to escape the conclusion that, notwithstanding the important and exciting developments in rapid diagnosis and in understanding pathophysiology that are likely to be seen in the next 10–15 years, we will continue to need to make a microbiological diagnosis in the septic patient. We will want to be able to do it more quickly, more accurately, and with greater precision than we can now, but simply to ignore it will not be an option. It would be wonderful to have a 'magic bullet' that we could use in any potentially infected patient, secure in the knowledge that it would be effective, irrespective of the organism. Unfortunately, like all magic, that is likely to remain firmly in the world of fantasy.

References

1. Cohen J (2002) The immunopathogenesis of sepsis. Nature 420:885–891
2. Hotchkiss RS, Karl IE (2003) The pathophysiology and treatment of sepsis. N Engl J Med 348:138–150
3. Martin GS, Mannino DM, Eaton S, Moss M (2003) The epidemiology of sepsis in the United States from 1979 through 2000. N Engl J Med 348:1546–1554
4. Padkin A, Goldfrad C, Brady AR, et al (2003) Epidemiology of severe sepsis occurring in the first 24 hrs in intensive care units in England, Wales, and Northern Ireland. Crit Care Med 31:2332–2338
5. Vincent J-L (2003) Nosocomial infections in adult intensive-care units. Lancet 361:2068–2077
6. Calandra T, Cohen J (2005) The ISF consensus conference on definitions of infection on the intensive care unit. Crit Care Med 33:1538–1548
7. Garnacho-Montero J, Garcia-Garmendia JL, Barrero-Almodovar A, et al (2003) Impact of adequate empirical antibiotic therapy on the outcome of patients admitted to the intensive care unit with sepsis. Crit Care Med 31:2742–2751
8. Dellinger RP, Carlet J, Masur H, et al (2004) Surviving sepsis campaign guidelines for management of severe sepsis and septic shock. Intensive Care Med 30:536–555
9. Cohen J (2003) Recent develpoments in the identification of novel therapeutic targets for the treatment novel therapeutic targets for the treatment of patients with sepsis and septic shock. Scand J Infect Dis 35:690–696
10. Simon L, Gauvin F, Amre DK, et al (2004) Serum procalcitonin and C-reactive protein levels as markers of bacterial infection: a systematic review and meta-analysis. Clin Infect Dis 39:206–217
11. Golden SM, Stamilio DM, Faux BM, et al (2004) Evaluation of a real-time fluorescent PCR assay for rapid detection of Group B Streptococci in neonatal blood. Diagn Microbiol Infect Dis 50:7–13
12. Artz LA, Kempf VA, Autenrieth IB (2003) Rapid screening for Streptococcus agalactiae in vaginal specimens of pregnant women by fluorescent in situ hybridization. J Clin Microbiol 41:2170–2173
13. Marlowe EM, Hogan JJ, Hindler JF, et al (2003) Application of an rRNA probe matrix for rapid identification of bacteria and fungi from routine blood cultures. J Clin Microbiol 41:5127–5133
14. Worthington T, Lambert PA, Traube A, Elliott TS (2002) A rapid ELISA for the diagnosis of intravascular catheter related sepsis caused by coagulase negative staphylococci. J Clin Pathol 55:41–43
15. Rider TH, Petrovick MS, Nargi FE, et al (2003) A B cell-based sensor for rapid identification of pathogens. Science 301:213–215
16. Sivadon V, Rottman M, Quincampoix JC, et al (2004) Use of sodA sequencing for the identification of clinical isolates of coagulase-negative staphylococci. Clin Microbiol Infect 10:939–942
17. Johnsson D, Molling P, Stralin K, Soderquist B (2004) Detection of Panton-Valentine leukocidin gene in Staphylococcus aureus by LightCycler PCR: clinical and epidemiological aspects. Clin Microbiol Infect 10:884–889
18. Gillet Y, Issartel B, Vanhems P, et al (2002) Association between Staphylococcus aureus strains carrying gene for Panton-Valentine leukocidin and highly lethal necrotising pneumonia in young immunocompetent patients. Lancet 359:753–759
19. Hervás F (2004) Chip-mediated techniques: how close are we to generalised use in the infectious diseases clinic? Clin Microbiol Infect 10:865–867
20. Warren DK, Liao RS, Merz LR, et al (2004) Detection of methicillin-resistant Staphylococcus aureus directly from nasal swab specimens by a real-time PCR assay. J Clin Microbiol 42:5578–5581

21. Rolain JM, Mallet MN, Fournier PE, Raoult D (2004) Real-time PCR for universal antibiotic susceptibility testing. J Antimicrob Chemother 54:538–541
22. Pea F, Porreca L, Baraldo M, Furlanut M (2000) High vancomycin dosage regimens required by intensive care unit patients cotreated with drugs to improve haemodynamics following cardic surgical procedures. J Antimicrob Chemother 45:329–335
23. Reller LB (1986) The serum bactericidal test. Rev Infect Dis 8:803–808
24. Kaltsas P, Want S, Cohen J (2005) Development of a time to positivity assay as a tool in the antibiotic management of septic patients. Clin Microbiol Infect 11:109–114
25. Opal SM, Cohen J (1999) Are there fundamental differences of clinical relevance between Gram positive and Gram negative bacterial sepsis? Crit Care Med 27:1608–1616
26. Corona A, Wilson AP, Grassi M, Singer M (2004) Prospective audit of bacteraemia management in a university hospital ICU using a general strategy of short-course monotherapy. J Antimicrob Chemother 54:809–817
27. Gruson D, Hilbert G, Vargas F, et al (2003) Strategy of antibiotic rotation: long-term effect on incidence and susceptibilities of Gram-negative bacilli responsible for ventilator-associated pneumonia. Crit Care Med 31:1908–1914
28. Wallis RS, Broder MS, Wong JY, et al (2004) Granulomatous infectious diseases associated with tumor necrosis factor antagonists. Clin Infect Dis 38:1261–1265
29. Charles PG, Grayson ML (2004) The dearth of new antibiotic development: why we should be worried and what we can do about it. Med J Austr 181:549–553
30. Spellberg B, Powers JH, Brass EP, et al (2004) Trends in antimicrobial drug development: implications for the future. Clin Infect Dis 38:1279–1286

Immunological Monitoring, Functional Genomics and Proteomics

E. Abraham

Introduction

Outcome from critical illness is affected not only by the nature of the physiologic insult, such as the severity of multisystem trauma or the site and microbiology of infection, but also by the individual patient's response. While genetics is the fundamental underpinning that determines cellular activation and host mechanisms that are initiated by pathophysiologic events, such as sepsis, blood loss, or tissue injury, clearly such responses are also modulated by events distinct from genetic background. Such external factors include pharmacologic and other interventions, such as blood transfusion and even the mode of mechanical ventilation, utilized to treat the patient.

Monitoring cellular function and responses in the future will involve not only determination of parameters of intracellular activation, but also the expression of genes and proteins in response to critical illness and its treatment. Some techniques currently used, including enzyme-linked immunosorbent assay (ELISA), will permit rapid analysis of patterns of cellular activation in the future, allowing determination not only of cellular response to the factors initiating the intensive care unit (ICU) hospitalization, but also of how such cellular alterations change during the course of hospitalization, in response to therapeutic interventions or the progression of disease. While techniques that measure specific parameters of cellular function may be useful in monitoring a patient's condition, a more global determination can be achieved by assessing alterations in the expression of genes (genomics) and proteins (proteomics) among distinct cellular populations and relevant anatomic compartments. For example, knowing how neutrophils or macrophages increase or decrease the expression of groups of genes relating to apoptosis or inflammation, or monitoring the concentrations of large numbers of anti-apoptotic or pro-inflammatory proteins in plasma or bronchoalveolar lavage (BAL) fluid will permit assessment of host response to critical illness, and also will guide therapies to generate appropriate counter-regulatory events aimed at improving outcome in the critically ill patient.

Currently available gene arrays provide assessment of almost all of the human genome. Similarly, proteomic techniques permit measurement of alterations in thousands of proteins in serum, BAL fluid, cell extracts, or other relevant samples. While it would seem that the ability to determine alterations in such large numbers of genes and proteins would reduce the utility of measurement of specific steps in cellular activation or function, genomic and proteomic techniques remain qualitative and, for the foreseeable future, additional measures to assess quantitative changes in such parameters will continue to be required in monitoring ICU patients.

Because of the large numbers of genes and proteins that are involved in cellular alterations associated with critical illness, the goals for this chapter can only be to provide some insights into the techniques available, and their potential utility in monitoring patients at present and in the future. Examples of pathways and measurements will be presented, but by necessity these can only reflect what is known now. Where appropriate, though, estimates of future techniques for monitoring cellular activation parameters will be discussed.

Monitoring Immunologic Mediators in Blood and other Fluids

Cells can be activated through interaction with endogenously generated stimuli, such as reactive oxygen species, cytokines, and complement fragments, and by antigens that are not normally found in humans. Among this latter class are components of bacteria, viruses, protozoa, and fungi, such as lipopolysaccharide (LPS), flagellin, and hemagglutins. Interaction of endogenous or exogenous mediators with membrane based receptors initiates a cascade of intracellular signaling events, primarily involving the phosphorylation and activation of kinases that leads to assembly of the transcriptional apparatus on the promoter regions of genes, followed by expression of the genes and their encoded proteins. Reactive oxygen and nitrogen species are able to cross the cell membrane in a rapid fashion and also can lead to activation of similar intracellular signaling pathways, but without interaction with receptors.

Regulation of cellular activation can occur at multiple steps, starting with generation of the mediators that initially interact with receptors or initiate discrete intracellular signaling events through receptor independent mechanisms, and concluding with the actual production and secretion of proteins. Monitoring each of these stages in cellular activation is becoming increasingly available at present, but often these techniques are only available in research laboratories, and cannot be performed with the rapidity necessary for use in clinical settings. However, improved technology is to be expected over the next 10 years, allowing these measurements to be used in the assessment and management of ICU patients.

Techniques presently available to measure concentrations of immunomodulatory substances, including cytokines and bacterial products, in blood, urine, BAL fluid, and other fluids include quantitative Western blotting, ELISA, chemoluminescent assays using cell populations, cytometric bead arrays, and flow cytometry based assays. Classic methodologies, such as Western blotting and ELISA, are slow, taking hours or even days to yield results. Newer methods, such as flow cytometry or cytometric bead assays in whole blood, can produce results in less than an hour. Techniques using calibrated sensors presently provide continuous, real time measurements at the bedside for electrolytes and other routine clinical variables. Adaptation of such probes to provide similar continuous readouts of circulating mediators, such as cytokines, is technologically feasible and will be available by 2015.

A major impediment to determining concentrations of multiple circulating mediators has been the volume of sample required for ELISA or other presently available techniques. For example, volumes of 100–200 µl are classically required for ELISA. Recent advances using cytometric bead assays or flow cytometry allow the measurement of as many as 20 cytokines in much smaller volumes, such as 100 µl. Such techniques provide rapid turnaround time for samples, and will permit panels of cytokines and other mediators, associated with outcome and response to therapy in critical illness, to be determined with sufficiently small volumes of blood or other relevant fluid samples so that analyses can be performed frequently enough, e.g., 3–6 times per day, to assess response of such measures to therapy.

Although presently used techniques to measure cytokines and other circulating inflammatory mediators often take hours, or even longer, to yield results, the number of parameters that can be measured continues to increase. At least 31 cytokines have been identified. Leukotrienes, complement fragments, circulating cytokine and other receptors, anti- and pro-apoptotic proteins, as well as other factors that participate in immune regulation have been characterized and shown to be present in abnormal concentrations in critically ill patients. The technical ability to measure multiple parameters in the future will be of little use clinically unless we have a better understanding of the relative importance of such measurements. Therefore, an important question is how to identify which of these mediators are important to measure and actually play a pathologic role in critically ill patients or are of use as prognostic markers. In addition, an important advance for the future will be in using multivariate analyses to define the importance of changes in panels of mediators. Rather than the clinician making decisions based on a limited number of parameters, as done at present, confirmatory results using determinations of multiple measures will permit a better understanding of each patient's pathophysiologic state and will enable more precise tailoring of therapies.

Monitoring Parameters of Cellular Activation

Assessment of activation of intracellular signaling pathways, involving kinases and transcriptional factors, has classically been time consuming, using Western blots and electrophoretic mobility shift assays (EMSA), to determine levels of the active, phosphorylated form of kinases or of nuclear concentrations of transcriptional factors, such as nuclear factor-kappa B (NF-κB) [1–4] Determination of actual kinase activity is cumbersome, and involves immunoprecipitation of kinases and then use of radiolabeled substrate in the measurement of the ability of the precipitated kinase to phosphorylated a relevant substrate. Recent advances have generated ELISA kits that directly measure amounts of phosphorylated kinases or transcriptional factors in whole cell or nuclear extracts. In addition, there are now a number of flow cytometry based assays that permit rapid measurement of nuclear concentrations of transcriptional factors, such as NF-κB. It is reasonable to envisage further development of techniques to measure the activation states of multiple kinases and transcriptional factors.

At present, there is only limited evidence linking kinase and transcriptional factor activation to outcome in critically ill patients. Several studies have shown that increased nuclear concentrations of NF-κB in neutrophils or peripheral blood mononuclear cells in patients with sepsis or acute lung injury (ALI) are associated with a worse clinical outcome [5–9]. Similar findings for the kinases p38 and Akt indicate that greater activation of these signaling molecules correlates with prolonged time on the ventilator or mortality [5, 8, 10]. Initial studies also indicate that patients whose neutrophils demonstrate no activation of NF-κB or Akt in response to culture with LPS, have a better clinical outcome than those who show further activation after *in vitro* stimulation [8]. Such results suggest that underlying stable cellular phenotypes may exist and determine the course in critical illness. In particular, these findings indicate that individuals whose neutrophils respond poorly to relevant stimuli, such as bacterial products, are less likely to have dysregulated, overly exuberant inflammatory responses that lead to ALI and other organ dysfunctions when they become infected. In contrast, individuals with more reactive neutrophils tend to have severe clinical courses, associated with increased morbidity and mortality, when infected or when exposed to other relevant pathophysiologic conditions, such as severe multi-system trauma.

The ability to assess multiple parameters relating to cellular activation will not only permit identification of patients at increased risk for poor outcome, but also will be highly useful for guiding therapy. For example, increased activation of the kinase, Akt, not only predicts a worse clinical outcome, but also appears to participate in modulating pathogenic downstream events, such as enhanced transcription of NF-κB-dependent pro-inflammatory genes [5, 8, 11–18]. In part, this action of Akt is due to its ability to enhance phosphorylation of the p65 subunit of NF-κB, an event known to be important in maximizing the transcriptional activity of NF-κB. Rapid assessment of Akt phosphorylation, as well as downstream events known to be affected by Akt, including phosphorylation of the p65 NF-κB subunit, therefore could be used to identify high risk patients who would benefit from therapies specifically aimed at inhibiting Akt.

Improvements in diagnostic tests that enable rapid assessment of the activation status of intracellular signaling pathways will be highly useful not only for determining therapies for critically ill patients, but also for designing interventional studies in such patients. At present, many therapeutic interventions, such as the use of recombinant human activated protein C, are utilized based on clinical or physiologic parameters, such as APACHE II scores [19, 20]. Future therapies, aimed at specific steps in cellular activation, can be chosen based on whether the intracellular pathway of interest is actually altered, using direct assessment of relevant cellular parameters. For example, consider a trial testing an inhibitor of NF-κB. In such a trial, it will be valuable to treat only those patients who actually show evidence of increased activation of NF-κB. Including patients selected by less direct measures, who may not actually have the desired level of activation of NF-κB, could dilute out any potential therapeutic effect of such an inhibitor, because these patients do not have the appropriate cellular abnormality.

In addition to technical issues that limit the turnaround time for assays of intracellular signaling events, access to and isolation of relevant cell populations also is a problem with such assays at present. For example, isolation of neutrophils from peripheral blood requires sedimentation or centrifugation in isolation media while purification of alveolar macrophages necessitates adhesion to plastic cultureware surfaces. Other cell populations of interest, such as cells from the liver or kidney, are not obtainable in patients without invasive surgical procedures. New radiologic techniques that permit non-invasive labeling and imaging of intracellular events in specific cell populations are presently available in experimental settings and can be expected to move to the clinical arena in the next 10 years. For example, metabolic parameters relating to intracellular kinase activation in alveolar macrophages have been determined using positron emission tomography (PET) in experimental models of endotoxin- and infection-induced pulmonary inflammation [21–23]. While such methodologies cannot be expected to provide assessment of a large number of intracellular parameters, they still should be highly useful in defining cellular abnormalities that can be addressed by application of specific therapies.

Functional Genomics

Gene arrays with the most recently produced chips permit determination of upregulation and downregulation of genes that encompass almost the entire human genome (Fig. 1). Present arrays permit assessment of more than 12,000 genes [24–26]. The technique, while powerful because of its ability to provide insights into alterations in large numbers of genes, is also limited in the clinical evaluation of critically ill patients for a number of reasons. Cell populations of interest need to be isolated by techniques that often involve collection of blood or biopsy samples and then purification of cellular populations. After the cellular populations of interest are collected, RNA from the cells must be purified and then applied to the chips. Actual performance of gene arrays, with appropriate controls, requires several hours by highly skilled personnel, followed by an intensive analytic period, using univariate and multivariate permutation software. The results generated are primarily qualitative in nature, and major findings usually need to be verified with quantitative polymerase chain reaction (PCR).

Recent studies with gene arrays have focused on patterns of gene expression that differ in critically ill patients with sepsis, trauma, or ALI [24, 27–31]. Such studies have shown parallel alterations in multiple genes involved in specific cellular functions, such as apoptosis, differentiation, or inflammation. In large part, these initial studies have produced results that are consistent with those found when multiple mediators are measured with ELISA or PCR techniques.

There are two areas in which gene arrays may provide powerful insights into pathophysiologic mechanisms involved in critical illness. First, because of the information that this technique yields concerning alterations involving large numbers of genes, it can generate more extensive insights into abnormalities in cellular functions than do assays that measure multiple discrete measures of cellular activation. Patterns in gene arrays can therefore provide important confirmatory information about prognosis, and also about cellular pathways that may be involved in critical illness. A second important function of arrays is in providing novel insights into genes that may be involved in pathophysiologic processes, but whose participation was not previously recognized. This 'discovery' potential of gene arrays is a powerful technique for identifying potential new targets for drug discovery and intervention in critically ill patients.

An example of the power of gene arrays in showing novel pathways for cellular activation was shown in experiments where human neutrophils were stimulated with either LPS or the novel proinflammatory mediator, high mobility group box protein 1 (HMGB1) [32]. In these studies, the patterns of genes whose expression was altered after exposure of neutrophils to HMGB1 was different from that seen after LPS stimulation (Fig. 2). Such experiments indicated that

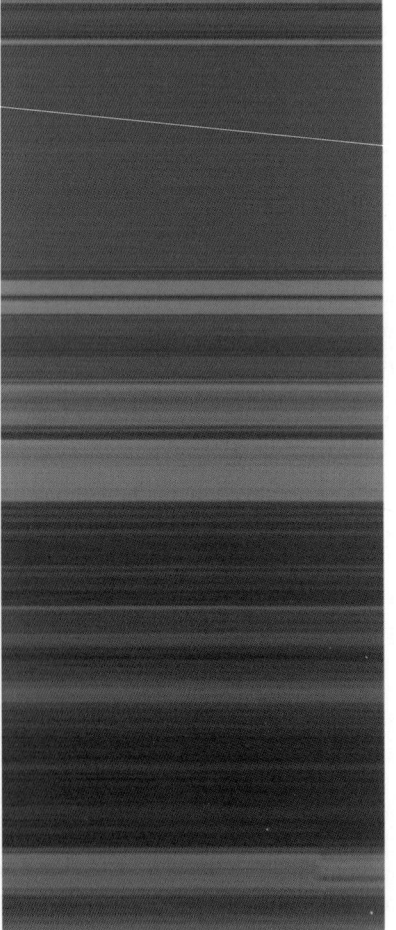

Fig. 1. Gene expression patterns among 12,626 human genes examined. Genes upregulated above control levels are shown in light gray, with greater fold increases as brighter lines. Dark gray represents no change from baseline levels of expression.

cellular activation induced by exposure to HMGB1 was different from that produced by LPS. As LPS is known to interact with the Toll-like receptor 4 (TLR4), these studies suggested that HMGB1 utilized receptors other than TLR4 or, if TLR4 was the primary HMGB1 receptor, then the pathways for cellular activation through TLR4 were different from those activated by LPS. Subsequent experiments showed that although TLR4 was involved in HMGB1 signaling, TLR2 and the receptor for advanced glycation endproducts (RAGE) also could interact with HMGB1 and lead to cellular activation [33].

In critically ill patients, gene arrays using peripheral blood mononuclear cells or neutrophils have shown patterns of alterations that correlate with outcome. For example, in recent studies from our laboratory, neutrophils from BAL fluid obtained from healthy volunteers exposed to pulmonary endotoxin showed different patterns of gene expression compared to peripheral blood neutrophils obtained at the same time. Subsequent analyses demonstrated that patients with

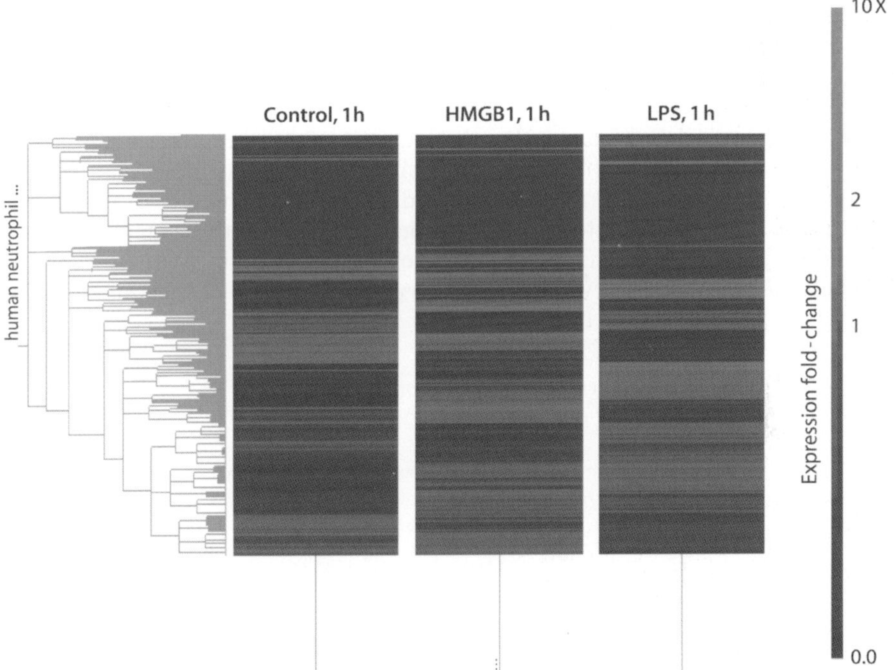

Fig. 2. Hierarchical cluster images showing gene expression patterns among 12,626 human genes examined (using Affymetrix GeneChip Human Genome U95AV2 arrays) after culture of human neutrophils with high mobility group box 1 (HMGB1) protein or lipopolysaccharide (LPS) for 1 hour. Genes that showed >2-fold changes in control vs. HMGB1 or control vs. LPS were subjected to clustering analysis (Gene Spring 4.07 program; Silicon Genetics, Redwood City, CA) The fold changes were based on comparison with internal standards, including β-actin. Each sample was loaded on separate chips and was run separately with its own control. Upregulated genes are shown in light gray, with greater fold increases being presented as brighter lines. From [32] with permission

more severe clinical outcome from ALI had circulating neutrophils whose patterns of gene expression more closely resembled those of lung neutrophils from the endotoxin exposed volunteers than the expression profiles found in peripheral blood neutrophils from healthy individuals.

Proteomics

Standard methodology for identifying alterations in protein expression in critical illnesses has utilized ELISA or Western blotting, but these techniques are time consuming and can only be used for the analysis of a very limited number of proteins. Recently, improvements in protein separation techniques, using two-dimensional electrophoresis (2-DE), combined with methodology that permits identification of proteins using matrix-assisted laser desorption/ionization time-of-flight mass spectrometry (MALDI-TOF MS) have made possible the determination of alterations in multiple proteins [34–36]. These proteomics techniques have been used to phenotype lung cancers, as well as alterations in protein patterns in BAL fluid from smokers, and patients with pulmonary disorders, including cystic fibrosis and ALI [35]. Table 1 shows a comparison of the different techniques.

Using a spot, isolated from a 2D gel, MALDI-TOF MS generates a pattern of proteins, characterized by peaks and intensities with precise molecular weight. In this technique, the spot must be excised, then proteolytically digested, extracted and then loaded onto a MALDI target plate. All of these steps are time consuming, and labor intensive. Protein profiles generated by MALDI-TOF can then be analyzed using software that performs hierarchical clustering analysis,

Table 1. Comparison of different techniques for protein analysis

	ELISA	2DE	MALDI-TOF	Photoaptamers
Sensitivity	high	low	medium	medium/high
Direct identification of markers	N/A	Yes	No	Yes
Detects unknown biomarkers	No	Yes	Yes	No
Throughput	medium	Very Low	High	High
Advantages/ disadvantages	Well described, difficult to develop	Well described, good for post-translational modifications, very labor intensive, additional steps for protein identification	Can be automated, additional steps for protein identification	Flexible format, limited number of analytes

similar to that used for gene arrays. A disadvantage is that the identities of the biomarkers are not immediately known. To address this problem, photoaptamer arrays have been developed. Photoaptamers are synthetic molecules of DNA that selectively bind to proteins and are capable of identifying specific proteins. While photoaptamers are presently available for only a limited number of proteins, their numbers are likely to expand hugely over the next several years, allowing rapid characterization of specific proteins and their alterations in plasma, BAL fluid, and other samples.

A new technique uses surface enhanced laser desorption/ionization time-of-flight mass spectrometry (SELDI-TOF) and permits high throughput to identify protein biomarkers in plasma, BAL fluid, and other fluids. An additional chromatographic technique that reduces sample time preparation and permits quantitative proteomics is isotype ratio mass spectrometry (IRMS). At the present time, the most advanced IRMS technique is the isotope-coded affinity tagging (ICAT) technology, which relies on differential labeling of reduced cysteine residues of proteins. ICAT has important limitations, since only cysteine-containing peptides are labeled [37, 38]. It is expected that methods for quantitative proteomics that have greater generalizability than ICAT will become available in the future and also that their utility will move from the research laboratory to become more directly applicable to assessment of alterations in critically ill patients.

Similar to genomics, there are issues with proteomics that hinder analysis at present, but are likely to be addressed in the future. Among the major concerns is the variability of results generated with present techniques. Multiple factors have an impact on the quality of proteomic data, including sample preparation and handling, instrument variability, and consistency of algorithms used for data analysis. An additional concern is the identification of proteins present in very low concentrations.

In recent studies, 2DE and two-dimensional differential gel electrophoresis (DIGE) were used to study patients with ALI [34]. More than 300 distinct protein spots were visualized in BAL fluid from normal subjects and ALI patients. Using MALDI-TOF MS, 158 of these spots could be identified. There were multiple qualitative changes in the BAL fluid of patients with ALI. Among these differences were the presence of seven distinct surfactant protein A isoforms in normal volunteers, but the presence of such isoforms in only one of the ALI patients. Another difference was the presence of α_1-antitrypsin in the BAL fluid of all normal subjects, but in only half of the ALI patients. There were also a number of proteins, such as haptoglobulin, that were present in truncated forms in BAL fluid from patients with ALI, unlike their status in BAL fluid from normal volunteers. Most of the BAL fluid proteins identified in ALI patients were plasma proteins, consistent with enhanced capillary, endothelial, and epithelial permeability being present in ALI. However, the modification of proteins in BAL fluid indicates that degradation appears to occur after transudation of plasma proteins into the airspace.

Such results indicate that proteomics may be useful not only in identifying differences in the concentrations of proteins in plasma, BAL fluid, and other samples from critically ill patients, but may also demonstrate alterations in proteins that were not previously appreciated. Proteomics is also able to identify concentrations of proteins that are phosphorylated or otherwise modified through the effects of kinases or other intracellular signaling mechanisms. Identification of alterations in the concentrations of proteins or in the configuration of proteins associated with critical illness is likely to be highly useful in predicting outcome for patients with ALI, sepsis, and other critical illnesses. In addition, proteomics techniques are likely to reveal alterations in important cellular pathways that contribute to the pathogenesis of organ dysfunction and mortality in these settings.

Like genomics, proteomics promises to allow identification at risk for poor outcomes in critical illness and can be used to titrate specific therapies in such patients. A benefit for proteomics is that one is measuring actual protein levels, rather than gene expression, as is the case with genomics. Because post-transcriptional events modulate protein generation, there are often differences found between alterations in mRNA levels detected by gene arrays or quantitative PCR and actual protein expression. For this reason, proteomics may provide a more useful technique for monitoring cellular alterations present in critical illness. Despite the advances in proteomics that have been made in recent years, future use of this technique in critical care will depend on further development of techniques with short turn-around times that can identify and quantify a more complete range of proteins in biologic fluids and that also can be widely used in clinical laboratories.

Conclusion

While techniques allowing evaluation of a limited number of biomarkers, such as cytokines, have generated insights into the pathophysiology of critical illness, new techniques, including genomics and proteomics, that permit the analysis of large numbers of genes or proteins promise to provide increasingly sophisticated information useful in outcome prediction as well as in choosing therapies for critically ill patients. Coupled with greater understanding of the intracellular pathways that are affected in critical illness, genomics and proteomics will not only allow early identification of patients who are at risk for a more severe clinical course, but will also permit institution of appropriate therapies before organ system dysfunction develops. Such methodologies are presently limited by the complexity of sample preparation and analysis. A major issue with the huge amount of information generated by these techniques will be to develop informatics systems that will permit appropriate clinical decision-making. However, future developments should permit genomics and proteomics to enter into the routine diagnostic evaluation and therapeutic monitoring of ICU patients.

References

1. Abraham E (2000) NF-κB activation. Crit Care Med 28: N100–104
2. Christman JW, Lancaster LH, Blackwell TS (1998) Nuclear factor kappa B: a pivotal role in the systemic inflammatory response syndrome and new target for therapy. Intensive Care Med 24:1131–1138
3. Christman JW, Sadikot RT, Blackwell TS (2000) The role of nuclear factor- B in pulmonary diseases. Chest 117:1482–1487
4. Fan J, Ye RD, Malik AB (2001) Transcriptional mechanisms of acute lung injury. Am J Physiol Lung Cell Mol Physiol 281:L1037–1050
5. Abraham E (2003) Nuclear factor-κB and its role in sepsis-associated organ failure. J Infect Dis 187 (Suppl 2):S364–369
6. Arnalich F, Garcia-Palomero E, Lopez J, et al (2000) Predictive value of nuclear factor κB activity and plasma cytokine levels in patients with sepsis. Infect Immun 68:1942–1945
7. Bohrer H, Qiu F, Zimmermann T, et al (1997) Role of NFκB in the mortality of sepsis. J Clin Invest 100:972–985
8. Yang KY, Arcaroli JJ, Abraham E (2003) Early alterations in neutrophil activation are associated with outcome in acute lung injury. Am J Respir Crit Care Med 167:1567–1574
9. Adib-Conquy M, Adrie C, Moine P, et al (2000) NF-κB expression in mononuclear cells of patients with sepsis resembles that observed in lipopolysaccharide tolerance. Am J Respir Crit Care Med 162:1877-1883
10. Rosengart MR, Nathens AB, Arbabi S, et al (2003) Mitogen-activated protein kinases in the intensive care unit: prognostic potential. Ann Surg 237:94–100
11. Abraham E (2003) Neutrophils and acute lung injury. Crit Care Med 31:S195–199
12. Ardeshna KM, Pizzey AR, Devereux S, Khwaja A (2000) The PI3 kinase, p38 SAP kinase, and NF-kappaB signal transduction pathways are involved in the survival and maturation of lipopolysaccharide-stimulated human monocyte-derived dendritic cells. Blood 96:1039–1046
13. Beraud C, Henzel WJ, Baeuerle PA (1999) Involvement of regulatory and catalytic subunits of phosphoinositide 3-kinase in NF-κB activation. Proc Natl Acad Sci U S A 96:429–434
14. Kane LP, Shapiro VS, Stokoe D, Weiss A (1999) Induction of NF-κB by the Akt/PKB kinase. Curr Biol 9:601–604
15. Madrid LV, Mayo MW, Reuther JY, Baldwin AS Jr (2001) Akt stimulates the transactivation potential of the RelA/p65 subunit of NF-κB through utilization of the Ikappa B kinase and activation of the mitogen-activated protein kinase p38. J Biol Chem 276:18934-18940
16. Ozes ON, Mayo LD, Gustin JA, et al (1999) NF-κB activation by tumour necrosis factor requires the Akt serine-threonine kinase. Nature 401:82–85
17. Strassheim D, Asehnoune K, Park JS, et al (2004) Phosphoinositide 3-kinase and Akt occupy central roles in inflammatory responses of Toll-like receptor 2-stimulated neutrophils. J Immunol 172:5727–5733
18. Yum HK, Arcaroli J, Kupfner J, et al (2001) Involvement of phosphoinositide 3-kinases in neutrophil activation and the development of acute lung injury. J Immunol 167:6601–6608
19. Bernard GR, Vincent JL, Laterre PF, et al (2001) Efficacy and safety of recombinant human activated protein C for severe sepsis. N Engl J Med 344:699–709
20. Ely EW, Laterre PF, Angus DC, et al (2003) Drotrecogin alfa (activated) administration across clinically important subgroups of patients with severe sepsis. Crit Care Med 31:12–19
21. Chen DL, Mintun MA, Schuster DP (2004) Comparison of methods to quantitate 18F-FDG uptake with PET during experimental acute lung injury. J Nucl Med 45:1583–1590
22. Richard JC, Zhou Z, Chen DL, et al (2004) Quantitation of pulmonary transgene expression with PET imaging. J Nucl Med 45:644–654

23. Richard JC, Zhou Z, Ponde DE, et al (2003) Imaging pulmonary gene expression with positron emission tomography. Am J Respir Crit Care Med 167:1257–1263
24. Cobb JP, Laramie JM, Stormo GD, et al (2002) Sepsis gene expression profiling: murine splenic compared with hepatic responses determined by using complementary DNA microarrays. Crit Care Med 30:2711–2721
25. Fessler MB, Malcolm KC, Duncan MW, Worthen GS (2002) Lipopolysaccharide stimulation of the human neutrophil: an analysis of changes in gene transcription and protein expression by oligonucleotide microarrays and proteomics. Chest 121:75S–76S
26. Pombo A (2003) Cellular genomics: which genes are transcribed, when and where? Trends Biochem Sci 28:6–9
27. Cariou A, Chiche JD, Charpentier J, et al (2002) The era of genomics: impact on sepsis clinical trial design. Crit Care Med 30:S341–348
28. Chung TP, Laramie JM, Province M, Cobb JP (2002) Functional genomics of critical illness and injury. Crit Care Med 30:S51–57
29. Cobb JP, O'Keefe GE (2004) Injury research in the genomic era. Lancet 363:2076–2083
30. Feezor RJ, Moldawer LL (2003) Genetic polymorphisms, functional genomics and the host inflammatory response to injury and inflammation. Nestle Nutr Workshop Ser Clin Perform Programme 8:15–32
31. Leikauf GD, McDowell SA, Bachurski CJ, et al (2001) Functional genomics of oxidant-induced lung injury. Adv Exp Med Biol 500:479–487
32. Park JS, Arcaroli J, Yum HK, et al (2003) Activation of gene expression in human neutrophils by high mobility group box 1 protein. Am J Physiol Cell Physiol 284:C870–C879
33. Park JS, Svetkauskaite D, He Q, et al (2004) Involvement of Toll-like receptors 2 and 4 in cellular activation by High Mobility Group Box 1 protein. J Biol Chem 279:7370–7377
34. Bowler RP, Duda B, Chan ED, et al (2004) Proteomic analysis of pulmonary edema fluid and plasma in patients with acute lung injury. Am J Physiol Lung Cell Mol Physiol 286: L1095–1104
35. Hirsch J, Hansen KC, Burlingame AL, Matthay MA (2004) Proteomics: current techniques and potential applications to lung disease. Am J Physiol Lung Cell Mol Physiol 287:L1-23
36. Liu XW, Lu FG, Zhang GS, et al (2004) Proteomics to display tissue repair opposing injury response to LPS-induced liver injury. World J Gastroenterol 10:2701–2705
37. Griffin TJ, Han DK, Gygi SP, et al (2001) Toward a high-throughput approach to quantitative proteomic analysis: expression-dependent protein identification by mass spectrometry. J Am Soc Mass Spectrom 12:1238–1246
38. Gygi SP, Rist B, Gerber SA, et al (1999) Quantitative analysis of complex protein mixtures using isotope-coded affinity tags. Nat Biotechnol 17:994–999

Improving Organ Function

M. Singer

Introduction

Our vastly improved ability to support failed organs over the past three decades should be balanced by the stark realization that outcomes have not improved commensurately. For example, crude mortality rates from infectious diseases in the United States have not altered since before the inception of intensive care [1] Clearly, there has been a significant change in case-mix that can be used in part-mitigation. Many patients being routinely admitted and aggressively treated in intensive care units (ICUs) in 2005 would not have been contemplated for such a degree of intervention twenty years previously. Advanced age, severe immuno-suppression and a poor underlying prognosis are no longer absolute contraindications to ICU admission. Provision of intensive care is steadily increasing worldwide and there is no political will at present to curb this growing demand. Current growth rates in the requirement for intensive care, compounded in many cases by the ability to prolong death for weeks if not months, and a finite staff resource with the appropriate level of expertise, requires us to re-evaluate current management practices to improve both our quality of care and our efficiency.

A minority of ICU patients consumes approximately half the total resource in terms of bed days [2]. The relatively short-lived acute inflammatory phase of multi-organ dysfunction is often followed by a prolonged period of established organ failure with a continued need for mechanical and/or drug support, close monitoring and nursing care. These periods are punctuated by further bouts of infection plus other causes of inflammation and cardio-respiratory instability. These downturns serve to prolong the organ dysfunction still further, and/or provide the excuse for withholding or withdrawing life-sustaining treatments.

Advances in pharmacological treatments are heavily trumpeted but, in real terms, have limited impact. For example, use of activated protein C in the UK is currently limited to approximately 2-3% of total ICU admissions. Given a number-needed-to-treat of 10 to save a life of the more severe septic patient cohort (i.e., APACHE II >24), few additional survivors will emerge as a consequence. Clearly, there could be an advantage to the individual patient from such a treatment, yet major reductions in overall ICU mortality will only be seen with generic treatments that are applicable across a significant proportion of the ICU population.

It could be reasonably argued that the recent large multicenter studies showing the biggest overall improvement to a general ICU cohort are those involving reduced intervention, such as a lower hemoglobin threshold for blood transfusion [3] or reduced tidal volumes [4]. This signals an important point that will be expanded further in this chapter, namely an increased recognition of the potential harm we are inflicting on our patients by current 'established' therapies. I would extend this beyond mechanical ventilation and blood to encompass sedation, antibiotics, nutrition, inotropes and antipyretics as but five common examples.

This chapter will be structured into four components and I will unashamedly adopt a philosophical slant. First, I will briefly address the simple but crucial question as to what process exists whereby systemic inflammation leads to multi-organ failure (MOF)? This is a fundamental point that we have failed to properly consider over several decades. Indeed, many of the assumptions currently harbored are not borne out by the existing literature. Improved understanding of these 'organ failure' inducing pathways will clearly lead to more appropriate treatments, both in terms of timing and mechanism of action. Second, I will suggest that MOF may actually be misunderstood and could well represent a last-ditch adaptive response by which the organs retain the potential to recover normal functioning after passage of the acute systemic inflammatory insult [5]. Third, I will address the possibility that many of our current therapies may contribute to the development and/or delayed resolution of organ dysfunction. Last, I will attempt to predict how organ dysfunction will be managed 10 years from now, and this will encompass the first three points.

How Does Systemic Inflammation Lead to Multi-Organ Failure?

An acute insult such as infection, trauma or hemorrhage can provoke an acute, exaggerated systemic inflammatory response. Clearly, there are genetic, exogenous and other endogenous factors that determine why some individuals are affected more than others, and why different various combinations of organ dysfunction occur. Our current knowledge base does not as yet permit identification of high-risk individuals other than the recognition that patients with chronic organ disease are, in general, more susceptible.

The excess production of inflammatory mediators leads to activation of multiple systems within the body, including immune, coagulation, hormonal, metabolic and bioenergetic pathways. The circulation is affected early on, both at the macro- and microcirculatory level. Myocardial depression, endothelial activation, increased capillary leak, intravascular coagulation, adherent neutrophils and generalized loss of vascular tone are well-established phenomena. However, these standard textbook descriptions belie certain facts, particularly in the human being as opposed to the short-term, aggressive and often lethal animal models upon which much of our knowledge of pathophysiology is based. For example, acute tubular necrosis is a misnomer as the failed kidney in MOF usually looks remarkably normal; disseminated intravascular coagulation (DIC) – particularly apparent with meningococcal sepsis – is a predominantly dermal phenomenon with deeper organs essentially unaffected; lactic acidosis in sepsis is not generally an ischemic phenomenon; while the overall loss of vascular tone camouflages multiple areas of microvascular vasoconstriction within different organs.

Microvascular disruption has been elegantly demonstrated in sepsis, the degree of which has been associated with subsequent mortality [6]. However, the traditional concept of a disrupted microvasculature leading to tissue hypoxia, widespread cell death and organ dysfunction/failure is undermined and contradicted by a number of reproducible findings in both patients and animal models. First, tissue oxygen tensions are raised in established sepsis-induced organ failure, and this has been demonstrated in organs as varied as skeletal muscle, gut and bladder [7–9]. Second, these failed organs look remarkably normal despite severe functional and biochemical abnormality [10, 11]. Hotchkiss et al. [10] sampled multiple tissue biopsies soon after death in patients with MOF, specifically seeking evidence of necrosis and/or apoptosis. Apart from a small degree of apoptosis found in spleen, gut epithelium, and lymphocytes, they highlighted the relative normality and remarkable lack of cell death in organs that may have been totally dysfunctional pre-mortem. Third, recovery of organ function occurs within days to weeks, well beyond the regenerative capacity of many of these tissues.

A new paradigm of organ failure must therefore be developed which encompasses microvascular disruption though necessarily excludes large-scale cell death as a direct cause of organ dysfunction. We, and others, have demonstrated mitochondrial dysfunction in multiple organs in both patients and laboratory models [11, 12]. The rate of onset appears to be dictated by the severity of insult as contradictory results have been reported in short-term studies. However, all models lasting in excess of 16 hours uniformly show ultrastructural damage and/or biochemical dysfunction manifest as decreased respiratory enzyme activity or ATP levels [13]. Similar findings have been made in muscle biopsies taken from patients in septic shock [12]. Of note, patients undergoing tight glycemic control showed preservation of hepatic mitochondrial ultrastructure and function, in marked contradistinction to patients conventionally managed in terms of blood sugar control [14].

The presence of mitochondrial dysfunction implies a decrease in energy production. In health, glycolytic generation of ATP accounts for <5% of total energy production with the remainder arising from mitochondrial respiration. In disease states such as heart failure where oxygen supply is limited, the glycolytic contribution will increase though only by a relatively small amount. It is thus reasonable to assume that ATP production is compromised. The corollary of this reduction in energy availability is a direct down-regulatory effect on metabolism. As a consequence, the various physiological and biochemical processes of the cell become compromised. If severe enough, this will lead to clinically manifest organ dysfunction and failure.

At present, the link between mitochondrial dysfunction and organ failure is only by association. Direct causation has yet to be established. There appears to be a parallel deterioration during the onset of critical illness and a concurrent improvement seen on disease resolution. There is also good direct and circumstantial evidence to suggest plausible mechanisms for mitochondrial dysfunction. First, excess production of nitrogen and oxygen reactive species will directly inhibit mitochondrial activity [15] and sepsis is the condition *par excellence* associated with increased whole body generation of nitric oxide (NO). Second, mitochondria are under direct hormonal regulatory control. Many of the effects of the thyroid hormones, for instance, are mediated through changes in mitochondrial activity. In prolonged sepsis, down-regulation in endocrine activity is well recognized, for example, relative adrenal deficiency, hypoleptinemia and the low T3 syndrome [16–18]. It is thus reasonable to assume that this downturn may impact upon energy production in prolonged sepsis. Third, the microvascular disturbance seen particularly in early, unresuscitated sepsis will also influence cellular oxygen availability and thus mitochondrial respiration. In contrast to cardiac arrest, the reduction in oxygen transport will not be so massive or abrupt with sepsis or other inflammatory insults. The cells thus have some time to adapt to hypoxia induced by hypovolemia, hypoxemia, microvascular flow redistribution, increased capillary leak and myocardial depression. This includes an augmented production of reactive oxygen and nitrogen species and cytokine production. Thus, tissue hypoxia has an amplifying effect on the initiating inflammatory insult.

This synergism between inflammation and tissue hypoxia could reasonably explain the improved outcome shown by the early goal-directed therapy approach reported by Rivers et al. [19], and the failure of a similar approach in patients with established MOF [20, 21]. The persistence of an abnormal microvasculature in prolonged sepsis could arguably be a reactive phenomenon. The decrease in cellular metabolism will reduce oxygen requirements; the tissue PO_2 is thus high so there is little need for the microcirculation to deliver unnecessary oxygen.

Could 'Multi-Organ Failure' Represent a Last-Ditch Adaptive Response?

If the cell continues to function normally in the face of mitochondrial dysfunction, ATP stores would be rapidly depleted. Below a certain threshold this is a recognized trigger for stimulating necrotic or apoptotic death pathways. The failure of this to occur suggests a reduction in energy-consuming cellular processes that preserve the ATP supply-demand balance, thereby maintaining the ATP level. Indeed, we reported this finding in muscle biopsies taken from patients in septic shock who subsequently survived [12], and have recently reported similar findings in muscle and liver in a long-term rodent model of fecal peritonitis [11]. This is analogous to the hibernation occurring with prolonged myocardial ischemia, and the numerous correlates seen in nature including cold weather hibernation, hot weather estivation and bacterial dormancy.

This suggests the fascinating concept that MOF may actually be a good thing [5]! If the patient is able to withstand the acute inflammatory insult, it would indeed be a Pyrrhic victory if the organs failed to recover and he/she died as a result. Yet we recognize that organs that were normal before the initiating inflammatory event, and were not irreparably harmed by the insult itself, will usually regain normal functioning unless iatrogenic complications ensue. A large Scottish audit of patients with previously normal renal function who survived their critical illness yet required acute renal replacement therapy revealed that only 1.5% required long-term dialysis [22].

It may be pertinent to consider MOF as a three-phase process with multiple interactions between inflammatory, immune, hormonal, bioenergetic, metabolic, and other pathways. Initially, the organism will meet an acute inflammatory insult 'head-on'. This 'acute phase response' is well-recognized with an increase in pro-inflammatory mediators, immune stimulation, stress hormones, mitochondrial and metabolic activity all individually reported. The temporal relationship between these different pathways still needs to be established. A proportion of patients will die in this phase due to the consequences of overwhelming inflammation. The majority of deaths, however, occur in the subsequent downturn phase. In the face of a prolonged and severe inflammatory insult there is reduced activity in all of the above pathways with immune paresis [23], endocrine downregulation [24], metabolic suppression [25], and the bioenergetic shutdown described previously. The patient is thus more susceptible to secondary bouts of infection and inflammation, and perhaps less well able to respond. The final phase represents recovery, with restoration of organ function, an increase in energy expenditure and a general anabolic state with enhanced protein synthesis.

The Covert Harm from Established Therapies

We blithely assume that our current therapies and management strategies confer benefit, otherwise we would not be using them. Unfortunately, the evidence base for much of what we do in intensive care is rather paltry. More than half the recommendations within the Surviving Sepsis Campaign guidelines [26] were graded 'E', i.e., only supported by anecdote, uncontrolled or historically controlled case series and studies, and expert opinion. Many of the original papers upon which the recommendations were based are also of dubious merit. Thus, it is highly likely that practice in the future will differ considerably from contemporary practice. In much the same way that we scoff at what we were doing way back in 1995 (Table 1), we are likely to be denigrating many of our current ideas in the future – and rightly so.

We are increasingly recognizing that 'less is best'. Most of the major advances in recent years have arisen from this concept. The Canadian multicenter triallists showed how a transfusion trigger of 7 g/dl improved outcomes compared to a 10 g/dl trigger point [3]. Likewise, the ARDS-NET group demonstrated significant outcome benefit from lower tidal volumes (approximating 6–7 ml/kg) [4]. Intuitively, we are using less sedation and, in many countries, shorter courses of antibiotics as the perception takes hold (albeit in the absence of much hard data) that earlier weaning and a lower antibiotic load reduce complications and hospital stay.

We have perhaps failed to properly consider the notion that many of our standard therapies may, in fact, be covertly harmful and may act counter to the body's attempts to adapt to a prolonged, acute illness. In heart failure, for example, there is increasingly compelling evidence that two of our mainstay treatments over the past two decades, dobutamine and phosphodiesterase inhibitors,

Table 1. Examples of changing fashions 1995-2005

	Example	1995	2005
Respiratory	tidal volume	10 ml/kg	5–6 ml/kg
	steroids for ARDS	rarely used	increasing use
	nitric oxide inhalation	fashionable	limited use
Hemodynamic	O_2 delivery/ consumption	'supranormal'	normal
	vasopressin	not used	fashionable
Sepsis (until 1993)	expensive immunotherapy	HA-1A anti-endotoxin antibody	activated Protein C
	steroids	derided	in vogue
Hematological	transfusion threshold	10 g/dl	7 g/dl
Renal	hemofiltration	10 ml/kg, lactate buffer	high-flow, bicarbonate
Monitoring	pulmonary artery catheter	gold standard	on the wane
	gastric tonometry	fashionable	forgotten
Endocrine	glycaemic control	glucose <10 mmol/l	4–7 mmol/l
Gastrointestinal	gastric protection	sucralfate, ranitidine	omeprazole

actually worsen long-term outcomes [27, 28]. A variety of mechanisms have been proposed including increased fatty acid oxidation, arrhythmogenesis, and decreased cardiac efficiency. Norepinephrine and dobutamine have also been shown to accelerate both Gram-positive and Gram-negative bacterial growth [29, 30] while dopamine is a potent suppressor of prolactin secretion, even at low doses [31].

All sedatives commonly in use today have potent effects, at least *in vitro,* on immune function [32-34] while a single dose of etomidate can compromise adrenal function in critically ill patients for at least 24 hours [35]. Sedatives also affect mitochondrial function *in vitro* and this may be amplified in sepsis or other conditions with increased levels of NO [36]. Likewise, antibiotics affect *in vitro* mitochondrial activity and biogenesis, though at concentrations equivalent to *in vivo* therapeutic levels [37, 38]. If the hypothesis that organ failure is related to mitochondrial dysfunction is borne out, then recovery will depend upon new mitochondrial protein formation, a process that could be delayed by antibiotics, sedatives, hormonal modulators, and so forth.

The harmful effects from blood transfusion suggested by the prospective TRICC study and other, non-randomized studies [39] may potentially arise from effects on the recipient's immune response. This is implied by the recent study by Hebert and colleagues who found better outcomes in patients transfused with leukoreduced blood [40]. Similarly, the benefits of lower tidal volume ventilation may be related to reduced production of local and systemic cytokines [41].

This concern of unrecognized detriment can be transmitted to many other areas of intensive care medicine that we perhaps take for granted. For example, we make no attempt to modulate nutritional inputs and constituents in the different phases of an acute illness, and the trend to an increased mortality found by many of the immunonutrition trials [42, 43] should not necessarily be dismissed as chance findings. The gut that is not absorbing enteral feed is driven with prokinetics and persisting attempts to establish an adequate nasogastric intake. What are the consequences of enterally feeding a patient with a bloated, distended and painful abdomen? They are unlikely to be positive. Likewise, as an article of faith we treat pyrexia as patients feel better and vasopressor requirements are often reduced. However, there are numerous experimental studies to suggest that an important protective response may be overridden by our attempts to normalize temperature. The vogue for corticosteroid therapy waxes and wanes; currently, it is fashionable for catecholamine-resistant septic shock and acute respiratory distress syndrome (ARDS). However, reports of an increased incidence of myopathy in which high-dose steroids are implicated (Bernard et al NIH NHLBI ARDS Network: Report on ongoing clinical trials. Presented at: Annual meeting of the American Thoracic Society; May 24, 2004; Orlando) should encourage some caution until we better understand when, how much, for how long and to whom steroids should be prescribed.

Management in the Future

By 2015, I am confident that advances in our understanding of the disease processes underlying critical illness and organ failure will considerably alter much of our current practice. This will be augmented by major developments in bedside monitoring technology that will enable more individualized interventions at the appropriate time as we gain a better grasp of underlying immune, hormonal, bioenergetic and metabolic function. I feel that we will be intervening less and tolerating greater degrees of abnormality, be it for hypotension, hypoxemia, acidosis, etc. I am less confident that major blockbusting anti-inflammatory therapies will arise over the next decade that will significantly impact upon large numbers of critically ill patients. However, we should be starting to focus more upon prophylactic measures, particularly in the high-risk elective surgical patient and in the period of acute illness before admission to the ICU. We will also be developing and trialling novel agents that will hasten the resolution of organ failure as it dawns on both clinicians and industry that this is now the major sticking point for many critically ill patients and the major drain on our limited resources. We can generally tide our patients through the acute inflammatory phase, yet the prolonged period of established organ failure punctuated by episodes of decompensation and further inflammation (e.g., nosocomial infection, bleeding) is where most of them die – or are allowed to die. Table 2 highlights

Table 2. Areas of potential practice in 2015

Diagnostic and monitoring tools	• rapid, bedside monitoring of inflammatory, immune, hormonal, metabolic and bioenergetic status, and a happy/unhappy intracellular milieu • rapid and reliable, non-invasive macro- and microcirculatory and tissue/cellular oxygen monitoring at whole body and regional level • rapid diagnosis of infection and identification of pathogen and antimicrobial sensitivities • ready availability of, and expertise with, portable diagnostic devices such as ultrasound and echo • improved monitoring of sedation, 'useful' sleep and neurological function • computer-aided diagnosis • servo-controlled delivery systems for targeted controlled infusions, e.g., for glycemic control, plasma antibiotic therapeutic levels
Prophylaxis	• rapid, goal-directed cardio-respiratory resuscitation of critically ill patients • goal-directed cardio-respiratory optimization of high-risk elective surgical patients • genetic identification of at-risk patients • non-antibiotic means of controlling/preventing infection • up-regulation of endogenous protective mechanisms, e.g., preconditioning, heat shock protein, heme oxygenase-1 induction • antioxidant supplementation, immunomodulation • viral transfection of protective proteins
Prevention of short/ long-term complications	• muscle wasting/weakness • ventilator-induced lung injury and lung fibrosis • neuropsychiatric complications
Reductionism	• acceptance of physiological/biochemical abnormality (e.g., blood pressure, hypoxemia, hypercapnia, Hb) titrated individually and temporally • reduction in overall use of sedation, antibiotics, inotropes, blood, etc.. but improved targeting • recognition and avoidance of currently accepted yet covertly harmful therapies, e.g. etomidate
Awakening 'sleeping' organs	• metabolic/mitochondrial switches to hasten resolution of organ failure
Modulation of metabolic, endocrine and immune pathways	• providing substrate to optimize efficiency of organ function and immune status, and to prevent autocannibalism • optimizing type and timing of substrate, hormone or immunotherapy to patient status – may involve up- or downregulation of endogenous pathways
Specific treatments, for example	• immunomodulation • alternative ventilatory techniques, surfactant, pulmonary fibrinolytics, • heart-friendly inotropes • hemoglobin substitutes • hemostatic agents to halt bleeding • non- or minimally invasive revascularization techniques

areas of potential development. I await with interest the accuracy of my predictions!

References

1. Armstrong GL, Conn LA, Pinner RW (1999) Trends in infectious disease mortality in the United States during the 20th century. JAMA 281:61–66
2. Padkin A, Goldfrad C, Brady AR, Young D, Black N, Rowan K (2003) Epidemiology of severe sepsis occurring in the first 24 hrs in intensive care units in England, Wales, and Northern Ireland. Crit Care Med 31:2332–2338
3. Hebert PC, Wells G, Blajchman MA, et al (1999) A multicenter, randomized, controlled clinical trial of transfusion requirements in critical care. Transfusion Requirements in Critical Care Investigators, Canadian Critical Care Trials Group. N Engl J Med 340:409–417
4. The Acute Respiratory Distress Syndrome Network (2000) Ventilation with lower tidal volumes as compared with traditional tidal volumes for acute lung injury and the acute respiratory distress syndrome. N Engl J Med 342:1301–1308
5. Singer M, De Santis V, Vitale D, Jeffcoate W (2004) Multiorgan failure is an adaptive, endocrine-mediated, metabolic response to overwhelming systemic inflammation. Lancet. 364:545–548
6. De Backer D, Creteur J, Preiser JC, Dubois MJ, Vincent JL (2002) Microvascular blood flow is altered in patients with sepsis. Am J Respir Crit Care Med 166:98–104
7. Vandermeer TJ, Wang H, Fink MP (1995) Endotoxemia causes ileal mucosal acidosis in the absence of mucosal hypoxia in a normodynamic porcine model of septic shock. Crit Care Med 23:1217–1226
8. Rosser DM, Stidwill RP, Jacobson D, Singer M (1995) Oxygen tension in the bladder epithelium increases in both high and low output endotoxemic sepsis. J Appl Physiol 79:1878–1882
9. Boekstegers P, Weidenhofer S, Kapsner T, Werdan K (1994) Skeletal muscle partial pressure of oxygen in patients with sepsis. Crit Care Med 22:640–650
10. Hotchkiss RS, Swanson PE, Freeman BD, et al (1999) Apoptotic cell death in patients with sepsis, shock, and multiple organ dysfunction. Crit Care Med 27:1230–1251
11. Brealey D, Karyampudi S, Jacques TS, et al (2004) Mitochondrial dysfunction in a long-term rodent model of sepsis and organ failure. Am J Physiol Regul Integr Comp Physiol 286:R491–R497
12. Brealey D, Brand M, Hargreaves I, et al (2002) Association between mitochondrial dysfunction and severity and outcome of septic shock. Lancet 360:219–223
13. Singer M, Brealey D (1999) Mitochondrial dysfunction in sepsis. Biochem Soc Symp 66:149–166
14. Vanhorebeek I, De Vos R, Mesotten D, Wouters PJ, De Wolf-Peeters C, Van den Berghe G (2005) Protection of hepatocyte mitochondrial ultrastructure and function by strict blood glucose control with insulin in critically ill patients. Lancet 365:53–59
15. Beltran B, Mathur A, Duchen MR, Erusalimsky JD, Moncada S (2000) The effect of nitric oxide on cell respiration: A key to understanding its role in cell survival or death. Proc Natl Acad Sci USA 97:14602–14607
16. Annane D, Sebille V, Troche G, Raphael JC, Gajdos P, Bellissant E (2000) A 3-level prognostic classification in septic shock based on cortisol levels and cortisol response to corticotropin. JAMA 283:1038–1045
17. Bornstein SR, Licinio J, Tauchnitz R, et al (1998) Plasma leptin levels are increased in survivors of acute sepsis: associated loss of diurnal rhythm, in cortisol and leptin secretion. J Clin Endocrinol Metab 83:280–283

18. Joosten KF, de Kleijn ED, Westerterp M, et al (2000) Endocrine and metabolic responses in children with meningoccocal sepsis: striking differences between survivors and non-survivors. J Clin Endocrinol Metab 85:3746–3753
19. Rivers E, Nguyen B, Havstad S, et al (2001) Early Goal-Directed Therapy Collaborative Group. Early goal-directed therapy in the treatment of severe sepsis and septic shock. N Engl J Med 345:1368–1377
20. Hayes MA, Timmins AC, Yau EHS, Palazzo M, Hinds CJ, Watson D (1994) Elevation of systemic oxygen delivery in the treatment of critically ill patients. N Engl J Med 330:1717–1722
21. Gattinoni L, Brazzi L, Pelosi P, et al (1995) A trial of goal-oriented hemodynamic therapy in critically ill patients. N Engl J Med 333:1025–1032
22. Noble JS, MacKirdy FN, Donaldson SI, Howie JC (2001) Renal and respiratory failure in Scottish ICUs. Anaesthesia 56:124–129
23. Docke WD, Randow F, Syrbe U, et al (1997) Monocyte deactivation in septic patients: restoration by IFN-gamma treatment. Nat Med 3:678–681
24. Van den Berghe G, de Zegher F, Bouillon R (1998) Acute and prolonged critical illness as different neuroendocrine paradigms. J Clin Endocrinol Metab 83:1827–1834
25. Kreymann G, Grosser S, Buggisch P, Gottschall C, Matthaei S, Greten H (1993) Oxygen consumption and resting metabolic rate in sepsis, sepsis syndrome, and septic shock. Crit Care Med 21:1012–1019
26. Dellinger RP, Carlet JM, Masur H, et al (2004) for the Surviving Sepsis Campaign Management Guidelines Committee. Surviving Sepsis Campaign guidelines for management of severe sepsis and septic shock. Crit Care Med 32:858–873
27. Cuffe MS, Califf RM, Adams KF Jr, et al (2002) Outcomes of a Prospective Trial of Intravenous Milrinone for Exacerbations of Chronic Heart Failure (OPTIME-CHF) Investigators. Short-term intravenous milrinone for acute exacerbation of chronic heart failure: a randomized controlled trial. JAMA 287:1541–1547
28. Cleland JG, Ghosh J, Freemantle N, et al (2004) Clinical trials update and cumulative meta-analyses from the American College of Cardiology: WATCH, SCD-HeFT, DINAMIT, CASINO, INSPIRE, STRATUS-US, RIO-Lipids and cardiac resynchronisation therapy in heart failure. Eur J Heart Fail 6:501–508
29. Lyte M, Freestone PPE, Neal CP, et al (2003) Stimulation of Staphylococcus epidermidis growth and biofilm formation by catecholamine inotropes. Lancet 361:130–135
30. Lyte M, Ernst S (1992) Catecholamine induced growth of Gram negative bacteria. Life Sci 50:203–212
31. Bailey AR, Burchett KR (1997) Effect of low-dose dopamine on serum concentrations of prolactin in critically ill patients. Br J Anaesth 78:97–99
32. Brand JM, Frohn C, Luhm J, Kirchner H, Schmucker P (2003) Early alterations in the number of circulating lymphocyte subpopulations and enhanced proinflammatory immune response during opioid-based general anesthesia. Shock 20:213–217
33. Helmy SA, Al-Attiyah RJ (2001) The immunomodulatory effects of prolonged intravenous infusion of propofol versus midazolam in critically ill surgical patients. Anaesthesia 56:4–8
34. Kelbel I, Koch T, Weber A, Schiefer HG, van Ackern K, Neuhof H (1999) Alterations of bacterial clearance induced by propofol. Acta Anaesthesiol Scand 43:71–76
35. Absalom A, Pledger D, Kong A (1999) Adrenocortical function in critically ill patients 24 h after a single dose of etomidate. Anaesthesia 54:861–867
36. Stevanato R, Momo F, Marian M, et al (2002) Effects of nitrosopropofol on mitochondrial energy-converting system. Biochem Pharmacol 64:1133–1138
37. Tune BM, Hsu CY (1990) The renal mitochondrial toxicity of beta-lactam antibiotics: in vitro effects of cephaloglycin and imipenem. J Am Soc Nephrol 1:815–821
38. Wilkie D (1977) Mitochondrial biogenesis: inhibitors of mitochondrial protein synthesis. Mol Cell Biochem 14:97–100

39. Rao SV, Jollis JG, Harrington RA, et al (2004) Relationship of blood transfusion and clinical outcomes in patients with acute coronary syndromes. JAMA 292:1555–1562
40. Hebert PC, Fergusson D, Blajchman MA, (2003) Clinical outcomes following institution of the Canadian universal leukoreduction program for red blood cell transfusions. JAMA 289:1941–1949
41. Ranieri VM, Suter PM, Tortorella C, et al (1999) Effect of mechanical ventilation on inflammatory mediators in patients with acute respiratory distress syndrome: a randomized controlled trial. JAMA 282:54–61
42. Heyland DK, Samis A (2003) Does immunonutrition in patients with sepsis do more harm than good? Intensive Care Med 29:669–671
43. Bertolini G, Iapichino G, Radrizzani D, et al (2003) Early enteral immunonutrition in patients with severe sepsis: results of an interim analysis of a randomized multicentre clinical trial. Intensive Care Med 29:834–840

The Profile and Management of Acute Respiratory Distress Syndrome

L. Gattinoni, P. Caironi, and E. Carlesso

Introduction

Since its first description almost 40 years ago [1], the acute respiratory distress syndrome (ARDS) has been intrinsically linked with its management. In fact, the appearance of ARDS, in its most severe form, is possible only when artificial ventilatory support is available to keep the patient alive. Thus, the 'natural history' of ARDS is the natural history of ARDS plus its ventilatory management. Therefore, we need to keep in mind that the profile and the management of this syndrome are interwoven. Nonetheless, in an attempt for clarity, we will try to discuss these two topics separately, considering the past, the present and, perhaps, the future.

Pathophysiological Profile

Gas Exchange

The past

The hypoxemia associated with ARDS was initially called 'refractory hypoxemia', as a normal value of arterial partial pressure of oxygen (PO_2) could not be reached even when delivering an inspiratory oxygen fraction (FiO_2) equal to 1.0. The mechanism of this hypoxemia has been the object of several investigations. An initial problem was to understand whether hypoxemia is caused by true right-to-left intrapulmonary shunt, i.e., blood flow perfusing non-ventilated (atelectatic and/or consolidated) lung regions, or by venous admixture, i.e., a combination of true intrapulmonary shunt and lung regions with low ventilation/perfusion (V/Q) ratios. The theoretical framework of the shunt equation still in use to compute intrapulmonary shunt is based on the three-compartment lung model of Riley and Cournand [2]: an ideal compartment with a V/Q equal to the mean average V/Q of the lung, another compartment with a V/Q equal to zero (shunt), and a third one with a V/Q equal to infinity (anatomical plus alveolar dead space). Unfortunately, this model does not allow discrimination between true intrapulmonary shunt and low V/Q lung compartments. In Riley's model, low V/Q lung compartments are split between both the ideal and the true intrapulmonary shunt compartment.

In the early 1980s, Wagner and colleagues [3] proposed a method based on the administration of six inert gases to the lungs to estimate V/Q distributions from 0 to infinity. By applying this procedure in 16 patients affected by ARDS, Dantzker and colleagues [4] found that arterial hypoxemia was primarily due to the true intrapulmonary shunt; the contribution of low V/Q areas to the development of hypoxemia was negligible. Moreover, it was recognized early that shunt fraction is strictly dependent on hemodynamics; a reduction in cardiac output decreases shunt fraction and vice versa [5, 6]. This phenomenon has been observed not only in patients with ARDS but also during cardiogenic pulmonary edema [7]. However, up to now, the underlying mechanism has not been fully elucidated [8]. The main role of true shunt in determining hypoxemia in ARDS patients, although derived from a very small population, has become a universal and well-accepted dogma. However, it is conceivable that, in some patients, low V/Q lung compartments substantially contribute to the observed hypoxemia, depending on the FiO_2 used. Measuring the true intrapulmonary right-to-left shunt using sulfur hexafluoride (SF_6), we found that a significant portion of the hypoxemia observed during acute respiratory failure was related to low V/Q lung regions rather than to true shunt, particularly among patients receiving FiO_2 between 0.4 and 0.6 [9]. Unfortunately, the assessment of V/Q distribution, which is difficult in the routine clinical setting, does not tell us anything about the regional anatomical distribution of lung areas with different V/Q ratios.

It is important to note that, up to the early 1990s, the main focus of all the investigations dealing with gas exchange during acute respiratory failure was oxygenation, while the other side of the gas exchange, i.e., the clearance of carbon dioxide (CO_2), was neglected.

The present

During the 1980s, in patients with ARDS, the arterial partial pressure of CO_2 (PCO_2) was targeted to values within normal range (35–45 mmHg). The price paid for achieving this target was the use of mechanical ventilation at high pressures and volumes. Recently, there has been increasing attention to the importance of CO_2 in ARDS under different perspectives. It has been known for a long time that, for the same minute ventilation, the PCO_2 increases with increasing duration of the syndrome, from early (1 week) to intermediate (2 weeks) and late ARDS (3 weeks or more) [10]. This progression is likely to reflect, more than what oxygenation does, the structural changes of the lung parenchyma, with appearance of fibrosis, bubbles and pseudocysts [10–12].

Alteration of CO_2 elimination, inferred from an increase in dead space, is not only associated with the time course of ARDS, but is considered a marker of the severity and a prognostic index in early ARDS, as shown by Nuckton and colleagues [13]. Moreover, we observed that when arterial PCO_2 (at the same minute ventilation) decreases in ARDS patients after a change from supine position to prone position, survival is longer than when PCO_2 increases after the same maneuver [14]. Also from this investigation, the arterial PCO_2 response seems to be a marker of the underlying condition of the lung. In the Nuckton et al. study [13], higher dead space was associated with higher mortality, suggesting severe structural changes of the lung, both considering ventilation (alveolar disruption) and perfusion (microthrombosis). The response of arterial PCO_2 to the prone position likely reflects the potential for recruitment, although the hypothesis needs to be proved.

Indeed, it is well established that high dead space is a marker of 'severity'. However, is high PCO_2 *per se* harmful? In the 1970s we did not have an answer to this question, as the arterial PCO_2 was maintained within the normal range with mechanical ventilator settings now considered harmful. The merit of the study by Hickling and colleagues, in the early 1990s, was the introduction of the concept of 'permissive hypercapnia', a procedure aimed to put the lung at rest by using mechanical ventilation with low pressures and volumes [15]. 'Lung rest' was first obtained by avoiding mechanical ventilation and clearing CO_2 with extracorporeal tools [16, 17]. Hickling et al. pursued a similar target, paying, as a price, a remarkable degree of hypercapnia. Nonetheless, despite theoretical discussions about their relative importance, hypercapnia and acidosis have never been shown to be harmful. Setting arterial PCO_2 at a higher level [18] and decreasing the 'price' of mechanical ventilation is nowadays the common strategy for mechanical ventilation.

Furthermore, it has been suggested that hypercapnia may be not only harmless, but even beneficial as 'therapeutic hypercapnia' [19]. The possible mechanisms of these effects are still speculative and we lack proof of similar findings in patients. However, there is increasing evidence of possible beneficial effects of hypercapnia in cell culture studies and experimental animal models [20]. Although we cannot recommend, at present, hypercapnia as a target, we may accept it as a side effect.

The future

We believe that, in the future, new techniques will allow a better understanding of CO_2 clearance and oxygenation in ARDS. For this purpose, the knowledge of the real anatomical relationships between ventilation and perfusion in the ARDS lung is necessary. Without this knowledge, in our opinion, a full elucidation of gas exchange rules and their alteration while modifying the conditions of the system is impossible. Combinations of different imaging techniques such as computed tomography (CT), positron emission tomography (PET) and nuclear magnetic resonance [21, 22], will be essential in achieving this goal.

Lung Mechanics

The past

Since the first description of ARDS, the lungs in this condition were considered to be 'stiff'. This term suggests that the pulmonary structure is stiffer than normal. Only in the middle 1980s, was it recognized that the lungs in ARDS are small rather than stiff; this is the 'the baby lung' concept. In ARDS, the elasticity of the ventilated lung structure is nearly normal, as measured by the specific compliance (the ratio of measured lung compliance and the measured end-expiratory gas volume) [23–25].

Lung mechanics during ARDS have been extensively studied in order to find a physiological rationale for the selection of positive end-expiratory pressure (PEEP). For this purpose, the pressure volume (PV) curve of the respiratory system has been considered the ideal tool. The initial model of the relationship between pressure and volume in ARDS was both simple and appealing. The initial part of the PV curve, up to the lower inflection point, indicates the pressure at which the lung is open. Accordingly, it has been suggested that the PEEP should be set at a level 2 cmH_2O higher than the lower inflection point, in order to maintain the lung open (minimal PEEP) [26–28]. This approach reached the height of its glory as part of the protocol of the 'lung protective strategy' proposed by Amato and colleagues in 1998 [29]. Second, the linear part of the PV curve (the inflation compliance) was thought to include the range of pressures in which the alveolar units normally inflate. Finally, the last part of the PV curve (above the upper inflection point) was thought to indicate the high pressures at which overstretching of the lung structures occurs. Although we doubt that the PV curve was largely used in clinical practice for PEEP selection, this approach has been widely accepted by the scientific community.

The present

Despite its simplicity and appeal, the physiological model underlying the approach mentioned above is inadequate. Mathematical models [25, 30] applied to pressure and volume data from patients [31] and observations obtained with CT in experimental animals [32] and ARDS patients [24, 33, 34] indicate that alveolar recruitment occurs along the entire PV curve, including points well above the upper inflection point. Indeed, the PV curve of the respiratory system, when expressed as a fraction of the inspiratory capacity, is indistinguishable from the pressure-recruitment curve, which represents alveolar recruitment, as a fraction of the maximal potential for recruitment, at the airway pressure applied (Fig. 1). Unfortunately, the pressure-recruitment curve and the PV curve do not tell us anything about the absolute potential for recruitment, which may be relevant for a proper setting of mechanical ventilation. From what we have discussed above, the '2 cmH_2O above lower inflection point' approach for setting the PEEP seems questionable, as the lower inflection point does not correspond to a condition when the lung is open. Moreover, most of the studies referred to the inflation limb of the PV curve, while PEEP should be referred to the expiratory limb [24]. Although not yet clinically applied, this new approach is now under investigation regarding its physiological framework [34, 35].

For many years, PV curve parameters were identified by eye. Recently, a more rigorous and promising approach has been proposed by Venegas and colleagues [30, 36]. The new analysis consists of fitting the PV curve data points (or pressure-recruitment points) with a sigmoidal function. The advantage of this approach is a more objective assessment of the data. The disadvantage is the modification of the traditional nomenclature. Thus, what Venegas defines as the inflection point is not the lower 'knee' of the curve, but, rather, the pres-

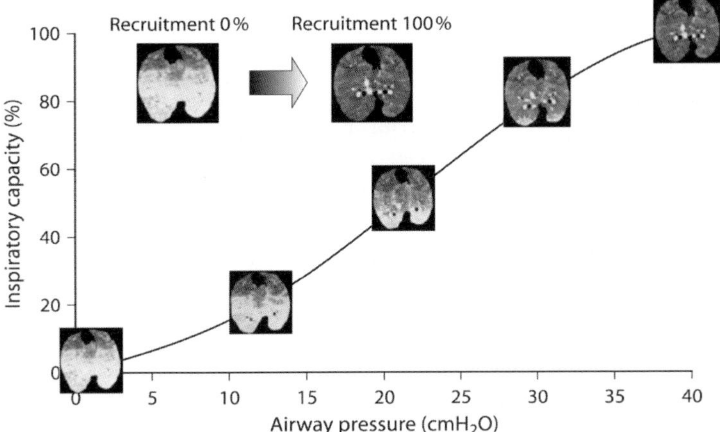

Fig. 1. Lung recruitment as a fraction of the applied airway pressure along the pressure volume curve of the respiratory system in an animal model of ARDS (oleic acid-induced lung injury in pigs – unpublished data from Quintel and Pelosi groups). As shown, alveolar recruitment occurs along the entire pressure volume curve, even above the lower and upper inflection point. Lung recruitment is expressed as a fraction of the maximal potential for recruitment, and is shown as CT scan images taken at the lung base at the corresponding airway pressure. Solid line represents pressure volume curve of the respiratory system, where volume is expressed as a percentage of the maximal inspiratory capacity. The data were fitted with a sigmoid function, according to Venegas and colleagues [30].

sure at which the maximal change of the curvature of the sigmoidal function occurs (i.e., the point of maximal compliance or the pressure at which the lung is inflated to 50% of its maximal capacity). A summary of the traditional and new nomenclature is presented in Table 1.

Until the middle 1990s, a change in the compliance of the respiratory system was believed to be caused mostly by changes in lung compliance, while the chest wall compliance was always considered normal. Nowadays, the importance of the chest wall in affecting the respiratory system mechanics is increasingly recognized [37, 38]. It has been found by our group and by other investigators that in ARDS patients with abdominal diseases, chest wall compliance is markedly reduced, due to increased intra-abdominal pressure [39, 40]. Intra-abdominal hypertension appears to be a common problem in critically ill patients, and it always is associated with decreased chest wall compliance [41]. Although it is extremely important to recognize decreased chest wall compliance in order to properly tailor ventilator settings, this observation has not yet affected routine practice.

Although respiratory mechanics in patients with ALI or ARDS are still widely investigated, a clear and definite relationship between lung mechanics assessment and clinical practice has not been found yet. What we believed in the past – mechanical ventilation should be tailored based on the inspiratory limb of the PV curve – does not have any rational physiological basis.

Table 1. Pressure volume curve nomenclature

Old nomenclature		
Starting compliance [23]	Cstart	Computed as the ratio between the first 100 ml on the inflation limb and the corresponding pressure
Inflation compliance [23]	Cinf	Slope of the most linear segment on the inflation limb of the pressure-volume curve
Lower inflection point [23]	Pflex, LIP	Intersection between Cstart and Cinf lines
Upper inflection point [71, 77]	UIP	Static end-inspiratory pressure after which compliance decreases more than 20% or 10% from the best compliance obtained
New nomenclature		
Inflection point [30, 78]	c, Pinf	Point of maximal compliance
Lower inflection point [30, 36]	Pcl	Lower corner point on inflation/deflation limb, calculated as c-2d or c-1.317d (d=linear portion of the curve/4)
Lower inflection point [79]	Pmci	Point of maximal compliance increase
Upper inflection point [30, 36]	Pcu	Upper corner point on inflation/deflation limb, calculated as c+2d or c+1.317d
Upper inflection point [79]	Pmcd	Point of maximal compliance decrease

The future

Fortunately, we cannot predict and describe the future, but we can express our wishes. In our opinion, in order to tailor the mechanical ventilation on a more physiological basis, we should know the main determinants of its damage to the lung. There are consistent data indicating that the first physical trigger of ventilator-induced lung injury (VILI) is excessive global and/or regional alveolar stress and strain [42]. Although monitoring the regional distribution of these parameters is beyond our actual technical possibilities, global alveolar stress and strain values may be estimated with rough surrogates. Alveolar stress, i.e., the tension developed onto the lung fiber skeleton when a pressure is applied, is quantitatively equal to the distending force of the lung (transpulmonary pressure). The continuous monitoring of transpulmonary pressure requires an esophageal balloon, which should be incorporated into the nasogastric tube. The rough equivalent of alveolar strain, i.e., the increase in lung volume relative to its resting position, requires the monitoring of end-expiratory lung volume (EELV). Adequate techniques (SF_6, oxygen/nitrogen analysis, helium dilution) have been available for many years for this purpose, but unfortunately they have never reached the market, likely because of a lack of interest by ICU physicians. We hope that the relationship between alveolar stress and strain will be monitored in the future. Probably, it will be sufficient to monitor either alveolar stress or alveolar strain alone, as the specific elastance (which links the two parameters) is nearly normal in lungs afflicted with ARDS [23, 24]. In our opinion, the following equation should be kept in mind for safe mechanical ventilation:

$$dP_L = El{,}spec * V_T / EELV$$

where dP_L is the variation of transpulmonary pressure, El,spec is the lung specific elastance, and V_T is the tidal volume.

Based on its physiological characteristics, the lung architecture receives excessive tension when the ratio between tidal volume and EELV is above 0.8, a level at which lung collagen fibers are fully distended [42]. It is conceivable that tailoring mechanical ventilation according to this physiological principle will make it safer.

Management and Side Effects

Mechanical Ventilation and Its Side Effects

The past

In the 1970s, the goal of mechanical ventilation was to maintain arterial PO_2 and PCO_2 within the normal ranges for these parameters. As previously discussed, these targets were reached by using high tidal volumes (12–15 ml/kg), and by setting PEEP between 5–10 cm H_2O. This approach was the 'state of the art' as stated by Pontoppidan, Geffin, and Lowenstein in the *New England Journal of Medicine* [43]. The recognized side effect of using such high values of tidal volume was hypocapnia, which was corrected by adding artificial dead space in order to achieve a normal arterial PCO_2. The main concern was oxygen toxicity, and the accepted dogma was to maintain FiO_2 below 0.6. In the same period, a new way of thinking had started, after the report by Hill and colleagues about the successful treatment of a young trauma patient with extracorporeal membrane oxygenation (ECMO) [44]. This new perspective led the National Institutes of Health to sponsor the first randomized clinical trial on ARDS. In this study, patients were randomized to receive standard therapy or long-term venous-arterial membrane lung oxygenation. The only modification of the ventilator setting in the treated group was reduction of FiO_2 aimed to decrease the oxygen toxicity, while the high tidal volumes and pressures were similar in treated and control patients. The mortality rate also was similar, being 90% in both groups [45].

The greatest debate, however, from about 1975 until about 1985 was the proper setting of PEEP. Suter and colleagues, in one of their famous papers [46], proposed that the best PEEP was that associated with the best oxygen transport, and this value was also associated with the best compliance. In France, Lemaire and colleagues [26] were the first to propose the concept of 'minimal PEEP' as the pressure 2 cmH_2O higher than the lower inflection point on the PV curve. On the other side of the Atlantic Ocean, in Florida, Kirby and colleagues [47] promoted the use of 'super-PEEP' as that at which the shunt fraction was reduced down to an average of 20%. It is impossible to quote all the contributions on this issue. The conclusion, however, is clear – we still do not know what level of PEEP should be applied. What we do know is that most ICU physicians treat ARDS patients with PEEP levels between 5 and 10 cmH_2O [48].

Another 'hot' topic in the 1980s was the hemodynamic profile during ARDS. The group from the Massachusetts General Hospital provided the best insights, carefully describing the development of pulmonary hypertension during ARDS and providing data about its physiological and pathological basis [49–53]. It is important to note that, as far as hemodynamics and gas exchange relationship is concerned, the oxygenation improvement mediated by hemodynamic changes caused by PEEP was well recognized in the 1980s but has been neglected in recent years.

The side effects of mechanical ventilation with high volumes and pressures have been recognized since the 1970s [54], and have been collectively named as 'barotrauma'. Several years later, an apparently different view of the problem was provided by the extensive work of Dreyfuss and colleagues, which focused the attention of the scientific community on lung distension (volume/strain) rather then lung tension (pressure/stress) [55]. As a result, the term 'volutrauma' gained popularity. In this context, the concept of lung rest evolved progressively. We first provided true lung rest [17] by removing CO_2 through extracorporeal membranes and ventilating the lung with 3–5 breaths per minute. When this technique was proposed, the 'baby lung' concept [56] and the 'sponge lung' concept [57] were ignored. Afterwards, with further advances in our knowledge about the pathophysiology of ARDS, lung rest became an accepted target and, along the same line of thinking, Hickling and colleagues proposed the idea of using low tidal volumes for ventilation (permissive hypercapnia) [15] for the 'gentle treatment' of the ARDS lung.

In the 1990s, physiological reasoning and experimental data led to the general concept of the 'lung protective strategy'. The theoretical basis of this approach was provided by Lachmann [58]. The biological effects of intratidal collapse and de-collapse were recognized in ex-vivo and in-vivo experimental models. Links between mechanical forces and inflammatory reactions were found in hundreds of papers (with some exceptions [59]) in cell cultures [60], in *ex vivo* [61] and *in vivo* experimental models [62], as well as in humans [63]. The inflammatory reaction consequent to mechanical forces was collectively named 'biotrauma'. By the late 1990s, the pathophysiological background for the present practice of mechanical ventilation was solid. Two concepts were clear: first, mechanical ventilation can injure the lung; second, avoiding intratidal collapse and de-collapse of alveolar units is beneficial.

The present

In this scenario, it is not easy to define the chronological beginning of 'the present'. In our opinion, we may date 'the present' from the paper by Amato and colleagues published in the *New England Journal of Medicine*, which represents the first clinical proof of the possible benefits of the lung protective strategy [29]. This paper had striking effects on the scientific community and stimulated further work. Indeed, we are living in the era of the lung protective strategy.

However, it is important to note that only the Amato study (on outcome) and the Ranieri study (on biotrauma) [63] really tested the lung protective strategy, which includes the control of both end-inspiratory and end-expiratory pressures (i.e., tidal volume or plateau pressure and PEEP). The following clinical trials separately investigated the effects of tidal volume and PEEP. The clinical trial conducted by the ARDS network clearly showed the advantages of gentle ventilation (6 ml/kg tidal volume) versus mechanical ventilation with high volumes (12 ml/kg tidal volume) [64]. This trial, however, compared two extreme tidal volumes. Other clinical trials comparing intermediate tidal volumes (7 versus 10–10.5 ml/kg) failed to show any differences [65–67].

Now, we have clinical and experimental evidence indicating that high tidal volume ventilation (12 ml/kg) is unsafe. Different questions and debatable answers may arise when discussing the ideal tidal volume: is it really 6 ml/kg? In our opinion, 6 ml/kg should not become a dogma for several reasons. First, what puts the lung at risk for injury is alveolar strain, i.e., the ratio of tidal volume and end-expiratory lung volume, and this ratio, in ARDS patients, is unrelated to body weight. As an example, the end expiratory lung volume in a hypothetical ARDS patient with an ideal body weight of 70 kg could be 500, 1000, 1500 ml, according to the severity of the disease. The alveolar strain resulting from 6 ml/kg tidal volume (420 ml) would be 0.84, 0.42, or 0.28, respectively. This is likely to be important for the development of VILI, but at the moment is not considered in standard care. Furthermore, it is not clear to us why we should use 6 ml/kg tidal volume in an ARDS patient with an intermediate lung compliance (which is an indirect estimate of the residual open lung [68]), and consequently a plateau pressure of about 25 cmH_2O at the tidal volume used. The use of low tidal volumes could induce unnecessary hypercapnia and force us to use heavy sedation, which may be clinically more harmful than a plateau pressure below 25 cmH_2O. These, of course, are only opinions, as we lack, at the moment, any direct proof that 6 is better than 8 or 10 ml/kg when the plateau pressure is limited. Moreover, it is important to highlight that the use of 6 ml/kg has not been widely implemented [69, 70], suggesting that in daily practice the problems caused by 6 ml/kg tidal volume ventilation are thought to be greater than the expected benefits [71–74]. Of note, the current recommendations for mechanical ventilation (published in the *New England Journal of Medicine*) [64] represent a complete reversal compared to the recommendations for mechanical ventilation advocated by experts in the 1970s (published in the *New England Journal of Medicine*) [43].

While the scientific community has reached a general consensus to avoid mechanical ventilation with high tidal volumes, the clinical approach to selecting PEEP is still in the fog. The recent ALVEOLI trial conducted by the ARDS network [75] failed to demonstrate any differences in outcome between ARDS patients treated with low PEEP (8.3 ± 3.2 cm H_2O) or high PEEP (13.2 ± 3.5 cm H_2O). In the era of the lung protective strategy, this result, possible methodological problems of the study notwithstanding [76], is disturbing. We may argue that the PEEP interval explored was too low, that the PEEP/FiO_2 scale was asymmetrical in the two arms of the study, and that the experimental design changed during the study. The real problem, in our opinion, is different. Most ICU scientists, at the moment, believe that the lung protective strategy is beneficial, and consequently all results contrary to this view are rejected. Indeed, there are only two alternatives: either the ALVEOLI study has been erroneously designed or the PEEP level, at least in the range explored, is really irrelevant for the outcome. We believe that we should be open to both possibilities. Certainly, the ALVEOLI study lacks a physiological rationale. We know that ARDS patients may have high or low potential for recruitment. It is possible that high PEEP will be beneficial in patients with high potential for recruitment and harmful in patients with low potential for recruitment. According to our knowledge of the pathophysiology of ARDS, the answer for PEEP benefit should be found in a study in which patients with high and low potential for recruitment are randomized separately to high and low PEEP levels. But again, we should also be prepared for the possibility that the level of PEEP is irrelevant for the outcome.

The future

The target for the future will be to make mechanical ventilation less harmful than it is today. This goal, however, implies an answer to a basic question: under this perspective, is opening the lung and keeping it open really the best strategy? In this case, high PEEP and low tidal volume would be the best ventilator setting, with possible re-evaluation of techniques, such as high frequency jet ventilation or high frequency oscillation. On the other hand, if we keep a portion of the lung always closed, low PEEP and low tidal volume strategies should be acceptable, as they would decrease the global alveolar stress and strain. In our opinion, only physiological studies can solve the dilemma between opening the lung and keeping it open or accepting some lung closure and keeping it closed.

Conclusion

Acute lung injury and ARDS are still a therapeutic challenge in intensive care, but great advances have been made in the last twenty years. However, if we have to summarize all the improvements in a single sentence, we can say that what we have learnt is that more gentle treatment of the inflamed lung improves outcome.

References

1. Ashbaugh DG, Bigelow DB, Petty TL, Levine BE (1967) Acute respiratory distress in adults. Lancet 2:319–323
2. Riley RL, Cournand A (1951) Analysis of factors affecting partial pressures of oxygen and carbon dioxide in gas and blood of lungs; theory. J Appl Physiol 4:77–101
3. Wagner PD, Saltzman HA, West JB (1974) Measurement of continuous distributions of ventilation-perfusion ratios: theory. J Appl Physiol 36:588–599
4. Dantzker DR, Brook CJ, Dehart P, Lynch JP, Weg JG (1979) Ventilation-perfusion distributions in the adult respiratory distress syndrome. Am Rev Respir Dis 120:1039–1052

5. Hedley-Whyte J, Pontoppidan H, Morris MJ (1966) The response of patients with respiratory failure and cardiopulmonary disease to different levels of constant volume ventilation. J Clin Invest 45:1543–1554
6. Lemaire F, Gastine H, Regner B, Teisseire B, Rapin M (1978) Perfusion changes modify intrapulmonary shunting (Qs/Qt) in patients with adult respiratory distress syndrome (ARDS). Am Rev Respir Dis 117:144 (abst)
7. Scheinman MM, Evans GT (1972) Right to left shunt in patients with acute myocardial infarction. A proposed mechanism. Am J Cardiol 29:757–766
8. Freden F, Cigarini I, Mannting F, Hagberg A, Lemaire F, Hedenstierna G (1993) Dependence of shunt on cardiac output in unilobar oleic acid edema. Distribution of ventilation and perfusion. Intensive Care Med 19:185–190
9. Pesenti A, Riboni A, Marcolin R, Gattinoni L (1983) Venous admixture (Qva/Q) and true shunt (Qs/Qt) in ARF patients: effects of PEEP at constant FIO2. Intensive Care Med 9:307–311
10. Gattinoni L, Bombino M, Pelosi P, et al (1994) Lung structure and function in different stages of severe adult respiratory distress syndrome. JAMA 271:1772–1779
11. Goodman LR (1996) Congestive heart failure and adult respiratory distress syndrome. New insights using computed tomography. Radiol Clin North Am 34:33–46
12. Rouby JJ, Lherm T, Martin DL, et al (1993) Histologic aspects of pulmonary barotrauma in critically ill patients with acute respiratory failure. Intensive Care Med 19:383–389
13. Nuckton TJ, Alonso JA, Kallet RH, et al (2002) Pulmonary dead-space fraction as a risk factor for death in the acute respiratory distress syndrome. N Engl J Med 346:1281–1286
14. Gattinoni L, Vagginelli F, Carlesso E, et al (2003) Decrease in PaCO2 with prone position is predictive of improved outcome in acute respiratory distress syndrome. Crit Care Med 31:2727–2733
15. Hickling KG, Henderson SJ, Jackson R (1990) Low mortality associated with low volume pressure limited ventilation with permissive hypercapnia in severe adult respiratory distress syndrome. Intensive Care Med 16:372–377
16. Gattinoni L, Agostoni A, Pesenti A, et al (1980) Treatment of acute respiratory failure with low-frequency positive-pressure ventilation and extracorporeal removal of CO2. Lancet 2:292–294
17. Gattinoni L, Pesenti A, Mascheroni D, et al (1986) Low-frequency positive-pressure ventilation with extracorporeal CO2 removal in severe acute respiratory failure. JAMA 256:881–886
18. Pesenti A (1990) Target blood gases during ARDS ventilatory management. Intensive Care Med 16:349–351
19. Laffey JG, Kavanagh BP (1999) Carbon dioxide and the critically ill–too little of a good thing? Lancet 354:1283–1286
20. Laffey JG, O'Croinin D, McLoughlin P, Kavanagh BP (2004) Permissive hypercapnia–role in protective lung ventilatory strategies. Intensive Care Med 30:347–356
21. Gattinoni L, Caironi P, Pelosi P, Goodman LR (2001) What has computed tomography taught us about the acute respiratory distress syndrome? Am J Respir Crit Care Med 164:1701–1711
22. Schuster DP, Kovacs A, Garbow J, Piwnica-Worms D (2004) Recent advances in imaging the lungs of intact small animals. Am J Respir Cell Mol Biol 30:129–138
23. Gattinoni L, Pesenti A, Avalli L, Rossi F, Bombino M (1987) Pressure-volume curve of total respiratory system in acute respiratory failure. Computed tomographic scan study. Am Rev Respir Dis 136:730–736
24. Gattinoni L, D'Andrea L, Pelosi P, Vitale G, Pesenti A, Fumagalli R (1993) Regional effects and mechanism of positive end-expiratory pressure in early adult respiratory distress syndrome. JAMA 269:2122–2127
25. Hickling KG (1998) The pressure-volume curve is greatly modified by recruitment. A mathematical model of ARDS lungs. Am J Respir Crit Care Med 158:194–202

26. Lemaire F, Harf A, Simonneau G, Matamis D, Rivara D, Atlan G (1981) [Gas exchange, static pressure-volume curve and positive-pressure ventilation at the end of expiration. Study of 16 cases of acute respiratory insufficiency in adults]. Ann Anesthesiol Fr 22:435–441
27. Matamis D, Lemaire F, Harf A, Brun-Buisson C, Ansquer JC, Atlan G (1984) Total respiratory pressure-volume curves in the adult respiratory distress syndrome. Chest 86:58–66
28. Pesenti A, Marcolin R, Prato P, Borelli M, Riboni A, Gattinoni L (1985) Mean airway pressure vs. positive end-expiratory pressure during mechanical ventilation. Crit Care Med 13:34–37
29. Amato MB, Barbas CS, Medeiros DM, et al (1998) Effect of a protective-ventilation strategy on mortality in the acute respiratory distress syndrome. N Engl J Med 338:347–354
30. Venegas JG, Harris RS, Simon BA (1998) A comprehensive equation for the pulmonary pressure-volume curve. J Appl Physiol 84:389–395
31. Jonson B, Richard JC, Straus C, Mancebo J, Lemaire F, Brochard L (1999) Pressure-volume curves and compliance in acute lung injury: evidence of recruitment above the lower inflection point. Am J Respir Crit Care Med 159:1172–1178
32. Pelosi P, Goldner M, McKibben A, et al (2001) Recruitment and derecruitment during acute respiratory failure: an experimental study. Am J Respir Crit Care Med 164:122–130
33. Crotti S, Mascheroni D, Caironi P, et al (2001) Recruitment and derecruitment during acute respiratory failure: a clinical study. Am J Respir Crit Care Med 164:131–140
34. Albaiceta GM, Taboada F, Parra D, et al (2004) Tomographic study of the inflection points of the pressure-volume curve in acute lung injury. Am J Respir Crit Care Med 170:1066–1072
35. Albaiceta GM, Taboada F, Parra D, Blanco A, Escudero D, Otero J (2003) Differences in the deflation limb of the pressure-volume curves in acute respiratory distress syndrome from pulmonary and extrapulmonary origin. Intensive Care Med 29:1943–1949
36. Harris RS, Hess DR, Venegas JG (2000) An objective analysis of the pressure-volume curve in the acute respiratory distress syndrome. Am J Respir Crit Care Med 161:432–439
37. Pelosi P, Cereda M, Foti G, Giacomini M, Pesenti A (1995) Alterations of lung and chest wall mechanics in patients with acute lung injury: effects of positive end-expiratory pressure. Am J Respir Crit Care Med 152:531–537
38. Mergoni M, Martelli A, Volpi A, Primavera S, Zuccoli P, Rossi A (1997) Impact of positive end-expiratory pressure on chest wall and lung pressure-volume curve in acute respiratory failure. Am J Respir Crit Care Med 156:846–854
39. Gattinoni L, Pelosi P, Suter PM, Pedoto A, Vercesi P, Lissoni A (1998) Acute respiratory distress syndrome caused by pulmonary and extrapulmonary disease. Different syndromes? Am J Respir Crit Care Med 158:3–11
40. Ranieri VM, Brienza N, Santostasi S, et al (1997) Impairment of lung and chest wall mechanics in patients with acute respiratory distress syndrome: role of abdominal distension. Am J Respir Crit Care Med 156:1082–1091
41. Malbrain ML, Chiumello D, Pelosi P, et al (2004) Prevalence of intra-abdominal hypertension in critically ill patients: a multicentre epidemiological study. Intensive Care Med 30:822–829
42. Gattinoni L, Carlesso E, Cadringher P, Valenza F, Vagginelli F, Chiumello D (2003) Physical and biological triggers of ventilator-induced lung injury and its prevention. Eur Respir J Suppl 47:15s–25s
43. Pontoppidan H, Geffin B, Lowenstein E (1972) Acute respiratory failure in the adult. 3. N Engl J Med 287:799–806
44. Hill JD, O'Brien TG, Murray JJ, et al (1972) Prolonged extracorporeal oxygenation for acute post-traumatic respiratory failure (shock-lung syndrome). Use of the Bramson membrane lung. N Engl J Med 286:629–634
45. Zapol WM, Snider MT, Hill JD, et al (1979) Extracorporeal membrane oxygenation in severe acute respiratory failure. A randomized prospective study. JAMA 242:2193–2196

46. Suter PM, Fairley B, Isenberg MD (1975) Optimum end-expiratory airway pressure in patients with acute pulmonary failure. N Engl J Med 292:284–289
47. Kirby RR, Downs JB, Civetta JM, et al (1975) High level positive end expiratory pressure (PEEP) in acute respiratory insufficiency. Chest 67:156–163
48. Esteban A, Anzueto A, Alia I, et al (2000) How is mechanical ventilation employed in the intensive care unit? An international utilization review. Am J Respir Crit Care Med 161:1450–1458
49. Zapol WM, Snider MT (1977) Pulmonary hypertension in severe acute respiratory failure. N Engl J Med 296:476–480
50. Zapol WM, Kobayashi K, Snider MT, Greene R, Laver MB (1977) Vascular obstruction causes pulmonary hypertension in severe acute respiratory failure. Chest 71:306–307
51. Tomashefski JF Jr, Davies P, Boggis C, Greene R, Zapol WM, Reid LM (1983) The pulmonary vascular lesions of the adult respiratory distress syndrome. Am J Pathol 112:112–126
52. Jones R, Zapol WM, Reid L (1983) Pulmonary arterial wall injury and remodelling by hyperoxia. Chest 83:40S–42S
53. Zapol WM, Jones R (1987) Vascular components of ARDS. Clinical pulmonary hemodynamics and morphology. Am Rev Respir Dis 136:471–474
54. Kumar A, Pontoppidan H, Falke KJ, Wilson RS, Laver MB (1973) Pulmonary barotrauma during mechanical ventilation. Crit Care Med 1:181–186
55. Dreyfuss D, Soler P, Basset G, Saumon G (1988) High inflation pressure pulmonary edema. Respective effects of high airway pressure, high tidal volume, and positive end-expiratory pressure. Am Rev Respir Dis 137:1159–1164
56. Gattinoni L, Pesenti A (1987) ARDS: the non-homogeneous lung; facts and hypothesis. Intensive Crit Care Digest 6:1–4
57. Bone RC (1993) The ARDS lung. New insights from computed tomography. JAMA 269:2134–2135
58. Lachmann B (1992) Open up the lung and keep the lung open. Intensive Care Med. 18:319–321
59. Dreyfuss D, Ricard JD, Saumon G (2003) On the physiologic and clinical relevance of lung-borne cytokines during ventilator-induced lung injury. Am J Respir Crit Care Med 167:1467–1471
60. Pugin J, Dunn I, Jolliet P, et al (1998) Activation of human macrophages by mechanical ventilation in vitro. Am J Physiol 275:L1040–L1050
61. Tremblay L, Valenza F, Ribeiro SP, Li J, Slutsky AS (1997) Injurious ventilatory strategies increase cytokines and c-fos m-RNA expression in an isolated rat lung model. J Clin Invest 99:944–952
62. Chiumello D, Pristine G, Slutsky AS (1999) Mechanical ventilation affects local and systemic cytokines in an animal model of acute respiratory distress syndrome. Am J Respir Crit Care Med 160:109–116
63. Ranieri VM, Suter PM, Tortorella C, et al (1999) Effect of mechanical ventilation on inflammatory mediators in patients with acute respiratory distress syndrome: a randomized controlled trial. JAMA 282:54–61
64. The Acute Respiratory Distress Syndrome Network (2000) Ventilation with lower tidal volumes as compared with traditional tidal volumes for acute lung injury and the acute respiratory distress syndrome. N Engl J Med 342:1301–1308
65. Brochard L, Roudot-Thoraval F, Roupie E, et al (1998) Tidal volume reduction for prevention of ventilator-induced lung injury in acute respiratory distress syndrome. The Multicenter Trail Group on Tidal Volume reduction in ARDS. Am J Respir Crit Care Med 158:1831–1838
66. Brower RG, Shanholtz CB, Fessler HE, et al (1999) Prospective, randomized, controlled clinical trial comparing traditional versus reduced tidal volume ventilation in acute respiratory distress syndrome patients. Crit Care Med 27:1492–1498

67. Stewart TE, Meade MO, Cook DJ, et al (1998) Evaluation of a ventilation strategy to prevent barotrauma in patients at high risk for acute respiratory distress syndrome. Pressure- and Volume-Limited Ventilation Strategy Group. N Engl J Med 338:355–361
68. Gattinoni L, Pesenti A, Baglioni S, Vitale G, Rivolta M, Pelosi P (1988) Inflammatory pulmonary edema and positive end-expiratory pressure: correlations between imaging and physiologic studies. J Thorac Imaging 3:59–64
69. Weinert CR, Gross CR, Marinelli WA (2003) Impact of randomized trial results on acute lung injury ventilator therapy in teaching hospitals. Am J Respir Crit Care Med 167:1304–1309
70. Young MP, Manning HL, Wilson DL, et al (2004) Ventilation of patients with acute lung injury and acute respiratory distress syndrome: has new evidence changed clinical practice? Crit Care Med 32:1260–1265
71. Roupie E, Dambrosio M, Servillo G, et al (1995) Titration of tidal volume and induced hypercapnia in acute respiratory distress syndrome. Am J Respir Crit Care Med 152:121–128
72. Feihl F, Perret C (1994) Permissive hypercapnia. How permissive should we be? Am J Respir Crit Care Med 150:1722–1737
73. Eichacker PQ, Gerstenberger EP, Banks SM, Cui X, Natanson C (2002) Meta-analysis of acute lung injury and acute respiratory distress syndrome trials testing low tidal volumes. Am J Respir Crit Care Med 166:1510–1514
74. Petrucci N, Iacovelli W (2004) Ventilation with smaller tidal volumes: a quantitative systematic review of randomized controlled trials. Anesth Analg 99:193–200
75. Brower RG, Lanken PN, MacIntyre N, et al (2004) Higher versus lower positive end-expiratory pressures in patients with the acute respiratory distress syndrome. N Engl J Med 351:327–336
76. Levy MM (2004) PEEP in ARDS–how much is enough? N Engl J Med 351:389–391
77. Nunes S, Uusaro A, Takala J (2004) Pressure-volume relationships in acute lung injury: methodological and clinical implications. Acta Anaesthesiol Scand 48:278–286
78. Markhorst DG, van Genderingen HR, van Vught AJ (2004) Static pressure-volume curve characteristics are moderate estimators of optimal airway pressures in a mathematical model of (primary/pulmonary) acute respiratory distress syndrome. Intensive Care Med 30:2086–2093
79. Pereira C, Bohe J, Rosselli S, et al (2003) Sigmoidal equation for lung and chest wall volume-pressure curves in acute respiratory failure. J Appl Physiol 95:2064–2071

The Ventilator of Tomorrow

L. Brochard, M. Dojat, and F. Lellouche

Introduction

The ventilator of our dreams does not exist. New technological tools have the potential to either move the ideal ventilator within our reach or make it recede into the distance. Technology is omnipresent in the ICU. The field of mechanical ventilation has benefited enormously from technological advances over the years, most notably since the development of computer science. Traditionally, the ventilator disregarded the patient's responses to mechanical ventilation, delivering a constant output until the ventilator's limits were reached. Modern ventilators can react to responses from the patient or respiratory system, thereby improving patient-ventilator synchrony, avoiding added work of breathing, and enhancing tolerance to assisted ventilation. This is achieved through closed-loop technology, in which the ventilator adapts its output in order to minimize the difference between ventilation results and predefined targets. The risks associated with mechanical ventilation have been extensively described, and decreased aggressiveness or invasiveness is now possible thanks to advanced monitoring systems and diverse ventilation modes that optimize patient-ventilator synchronization. These advances have grown out of improvements in physiological knowledge and progress in ventilation-output processing. The current surge of technological possibilities carries both the hope of priceless benefits for patients and the specter of major harm. One concern is that manufacturers, driven by commercial strategies, may make an increasing number of cosmetic changes that are based on simplistic physiological models and likely to disserve patients. Few of the new ventilation modes have proven clinical advantages [1], yet each of them increases the complexity of ventilators. Another concern is that the increased complexity of ventilator interfaces may multiply the number of setting errors. These two problems may lead to a third important source of harm, namely, a widening gap between the knowledge, understanding, and clinical skills of the average user and the complexity and sophistication of new machines. Clinicians, physiologists, and industrials must make every effort to minimize this inevitable risk.

What is Wrong With Mechanical Ventilation and Ventilators Today?

Ventilator-associated lung injury (VALI) is clearly a major threat in patients with the most severe forms of hypoxemic respiratory failure, i.e., acute lung injury (ALI) [2, 3]. When ventilatory settings are adjusted to optimize gas exchange, lung damage occurs, leading to poor outcomes [4, 5]. Thus, mechanical ventilation can be harmful to the patient, and trade-offs between gas exchange, hemodynamics, and lung distension must be made. Similar findings have been obtained in patients with asthma or obstructive lung disease [6, 7]. Surprisingly, the potential for ventilators to cause harm has often received limited attention from clinicians. Although the risk of lung damage can be decreased by simple measures (e.g., limiting plateau pressure and reducing tidal volume), lung protection remains a crucial objective that improved monitoring tools will help us to achieve.

During assisted ventilation, patient-ventilator asynchrony is being increasingly recognized as a sign that the ventilator is not meeting the patient's needs [8, 9]. Evidence from animal experiments shows a considerable impact of mechanical ventilation on diaphragm function and stresses the importance of maintaining some degree of spontaneous respiratory-muscle activity [10–13]. However, the actual synchrony provided by assisted modes is far from ideal and may not be optimal from the standpoint of preserving the respiratory muscles. Although it is difficult to evaluate the clinical consequences of asynchronies, such as missing efforts, double triggering, or prolonged inspiration, in most cases there is little reason to think that asynchrony will benefit the patient [14–17]. With non-invasive ventilation (NIV), poor synchrony may have direct adverse clinical effects [18].

Leaks are responsible for major dyssynchrony that may be difficult to recognize. For instance, in a patient with end-inspiration leaks, pressure-support ventilation may fail to synchronize with the end of the patient's inspiratory effort, as carefully analyzed by Calderini et al. [19]. In this situation, the ventilator may fail to detect the end-inspiratory off-switch, which may result in prolonged insufflation with major dyssynchrony. If leaks occur, the mask should be readjusted and the pressures reduced. In patients with persistent leaks and asynchrony, steps must be taken to minimize adverse effects on patient-ventilator interactions. During pressure-support ventilation, adjusting the cycling-off criterion or adding an inspiratory time limit helps to prevent the ventilator's inspiration from extending beyond the end of the patient's neural inspiration. These settings, however, may be difficult to access on the ventilator panel, absent, or available only indirectly. This is an interesting example of how manufacturers dealt with physiological and technical issues in a way that should benefit patients but that also creates new staff-training needs.

Asynchrony detection, on-line feedback to clinicians about the effects of current ventilatory settings or predicted effects of new settings, better technologies that minimize delays and response times, optimization of control of artifactual signals, or automatic ventilator driving in response to asynchrony are approaches that may deserve investigation in the future [20, 21]. Clearly, enhanced airway pressure control has considerably improved the sensitivity of inspiratory triggers but has also increased the risk of self-triggering. The extent to which clinicians should repeatedly optimize ventilatory settings may be difficult to determine. It is important, however, to realize that improper settings can generate major dyssynchrony, make the patient uncomfortable, and/or unnecessarily increase the work of breathing. Whether automated systems that make these adjustments based on reasonable physiological criteria will benefit both the patient and the clinician is therefore a crucial question for the future of intensive care medicine. Recently, Prinianakis et al. assessed a new automatic trigger that uses on-line flow waveform analysis [22]. They found improved trigger sensitivity with reduced work of breathing but more frequent auto-triggering. Other equivalent automatic systems have been incorporated into new ventilators but not evaluated. Automation of inspiratory cycling-off would also be helpful in improving patient-ventilator synchrony. This parameter is difficult to set, as optimal values may range from 1% to 85% of peak flow, according to the patient's respiratory mechanics [15]. Cycling-off based on automatic determination of time constants has been suggested [23], evaluated in a lung model [24], and implemented in a ventilator [25].

Specific shapes of the airway pressure and flow waveforms are related to patient-ventilator asynchronies [21] such as auto-triggering, ineffective efforts [8, 26, 27], short cycles [28], double cycles [29, 30], prolonged inspirations [28, 31], initial or final overshoot [21, 32], and premature termination [29]. Automatic recognition of these shapes followed by adjustment of the settings that cause them may deserve consideration. Figure 1 gives an example of numerous ineffective efforts that could be diagnosed by the ventilator, both from analysis of the flow signal or from esophageal pressure analysis. Figure 2 illustrates the problem of prolonged inspiration during noninvasive ventilation with leaks. The ventilator could perform similar detection automatically.

Undue prolongation of mechanical ventilation may result from failure to determine when the patient is ready to be separated from the ventilator. Furthermore, even a brief prolongation may lead to ventilation-related complications that require an additional period of mechanical ventilation [33]. Protocols for the so-called weaning phase have been found useful in some cases but unsuccessful in others, for many reasons including the difficulty in implementing such protocols into clinical practice [34, 35]. Closed-loop technology can be used to introduce weaning protocols or automated procedures into ventilatory modes.

Poor quality of the human-machine interface is another common problem. Excessive complexity is a more common cause than lack of technical options. Factors include complexity of ventilatory modes and monitoring, poor display legibility, or poor ergonomics to control the settings. Non-intuitive settings, a need for extensive training, and the non-standardized nomenclature used by manufacturers influence these factors.

What do we want from the Ventilator of Tomorrow?

Incorporation of modern monitoring tools is a first step toward improving the physiological approach to mechanical ventilation. Pressure volume (PV) curves

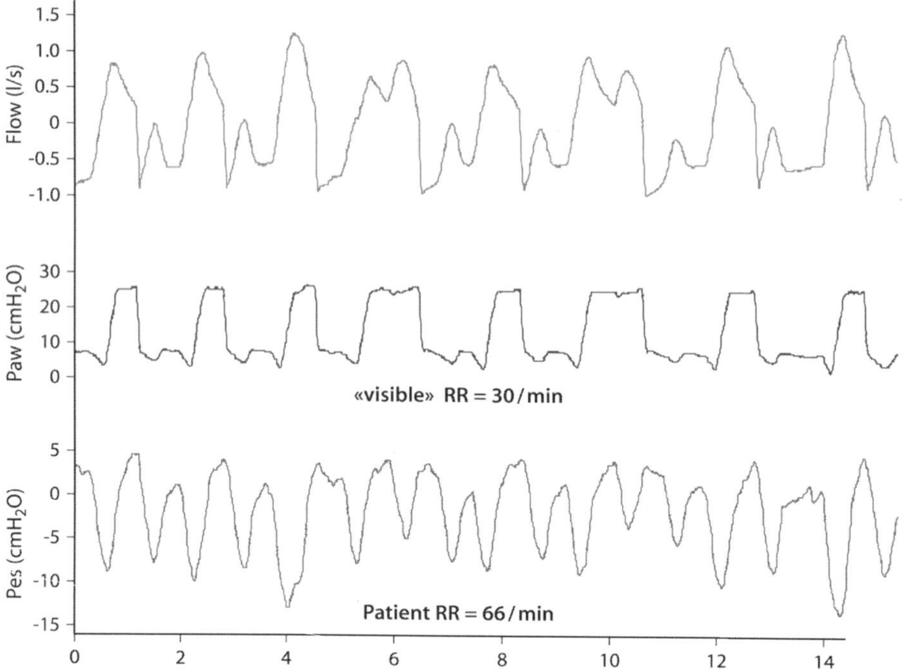

Fig. 1. An example of numerous ineffective efforts that are not detected by the ventilator from the airway pressure curve (Paw), but which could be detected from the flow signal (flow). There is a huge difference between the respiratory rate (RR) depicted by the ventilator's monitor and the true rate of the patient. The ventilator, from an automated analysis of the esophageal pressure signal (Pes), could also diagnose this and provide the two frequencies.

of the respiratory system, first used 30 years ago, are now being introduced into ventilator monitoring systems [36]. Unfortunately, a single PV measurement offers limited information, and generation of multiple loops, including tidal curves together with measurement of alveolar recruitment, will be important for optimizing ventilation in the most severely ill patients [37, 38].

Gas exchange monitoring has also improved considerably. Ironically, modern ventilators make little or no use of gas exchange monitoring, although blood gas abnormalities are the leading reason for clinician-driven changes in ventilatory settings. Little attention has been paid to monitoring carbon dioxide (CO_2) elimination in the intensive care. Today however, volumetric capnography can offer important insights into lung physiology and arterial PCO_2 trends can now be accurately assessed using transcutaneous measurements, even in adults [39–41].

Respiratory mechanics and work-of-breathing estimates may also help to improve ventilator settings [42, 43]. One difficulty is the need for semi-invasive measurements from esophageal (and gastric) probes, although a number of surrogates exist, such as occlusion pressure, also known as P0.1 [44]. Another common difficulty is the lack of precise or universally accepted threshold val-

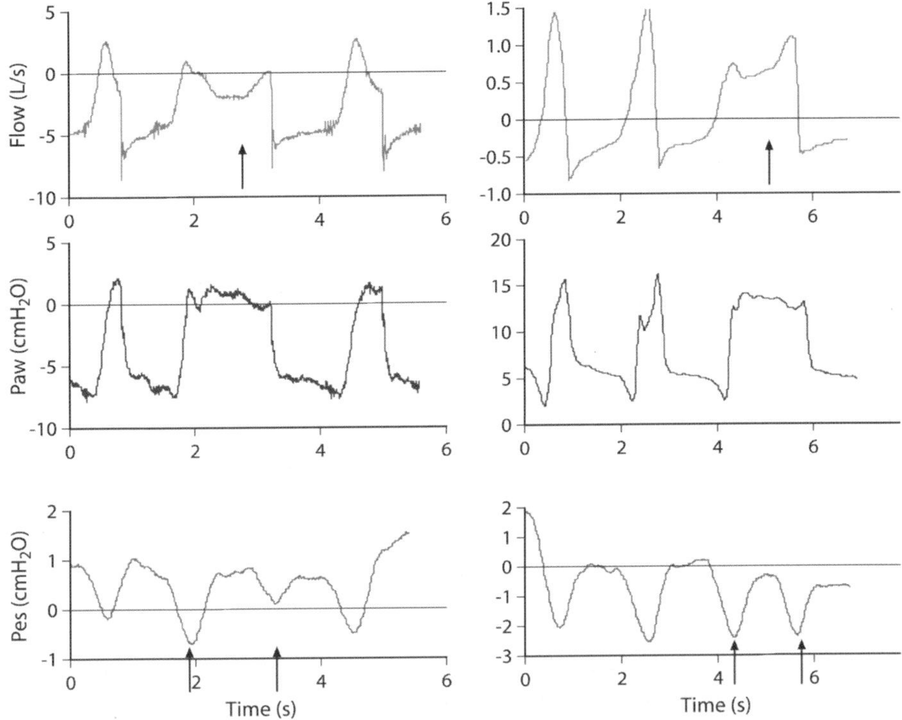

Fig. 2. Illustration of the problem of prolonged inspiration during non-invasive ventilation with leaks, as seen on the airway pressure tracing (Paw). The end of inspiration is not recognized and the insufflation time is prolonged well beyond the end of inspiration. The patient has time to expire and to take a second inspiration during the same breath, as indicated by arrows. The flow (flow) signal has a specific shape (arrow). The ventilator, from an automated analysis of the esophageal pressure signal (Pes), could also diagnose this and propose specific actions to the clinician, such as limiting the maximal inspiratory time.

ues. However, changes in measurement values over time can provide valuable information.

Working with gases that have different densities may have a number of advantages. A mixture of helium and oxygen can be used to measure and monitor lung volume. This mixture may also facilitate difficult ventilation and reduce work of breathing, especially during noninvasive ventilation [45–47]. It requires adequate calibration of transducers [48].

Sophisticated ventilation modes have been made possible by improvements in computer science [49, 50]. When the physiological and clinical knowledge needed to manage well-defined clinical situations is acquired, it can be embedded within a computer program that drives the ventilator using artificial intelligence techniques, such as production rules, fuzzy logic, or neural networks. These new techniques allow planning and control. Control is a local task that consists in determining what the immediate next step is. Planning is a strategic task aimed at regulating the time-course of the process. For control and planning, numerous techniques have been developed in the fields of control theory and artificial intelligence, respectively. The main difference between these two fields lies in the process models used. Control and planning are two complementary and essential tasks that must be combined to design multi-level controllers for automatically supervising complex systems such as mechanical ventilators. Because the driving process is based on complex physiological models, it is important to avoid both over-simplification and excessive complexity [51]. Strickland and Hasson attempted to develop a controller incorporating an active clinical strategy represented by production rules (IF conditions THEN actions), but their work was not followed by commercial development [52, 53]. Today, two control-and-planning systems are available for ventilators: adaptive support ventilation (ASV) [54, 55] and the Smart Care® system, an embedded version of the initial NeoGanesh system. ASV adapts breath frequency and pressure to deliver optimized ventilation, taking into account the optimal theoretical work of breathing, the need to minimize intrinsic positive end-expiratory pressure (PEEP), and safety limits. Clinical evaluation data remain limited [55]. The NeoGanesh (or Smart Care®) system drives the ventilator with pressure-support ventilation, keeps the patient within a zone of "respiratory comfort" as defined by respiratory parameters, and superimposes an automated strategy for weaning [56–58]. The designers of the knowledge-based NeoGanesh system intended to build a closed-loop system that 1) was efficient for automatically controlling mechanical support and planning of the weaning process, 2) could be evaluated with the goal of gradually improving its reasoning and planning capabilities, and 3) could be subjected at the bedside to performance measurements at each step of its operation. The NeoGanesh system is based on modeling of the medical expertise required to perform mechanical ventilation in pressure-support mode. It does not include mathematical equations of a physiological model. Several types of evaluation have been performed: i) to determine how well the system adapts the level of assistance to the patient's needs (evaluation of the control level), ii) to assess the extubation recommendation made by the system (evaluation of the strategic level), and iii) to estimate the impact on clinical outcomes. This system has been shown to reduce periods of excessive respiratory efforts and to predict the extubation time with considerable accuracy [57, 58]. It has been used safely during prolonged periods of mechanical ventilation [59] and has been shown recently to reduce the time spent on the ventilator [60].

Several parts of the ventilator are cumbersome, such as the screen and the humidification device (for heated humidifiers). In intensive care, monitoring the patient is essential but, rather than having several monitors for a given patient (respiratory monitoring, several screens for hemodynamic monitoring purposes, oximetry, transcutaneous or end-tidal CO_2, etc.), a single screen displaying all the information on the patient could improve the efficiency of the ICU workstation. The computer file could incorporate laboratory and radiology findings and protocols. The screen could be made separate from the ventilator, in order to decrease the bulk of the machine. Humidifiers could also be incorporated into the ventilator.

The ventilator interface could be improved [61]. Too many names and acronyms exist for each ventilation mode. Although utopian, a standardized nomenclature for modes, settings, and parameters would be highly desirable. This simple measure would improve the ventilator interface and facilitate the teaching of mechanical ventilation. Another utopian scheme consists in keeping only those ventilation modes that are truly innovative or useful and in eliminating modes that have not been proven beneficial or that might put patients at risk. For example, it is ironic to see that synchronized intermittent mandatory ventilation (SIMV) remains on all new ventilators, despite abundant evidence that this mode has many drawbacks and lengthens weaning [62–65].

What Can We Foresee for the Ventilator of Tomorrow?

Ventilator-driving systems based on the electromyographic (EMG) signal of the diaphragm can now be envisioned, given the promising results of animal and preliminary clinical studies [66, 67]. Neurally adjusted ventilatory assist offers the best possible synchrony between the patient's neural drive and the ventilatory assistance. This can eliminate delays generated by intrinsic PEEP or end-inspiration asynchronies. Also, the ventilatory signal can be made proportional to the ventilatory demand estimated from the diaphragm EMG [67]. Except in rare cases of uncoupling between the brain signal and the muscle signal, it is very close to brain-driven ventilation. The main limitation is the need for esophageal probe placement, but considerable work has been done to facilitate capturing of the signal.

Proportional-assist ventilation was described as having enormous potential for ventilating patients because it was the only modality specifically designed to adapt to changes in ventilatory demand [68]. Unfortunately, it requires continuous adjustment to respiratory mechanics. However, measurements of respiratory mechanics with adjustment of settings according to the results can now be done automatically [69, 70]. Although a bit further from the brain than the EMG signal, this method would provide an approximation of the diaphragm EMG approach without requiring an esophageal probe.

Work performed over the last few years at the LDS Hospital (Salt Lake City, Utah, USA) to develop computerized protocols is relevant here [71, 72]. The algorithm-oriented approach chosen for the LDS Hospital studies leads to a complex logic with intricate temporal aspects. The general principle consists in implementing ventilatory protocols using an open-loop approach in which the personnel interacts with the ventilator to resolve difficult problems in the most effective and standardized manner possible. Computerized tools can facilitate the representation, verification, and execution of such protocols.

Lastly, ventilator interfaces should be much more user-friendly and should offer advice to clinicians. When the ventilator detects asynchrony or inadequate settings, a dialogue should start with the user for the benefit of the patient. Modern ventilation should be more adept at meeting the patient's changing needs. At the same time, separation from the ventilator could be considered as soon as the risk of separation and subsequent extubation is deemed no greater than the risk of continuing the ventilatory assistance. All these actions require close monitoring and prompt adjustment of ventilatory settings to the patient's changing needs.

References

1. Branson RD, Johannigman JA (2004) What is the evidence base for the newer ventilation modes? Respir Care 49:742–760
2. Dreyfuss D, Saumon G (1998) From ventilator-induced lung injury to multiple organ dysfunction? Intensive Care Med 24:102–104
3. Dreyfuss D, Saumon G (1998) Ventilator-induced lung injury: lessons from experimental studies. Am J Respir Crit Care Med 157:294–323
4. ARDS Network (2000) Ventilation with lower tidal volumes as compared with traditional tidal volumes for acute lung injury and the acute respiratory distress syndrome. N Engl J Med 342:1301–1308
5. Ricard JD, Dreyfuss D, Saumon G (2002) Ventilator-induced lung injury. Curr Opin Crit Care 8:12–20
6. Pepe PE, Marini JJ (1982) Occult positive end-expiratory pressure in mechanically ventilated patients with airflow obstruction: the auto-PEEP effect. Am Rev Respir Dis 216:166–169.
7. Darioli R, Perret C (1984) Mechanical controlled hypoventilation in status asthmaticus. Am Rev Respir Dis 129:385–387
8. Leung P, Jubran A, Tobin M (1997) Comparison of assisted ventilator modes on triggering, patient effort and dyspnea. Am J Respir Crit Care Med 155:1940–1948
9. Nava S, Bruschi C, Rubini F, Palo A, Iotti G, Braschi A (1995) Respiratory response and inspiratory effort during pressure support ventilation in COPD patients. Intensive Care Med 21:871–879
10. Anzueto A, Peter JI, Tobin MJ, et al (1997) Effects of prolonged controlled mechanical ventilation on diaphragmatic function in healthy adult baboons. Crit Care Med 25:1187–1190
11. Sassoon CS, Caiozzo VJ, Manka A, Sieck GC (2002) Altered diaphragm contractile properties with controlled mechanical ventilation. J Appl Physiol 92:2585–2595
12. Sassoon CS (2002) Ventilator-associated diaphragmatic dysfunction. Am J Respir Crit Care Med 166:1017–1018
13. Sassoon CS, Zhu E, Caiozzo VJ (2004) Assist-control mechanical ventilation attenuates ventilator-induced diaphragmatic dysfunction. Am J Respir Crit Care Med 170:626–632
14. Rossi A, Appendini L (1995) Wasted efforts and dyssynchrony: is the patient-ventilator battle back? Intensive Care Med 21:867–870
15. Yamada Y, Du HL (2000) Analysis of the mechanisms of expiratory asynchrony in pressure support ventilation: a mathematical approach. J Appl Physiol 88:2143–2150
16. Hotchkiss J, Adams AB, Stone MK, Dries DJ, Marini JJ, Crooke PS (2002) Oscillations and noise: inherent instability of pressure support ventilation? Am J Respir Crit Care Med 165:47–53
17. Younes M, Kun J, Webster K, Roberts D (2002) Response of ventilator-dependent patients to delayed opening of exhalation valve. Am J Respir Crit Care Med 166:21–30
18. Brochard L (1993) Non invasive ventilation: practical issues. Intensive Care Med 19:431–432
19. Calderini E, Confalonieri M, Puccio PG, Francavilla N, Stella L, Gregoretti C (1999) Patient-ventilator asynchrony during noninvasive ventilation: the role of expiratory trigger. Intensive Care Med 25:662–667

20. Richard JC, Carlucci A, Breton L, et al (2002) Bench testing of pressure support ventilation with three different generations of ventilators. Intensive Care Med 28:1049–1057
21. Hess DR(2005) Ventilator waveforms and the physiology of pressure support ventilation. Respir Care 50:166–186
22. Prinianakis G, Kondili E, Georgopoulos D (2003) Effects of the flow waveform method of triggering and cycling on patient-ventilator interaction during pressure support. Intensive Care Med 29:1950–1959
23. Du HL, Ohtsuji M, Shigeta M, et al (2002) Expiratory asynchrony in proportional assist ventilation. Am J Respir Crit Care Med 165:972–977
24. Du HL, Amato MB, Yamada Y (2001) Automation of expiratory trigger sensitivity in pressure support ventilation. Respir Care Clin N Am 7:503–517
25. Branson R (2004) Understanding and implementing advances in ventilator capabilities. Curr Opin Crit Care 10:23–32
26. Nava S, Bruschi C, Rubini F, Palo A, Iotti G, Braschi A (1995) Respiratory response and inspiratory effort during pressure support ventilation in COPD patients. Intensive Care Med 21:871–879
27. Chao DC, Scheinhorn DJ, Stearn-Hassenpflug M (1997) Patient-ventilator trigger asynchrony in prolonged mechanical ventilation. Chest 112:1592–1599
28. Pertusini E, Lellouche F, Catani F, et al (2004) Patient-ventilator asynchronies during NIV: does level of pressure support matter? Intensive Care Med 30:S65 (abst)
29. Tokioka H, Tanaka T, Ishizu T, et al (2001) The effect of breath termination criterion on breathing patterns and the work of breathing during pressure support ventilation. Anesth Analg 92:161–165
30. Jubran A (1999) Inspiratory flow rate: more may not be better. Crit Care Med 27:670–671
31. Calderini E, Confalonieri M, Puccio PG, Francavilla N, Stella L, Gregoretti C (1999) Patient-ventilator asynchrony during noninvasive ventilation: the role of expiratory trigger. Intensive Care Med 25:662–667
32. MacIntyre N, Nishimura M, Usada Y, Tokioka H, Takezawa J, Shimada Y (1990) The Nagoya conference on system design and patient-ventilator interactions during pressure support ventilation. Chest 97:1463–1466
33. Ely EW, Baker AM, Dunagan DP, et al (1996) Effect on the duration of mechanical ventilation of identifying patients capable of breathing spontaneously. N Engl J Med 335:1864–1869
34. Ely EW, Bennett PA, Bowton DL, Murphy SM, Florance AM, Haponik EF (1999) Large scale implementation of a respiratory therapist-driven protocol for ventilator weaning. Am J Respir Crit Care Med 159:439–446
35. Krishnan JA, Moore D, Robeson C, Rand CS, Fessler HE (2004) A prospective, controlled trial of a protocol-based strategy to discontinue mechanical ventilation. Am J Respir Crit Care Med 169:673–678
36. Brochard L (1998) Pressure-volume curves. In: Tobin MJ (ed) Principles and Practice of Respiratory Monitoring. McGraw-Hill, Inc., New York, pp 579–616.
37. Rimensberger PC, Cheng A, Frndova H, Mannion D, Nakagawa S (2005) Ventilation with PEEP above the inflection point increases the risk of air leaks. Am J Respir Crit Care Med 151:A432 (abst)
38. Maggiore SM, Jonson B, Richard JC, Jaber S, Lemaire F, Brochard L (2001) Alveolar derecruitment at decremental positive end-expiratory pressure levels in acute lung injury: comparison with the lower inflection point, oxygenation, and compliance. Am J Respir Crit Care Med 164:795–801
39. Romero PV, Lucangelo U, Lopez Aguilar J, Fernandez R, Blanch L (1997) Physiologically based indices of volumetric capnography in patients receiving mechanical ventilation. Eur Respir J 10:1309–1315

40. Riou Y, Leclerc F, Neve V, et al (2004) Reproducibility of the respiratory dead space measurements in mechanically ventilated children using the CO2SMO monitor. Intensive Care Med 30:1461–1467
41. Rodriguez P, Lellouche F, Aboab J, Brun-Buisson C, Brochard L (2004) Transcutaneous arterial carbon dioxide partial pressure monitoring in ICU patients. Intensive Care Med 30:S168 (abst)
42. Cinnella G, Conti G, Lofaso F, et al (1996) Effets of assisted ventilation on the work of breathing: volume-controlled versus pressure-controlled ventilation. Am J Respir Crit Care Med 153:1025–1033
43. Tobin MJ, Van de Graaff W (1994) Monitoring of lung mechanics and work of breathing. In: Tobin MJ (ed) Principles and Practice of Mechanical Ventilation. McGraw-Hill, New York, pp 967–1004
44. Mancebo J, Albaladejo P, Touchard D, et al (2000) Airway occlusion pressure to titrate positive end-expiratory pressure in patients with dynamic hyperinflation. Anesthesiology 93:81–90
45. Jaber S, Fodil R, Carlucci A, et al (2000) Noninvasive ventilation with helium-oxygen in acute exacerbations of chronic obstructive pulmonary disease. Am J Respir Crit Care Med 161:1191–1200
46. Jaber S, Carlucci A, Boussarsar M, et al (2001) Helium-oxygen in the postextubation period decreases inspiratory effort. Am J Respir Crit Care Med 164:1–5
47. Tassaux D, Jolliet P, Roeseler J, Chevrolet JC (2000) Effects of helium-oxygen on intrinsic positive end-expiratory pressure in intubated and mechanically ventilated patients with severe chronic obstructive pulmonary disease. Crit Care Med 28:2721-2728
48. Tassaux D, Jolliet P, Thouret JM, Roeseler J, Dorne R, Chevrolet JC (1999) Calibration of seven ICU ventilators for mechanical ventilation with helium-oxygen mixtures. Am J Respir Crit Care Med 160:22–32
49. Brunner JX (2001) Principles and history of closed-loop controlled ventilation. Respir Care Clin N Am 7:341–362
50. Dojat M, Brochard L (2001) Knowledge-based systems for automatic ventilatory management. Respir Care Clin N Am 7:379–396
51. Sottiaux TM (2001) Patient-ventilator interactions during volume-support ventilation: asynchrony and tidal volume instability–a report of three cases. Respir Care 46:255–262
52. Strickland JH, Hasson JH (1991) A computer-controlled ventilator weaning system. Chest 100:1096–1099
53. Strickland JH, Hasson JH (1993) A computer-controlled ventilator weaning system. Chest 103:1220–1226
54. Brunner JX, Iotti GA (2002) Adaptive support ventilation (ASV). Minerva Anestesiol 68:365–368
55. Sulzer CF, Chiolero R, Chassot PG, Mueller XM, Revelly JP (2001) Adaptive support ventilation for fast tracheal extubation after cardiac surgery: a randomized controlled study. Anesthesiology 95:1339–1345
56. Dojat M, Brochard L, Lemaire F, Harf A (1992) A knowledge based system for assisted ventilation of patients in intensive care units. Int J Clin Monit Comput 9:239–250
57. Dojat M, Harf A, Touchard D, Laforest M, Lemaire F, Brochard L (1996) Evaluation of a knowledge-based system providing ventilatory management and decision for extubation. Am J Respir Crit Care Med 153:997–1004
58. Dojat M, Harf A, Touchard D, Lemaire F, Brochard L (2000) Clinical evaluation of a computer-controlled pressure support mode. Am J Respir Crit Care Med 161:1161–1166
59. Bouadma L, Lellouche F, Cabello M, et al (2005) A computer driven system to manage weaning during prolonged mechanical ventilation: a pilot study. Intensive Care Med (in press)

60. Lellouche F, Mancebo J, Jolliet P, et al (2004) Computer-driven ventilation reduces duration of weaning: a multicenter randomized controlled study. Intensive Care Med 30:S69 (abst)
61. Taille S, Lellouche F, Fartoukh M, Brochard L (2003) Évaluation de la simplicité d'utilisation de huit ventilateurs de réanimation. Réanimation 12:239S (abst).
62. Hess D (2001) Ventilator modes used in weaning. Chest 120:474S–476S
63. Brochard L, Rauss A, Benito S, et al (1994) Comparison of three methods of gradual withdrawal from ventilatory support during weaning from mechanical ventilation. Am J Respir Crit Care Med 150:896–903
64. Cook D, Meade M, Guyatt G, Griffith L, Booker L (2000) Criteria for weaning from mechanical ventilation. Evid Rep Technol Assess (Summ):1–4
65. Esteban A, Frutos F, Tobin MJ, et al (1995) A comparison of four methods of weaning patients from mechanical ventilation. Spanish Lung Failure Collaborative Group. N Engl J Med 332:345–350
66. Sinderby C, Navalesi P, Beck J, et al (1999) Neural control of mechanical ventilation in respiratory failure. Nature Med 5:1433–1436
67. Sinderby C (2002) Neurally adjusted ventilatory assist (NAVA). Minerva Anestesiol 68:378–380
68. Younes M (1994) Proportional assist ventilation. In: Tobin MJ (ed) Principles and Practice of Mechanical Ventilation. McGraw-Hill, Inc, New York, pp 349–369
69. Younes M, Webster K, Kun J, Roberts D, Masiowski B (2001) A method for measuring passive elastance during proportional assist ventilation. Am J Respir Crit Care Med 164:50–60
70. Younes M, Kun J, Masiowski B, Webster K, Roberts D (2001) A method for noninvasive determination of inspiratory resistance during proportional assist ventilation. Am J Respir Crit Care Med 163:829–839
71. East T, Böhm SH, Wallace CJ, et al (1992) A successful computerized protocol for clinical management of pressure control inverse ratio ventilation in ARDS patients. Chest 101:697–710
72. Morris AH, Wallace CJ, Menlovet RL, et al (1994) Randomized clinical trial of pressure-controlled inverse ratio ventilation and extracorporeal CO2 removal for adult respiratory distress syndrome. Am J Respir Crit Care Med 149:295–305

My NeuroICU 10 Years from Now

D. K. Menon

Introduction

In general, success in intensive care medicine has been predicated by the ability to buy time for a specific therapy to work, and for tissue repair to result in recovery of organ function. Unfortunately, this paradigm of intensive care medicine does not apply to many neurological diseases that come to critical care units. There are few specific therapies available for traumatic brain injury (TBI) or ischemic stroke, and the adult brain is thought to have limited capacity for repair.

Therapeutic Targets: Primary and Secondary Neuronal Injury Mechanisms

Classically, acute disorders of the central nervous system (CNS), and particularly of the brain, are best thought of as comprising two distinct sets of pathophysiological processes [1]. The first of these is primary neurological injury, which includes the physical impact in TBI, vascular occlusion and ischemia in ischemic stroke, and tissue disruption in intracerebral hemorrhage. Several preventive interventions are available to reduce the incidence and severity of these insults (seat belts and speed limits for TBI, antiplatelet drugs for ischemic stroke, and antihypertensive therapy for intracerebral hemorrhage). However, although these interventions deserve our wholehearted support, their implementation is outside the remit of critical care medicine.

Data from experimental models have shown, however, that several reactive processes are activated in response to primary injury, both within the brain, and systemically [1, 2]. These processes are responsible for secondary neuronal injury, and can have a major impact on outcome. Alterations in systemic physiology, such as hypoxia and hypotension and hyperglycemia, have been shown to worsen outcome in animal models, and in epidemiological analysis of clinical data sets. There is accumulating evidence (although not of Class I quality) that prevention or rapid correction of such physiological insults may improve clinical outcome in patients [3]. However, the concordance between experimental and clinical data is far less secure for secondary injury mechanisms that operate within the brain. There is a huge body of literature that shows benefit from drugs or other specific interventions that modulate such secondary neuronal injury mechanisms in experimental models. However, attempts to extrapolate these findings to clinical disease have been frustrating [4, 5].

The Limitations of Optimizing Systemic Physiology

Much of intensive care for these patients is therefore confined to supportive optimization of systemic physiology [3], but even this is a relatively crude process. We are only just beginning to understand the heterogeneity in pathophysiology among individual patients, and bedside techniques are lacking for determining responses to therapy in different parts of the injured brain. This is a particularly significant shortcoming in conditions such as TBI, where pathophysiology may be substantially discordant in different parts of the brain [6]. Furthermore, the brain is unforgiving in its tolerance to physiological insults. Neuronal injury is exacerbated by short epochs of systemic physiological decompensation that are unlikely to affect other organs. Finally, extracranial organ dysfunction and failure are common in severe neurological disease [7], with two undesirable consequences. First, extracranial organ dysfunction and failure may increase the incidence and severity of physiological insults, which worsen brain injury. Second, the demands of maintaining physiological targets appropriate for minimizing secondary neuronal injury may significantly conflict with modern approaches to supporting and treating systemic organ dysfunction.

Cause For Optimism and a Basis for Predicting the Future

While the discussion in previous sections underlines many of the difficulties associated with neurocritical care, there are clear causes for optimism.

Demonstration of the Efficacy of Neurocritical Care

A clutch of publications over the last two years attests to the efficacy of protocol driven neurocritical care in improving outcome. Patel et al. showed that establishment of an evidence-based head injury management algorithm resulted in significant improvements in outcome from severe head injury, when compared to historical controls [8], and similar results were reported by Elf et al. in a population that included all head injury admissions to critical care [9]. Significantly, while only Elf et al. [9] showed improvements in mortality, both papers reported clear improvements in the proportion of patients experiencing favorable outcomes (from 40.4 to 59.6% in severe head injury [8] and from 40 to 84% in all head injured patients [9]). These data suggest that good quality neurocritical care has its most consistent impact not on survival, but on the even more important goal of achieving better quality of survival. It is also clear that these results are best achieved by professional intensivists. Diringer et al., using data collected by Project Impact found that mortality following intracerebral hemorrhage was significantly increased (odds ratio 3.4; 95% CI 1.65–7.6) in units not staffed by a full time intensivist even when Glasgow Coma Scale (GCS) score, age, caseload, and unit size were accounted for [10]. Similarly, Varelas et al. [11] and Suarez et al [12] showed that care by a neurointensivist led team improved outcomes.

While these data do not clearly make the case for specialist neurointensive care units, evidence suggests that implementation of high quality protocol-driven management is more effective in some intensive care units (ICUs) than others. Bulger et al. [13] found that units that practiced more aggressive management along guidelines recommended by the Brain Trauma Foundation, such as placement of intracranial pressure (ICP) monitors in over 50% of such patients, achieved a significant reduction in the risk of mortality (hazard ratio 0.43; 95% CI 0.27–0.66), when compared to units that did not. Another recent publication, based on data collected as part of the National Acute Brain Injury Study: Hypothermia (NABISH) Trial [14] addressed a similar theme, and found no significant differences in the incidence or severity of episodes of intracranial hypertension among centres. However, there were significant differences in the maintenance of mean arterial pressure and cerebral perfusion pressure (CPP) targets, vasopressor usage, and tendency to dehydrate patients. Large units with many head injury admissions performed better, suggesting that management in these units was more sophisticated, and aimed to optimize cerebrovascular physiology in a more integrated fashion.

Better Knowledge of Pathophysiology May Contribute to Improved Outcomes

The commentaries and correspondence that accompany these papers make instructive reading. Kochanek et al. [15] make the point that neurointensive care is not simply a label, but a way of life. Clinical teams who frequently care for patients with acute brain insults are more likely to have knowledge regarding the impact of secondary physiological insults, and be more obsessive about minimizing their occurrence. Chesnut [16] makes the case for centers not just specializing in neurocritical care, but in the management of patients with TBI. There may be differences in outcome depending on whether patients are managed according to protocols that conform to different paradigms of neurocritical care [17, 18], but these clearly appear to be less important than those that result from being cared for by a clinical team, which understands the pathophysiology and has a professional interest in a given area of medicine. It is also important to note that specialization often attracts greater volumes of patients, and greater caseload is very likely to improve expertise in this area, as in others [19]. These considerations strongly suggest that the emergence of specialist neurocritical care units may represent not just another turf battle, but a development that answers a clinical need [20].

Better Knowledge Will Lead to Improved Individualization of Therapy

Improved understanding of pathophysiology has enabled us to understand mechanisms in human disease, and to identify how individual diseases differ from each other [21]. However, it is also important to understand the existence of inter-individual differences within a single disease category. Unsurprisingly, differences may arise from disease severity and co-morbidities, which predispose patients to worse clinical outcome, or make them prone to specific complications (both of the primary disease and its therapy). However, such individual differences may arise from more fundamental biological variation. For example, there is accumulating evidence that gender [22] and genotype [23, 24] may be important determinants of neurological outcome following head injury and cardiopulmonary bypass. Understanding how genetic polymorphisms modulate outcome may enable us to select patients for more intensive monitoring and physiological support, or even identify which patients are most likely to benefit from individual therapies. It is important to acknowledge that while genetic information may suggest a prominent role for an individual disease mechanism in a given patient, rational use of powerful therapies will require us to define when these processes are active within the time course of disease within patients, so that these interventions can be targeted at the appropriate time, and ideally titrated for maximum benefit within individual patients.

Understanding of Pathophysiology is Facilitated by Better Clinical Monitoring Tools.

The improved knowledge of pathophysiology amongst neurointensivists that Kochanek [15] and Chesnut [16] describe is the consequence of monitoring tools that allow us to document clinical physiology in translational medicine studies, rather than infer it (often incorrectly) from experimental studies in animal models. The last 20 years have seen substantial advances in the technology available for clinical monitoring in these patient groups. While the primary purpose of such advances must always be improved clinical care, the information that they provide has also advanced the practice of experimental medicine in the acutely injured brain.

Thus, ICP monitoring, jugular oximetry and transcranial Doppler ultrasound are now integral parts of many clinical protocols and management algorithms for head injury [25, 26], subarachnoid hemorrhage (SAH) [27], and (increasingly) ischemic stroke [28]. However, these tools also have enabled us to better understand the cerebrovascular pathophysiology and abnormal oxygen supply-dependency relationships that underpin many disease states. In addition, access to cerebrospinal fluid (CSF, from ventricular ICP catheters) and to blood directly draining the brain (from jugular bulb catheters) has allowed us to directly study events that occur in the cerebral microvasculature and extracellular fluid compartment [29, 30]. These results have provided us with a wealth of information regarding the neurobiology of human brain injury, and will inform the development and application of novel therapies.

More recently, the advent of near infrared spectroscopy (NIRS) [31], tissue oximetry probes [32], and cerebral microdialysis [30] has provided new information. Some of this information has confirmed previous understanding of

Table 1. Some techniques that image function in the injured brain

Functional imaging techniques	Abbreviation
Xenon computed tomography	Xe-CT
Dynamic contrast enhanced CT	Dyn CT
Perfusion weighted MRI	PWI
Diffusion weighted MRI	DWI
Blood oxygen level dependent functional MRI	BOLD fMRI
Positron emission tomography	PET

MRI: magnetic resonance imaging

disease mechanisms, while other results have led to entirely new paradigms of pathophysiology [33], which suggest the need for novel therapeutic strategies.

Perhaps the most exciting advances have been in the field of physiological imaging. X-Ray computed tomography (CT) made an enormous difference to clinical neuroscience when it was introduced in 1970s, and more recently, the clear benefits of magnetic resonance imaging (MRI) have revolutionized structural brain imaging [34]. Further dissemination of these techniques is vitally important, and the application of MRI to diseases such as head injury and ischemic stroke is still in development. However, such structural imaging may document disease progression in the brain at a stage when it is too late to intervene. Consequently, an enormous amount of interest has focused on techniques that image function (rather than structure) in the injured brain, and allow us to map spatially resolved physiology (Table 1) [34–38].

Of the techniques listed in Table 1, Xenon (Xe)-CT has been used to image cerebral blood flow (CBF) in many acute neurological diseases, while perfusion-weighted MRI (PWI) and diffusion-weighted MRI (DWI) have been used primarily to provide clinically relevant means of defining the core and penumbra in ischemic stroke. More recently positron emission tomography (PET) has been used to document ischemia and provide valuable insights regarding regional variations in physiology in head injury.

Insights from some Effective Therapies

Thrombolysis in ischemic stroke represents one specific therapy that has experienced clinical success [39], but does not, in the most commonly understood sense, provide an example of effective neuroprotection against secondary insults. However, it is important to point out that there are a few neuroprotective interventions that have been successful. These are important, since they provide evidence that neuroprotection against secondary injury is, at least in principle, an achievable goal. The list of such interventions includes nimodipine in aneurysmal SAH [40] and hypothermia in cardiac arrest [41, 42]. These examples are also intriguing, since both interventions have been shown to be ineffective in other settings in acute CNS insults, such as head injury [43, 44], where experimental studies would suggest efficacy. This discordance leads to one of two inferences; either our understanding of disease mechanisms in these diseases is wrong, or the side effects of these interventions may be differential in specific clinical populations.

In practice, such failures are probably a combination of both these circumstances. It is very likely that the individual disease mechanisms identified in experimental studies have different temporal patterns and significance in different clinical diseases, which can only be identified by high quality experimental medicine studies of pathophysiology in patients. However, there is accumulating evidence that neuroprotective interventions such as hypothermia may have significant side effects [45], which may substantially worsen outcome and negate any inherent neuroprotective effect of the intervention, unless they are adequately treated.

The Reversal of Therapeutic Nihilism

Perhaps the greatest benefit of the relatively modest successes that have been outlined in previous sections is their role in sustaining some clinical optimism, particularly in the face of repeatedly negative Phase III studies of neuroprotective agents over the last two decades [46]. This optimism has encouraged continued rapid referral and close clinical monitoring in conditions, such as head injury and stroke, providing clinical populations that are suitable for more realistically timed neuroprotective interventions. For example, only a small proportion of patients with ischemic stroke will reach hospital early enough to benefit from thrombolytic therapy within the classical time frame of three hours prescribed by the original National Institute of Neurological Disorders and Stroke (NINDS) study [47]. However, the attempt to meet such deadlines has encouraged more rapid hospital referral of conditions previously thought to merit only general supportive therapy. It is also important to point out that within hospital, such patients are now much more likely to be referred to ICUs, and over time, are likely to be seen in specialist neurocritical care units with specialist expertise in dealing with these problems.

It is also important to acknowledge that organizational changes in the delivery of health care may have significant impact in these areas, as in others. Thus, better organized trauma retrieval may be responsible for better outcome at a community-wide level [48], early referral of patients with ischemic stroke for thrombolysis is likely to improve outcome [49], while the implementation of rational protocols for clinical management may improve outcome within individual hospitals and ICUs [8, 9].

Recognition that the Brain has Capacity for Repair

The conventional view that the adult brain is incapable of repair has now been challenged [50]. We know that neural precursor cells exist in the human brain under normal circumstances, and that their turnover is substantially accelerated after acute neurological insults. Further, experimental studies show benefits from the administration of neuronal precursor cells, or even more excitingly, cord blood derived stem cells [51] or bone marrow stromal cells [52]. While some of these cells may contribute directly to neurogenesis, recent evidence suggests that a more prominent role may involve the secretion of trophic factors, which enhance angiogenesis and promote neurogenesis in endogenous stem cells, perhaps by downregulating repressor molecules and processes. In other settings, brain repair may depend on preventing neuronal death or damage through the action of neurotrophins, or through promotion of endogenous plasticity in surviving neurons, rather than the generation of new neurons. Also relevant is the exciting evidence that molecules (such as chemokines) that promote neuroinflammation and tissue injury, may also act as cues for recruitment of cells that participate in such repair mechanisms. If exploited, this phenomenon may solve one of the greatest problems that has faced cell based therapies in the CNS – that of targeting therapies to the site of injury without using invasive techniques.

More generally, it has been recognized that many of the intense inflammatory and reactive processes that may worsen neural injury in the acute phase, may actually promote recovery and repair when activated at relatively less intense levels in the chronic phase [50]. One of the challenges for the future must focus on being able to identify this dichotomy of effect for many of the processes we seek to antagonize, since inhibiting them to an inappropriate extent and at an inappropriate time may not only prevent benefit, but actually worsen tissue outcome.

Neurocritical Care in 2015: A synthesis

Epidemiological Drivers and Public Health Modifiers

Across the board, continuing improvements in emergency vehicle response, at least in Europe, will result in more rapid access to our patients. This change may have disparate effects. Early access to critical care may reduce the burden of secondary insults, and allow reduced neurological impact and possibly quicker discharge. However, it is also possible that such rapid response may allow patients who would have died in the prehospital phase to make it to hospital; these patients will have more severe disease or injury, and will demand greater ICU resources.

It is likely that the incidence of severe TBI will continue to decrease, both because of traffic legislation and safer vehicle design technology. However, the number of admissions with TBI to neuroICUs is likely to stay the same, or may even increase, as there is an increasing appreciation that close monitoring of physiology and protocol-driven therapy are beneficial in less severe head injury. It is well recognized that neurocognitive outcome can be extremely poor even after mild head injury [53] and that such patients may represent a significant socioeconomic burden. While these patients are less likely to require intensive care for their injury *per se*, the successful neuroprotective interventions may have side effects that require ICU care (e.g., mild hypothermia). While this would seem highly unlikely in the present context, attitudes may change if therapy was shown to have individual and societal benefits.

Conversely, there is likely to be a sharp increase in the number of patients admitted for specialist neurocritical care following ischemic stroke. There are already good data showing that protocol driven therapy in stroke units can improve outcome in this setting [54], but there is a clear need to understand whether the close physiological monitoring and stability achieved in critical care in other settings, such as in head injury, can have benefits in stroke. Thus far, any evidence of benefit (or even assessment of benefit) of such management has been limited [28], but improvements in bedside monitoring techniques may allow us to reconcile the hitherto opposing imperatives of continuous cerebrovascular monitoring and early ambulation. It is likely that the demonstrable efficacy of newer thrombolytic and neuroprotective interventions, coupled with increasing safety, may lead to use of these interventions in a larger proportion of patients with ischemic stroke, perhaps at longer intervals post stroke. In any case, the efficacy of conventional thrombolysis, coupled with better public education (e.g., the "Brain Attack Coalition" initiative [55]) is likely to result in a larger proportion of patients with ischemic stroke arriving in hospital early. What remains unclear is whether these patients will be cared for in specialized stroke units, or will require admission to critical care units. At a more general level, effective primary prevention may delay the age of onset of ischemic stroke, but changing public expectations mean that these older patients may well demand the full benefits of intensive care.

There is an increasing tendency to use non-operative techniques to manage intracranial hemorrhage. The International Subarachnoid Aneurysm Trial (ISAT) seemed to strongly support the use of interventional neuroradiology for aneurysmal SAH [56], while preliminary results from the Surgical Trial in Intracerebral Hemorrhage (STICH) have lead to greater reluctance to surgically evacuate intracerebral hematomas. The impact of these changes on neurocritical care remains unclear. At first sight, the reduced incidence of surgery might be expected to lead to a reduced requirement for postoperative critical care, but this view ignores several confounds. Coiling of aneurysms will not reduce morbidity associated with delayed ischemic neurological deficit (commonly referred to as vasospasm), and the fact that cisternal blood is not evacuated at surgery may theoretically increase its incidence. However, the perception that coiling is less invasive than surgery may lead to its use in older, sicker patients, who will require longer periods of intensive care if they have been offered the option of definitive therapy.

At a generic level, demographic changes will mean that more major neurosurgical procedures will be performed in older patients with several comorbidities, while improvements in operative techniques with result in more complex surgical interventions; this combination of circumstances suggests the need for increased critical care requirements.

Finally, the shape and nature of what happens to all critical care services will be dictated in large part by what happens to the hospitals in which they are sited. Across the United Kingdom, there has been increasing pressure to shift elective surgery to day-stay units, and to aim for early discharge of patients who do come in for inpatient procedures. Such rapid throughput has already compromised the ability of wards to care for patients who are even moderately sick. Indeed, in the United Kingdom, Outreach Teams from critical care units are becoming significantly involved in the care of patients on the wards, in an effort to avoid ICU admission and readmission (the 'bounce back' syndrome) [57]. If these trends continue, it is very likely that the critical care services will have to assume (at least partial) responsibility for the care of patients outside the ICU (sometimes referred to as critical care without walls). This approach is likely to be particularly relevant in patients with severe neurological disease, in whom depressed levels of consciousness, long term airway problems, and ventilatory insufficiency, increase the risk of extracranial morbidity and need for 'preventive' critical care.

Individualizing Therapy to Match Individual Host Responses

There is now clear evidence that genotype affects outcome from neurological insults, but this concept has, thus far, not resulted in any changes in the way individual patients receive critical care. The best studied genotypic influence on outcome involves the apolipoprotein E (ApoE) gene, which is not clearly tied to a particular pathophysiological mechanism. This situation could change in one of two ways. First, we may be able to elucidate the mechanisms by which possession of an ApoE*ε4* genotype actually modulates outcome; one possibility is the deposition of beta-amyloid [23]. Such knowledge would identify a subgroup of patients who are more likely to respond to interventions aimed at those mechanisms [58]. Conversely, we may find that host response genes that have been implicated elsewhere (in sepsis, for example) [59], have an important impact on outcome. If this were the case, we may find that a subset of patients with an enhanced inflammatory response respond preferentially to targeted anti-inflammatory interventions. Alternatively, we may find that patients with established functional polymorphisms in genes that modulate neurotransmitter production or breakdown, receptor affinity, or neurotrophin levels, have greater susceptibility to trans-synaptic neural injury, and a better chance of response to anti-excitotoxic drugs. Given these considerations, it seems plausible that at some stage in the future, patients admitted to neurocritical care will be rapidly genotyped for a clutch of key functional polymorphisms which modulate severity of disease (or at least individual disease mechanisms), and, as a corollary, have a higher chance of benefit from therapies aimed at such processes. Since such genotypic variations will be substantially confounded by disease or injury severity, detection of a high risk genotype may simply trigger, in the initial case, closer monitoring of key biomarker levels in such patients, for reasons of prognostication, early detection of deterioration, or therapy choice.

Better Monitoring Will Lead to Better Management

The title of this section is in some ways self evident, but the critical issue is how one defines better monitoring. In the past, more monitoring has always been assumed to be better, but we need to season this attitude with healthy skepticism. More monitoring may provide additional information, but whether this is an improvement or not depends on several attributes. We need to be certain that such information is accurate, relevant and useful, and that the risk-benefit ratio associated with its collection is positive. Achieving these requirements may require different approaches in different situations.

In general, there is an overriding imperative to move towards non-invasive monitoring, wherever this can be shown to be accurate and reliable. The insertion of intracranial probes for measuring ICP and tissue chemistry is, at present, unavoidable. While non-invasive estimation of CPP, using transcranial Doppler ultrasound, has been suggested [60], this is not fully reliable, and remains unsuitable for routine monitoring in patients ,who have, or are at high risk of having, intracranial hypertension. Similarly, although NIRS has had some success, it has not replaced jugular bulb oximetry for assessing the adequacy of cerebral oxygen delivery. It is very likely that these non-invasive technologies will evolve further, but I would estimate that clinically usable versions of these devices will be approaching wide spread testing, rather than routine clinical use by 2015. However, I would expect more rapid progress in two specific situations.

First, there is a substantial advantage to be gained from multiplexing invasive probes so that the risks of tissue injury are substantially reduced. I foresee many manufacturers offering a single probe with a variety of options, starting with a baseline of ICP plus temperature measurement, with the ability to also monitor PO_2, PCO_2 and pH, and possibly the incorporation of specific sensors that measure lactate and glucose levels. Such developments will increase the cost of composite probes, but ease of insertion and reduced insertion risk will make their evaluation far easier and more widespread, and if benefit is proven, widespread use may result in economies of scale, which reduce device costs.

Second, there may be situations where current non-invasive monitors may find use, despite their lack of precision. These include the prehospital or emergency room setting, or less severe disease (e.g., some patients with moderate head injury) where the likelihood of a positive finding does not justify the risks of invasive monitoring, but estimation of the probability of a pathophysiological process (e.g., intracranial hypertension) may significantly facilitate management. Current implementations of transcranial Doppler and NIRS for these applications remain cumbersome and require specially trained personnel. In the future, these tools will need to be far simpler, if their application in prehospital medicine can even be adequately assessed, let alone recommended. There remains, however, an undeniable (and as yet unfulfilled) need for better prehospital CNS monitoring in the unconscious patient. The development of such monitoring may also involve innovation in probe design that allows ambulatory monitoring. For example, the development of ambulatory transcranial Doppler monitoring may allow the monitoring of CBF in patients with ischemic stroke without the need for them to stay in bed.

Within the ICU itself, we need to make better use of the data that we do correct. Bedside multimodality monitoring has become complex; further increases in utility will only be possible if we find ways of integrating such information and improving its presentation. The use of expert systems may not only make intermediate pathophysiological inferences, but also suggest appropriate therapy [61]. For example, appropriate signal processing approaches to ICP and arterial waveforms can provide valuable information regarding the preservation of autoregulation and changes in autoregulatory thresholds. Further, an intelligent analysis of such information may allow individualization of such therapy.

In other settings, monitoring approaches may need to become more complex, rather than simpler. The detail provided by such complexity may result in better understanding of physiological processes; thus, PET, with measurement of regional oxygen extraction fraction has demonstrated true ischemia, when simpler techniques such as Xe-CT, even when combined with jugular oximetry, were unable to distinguish this abnormality from reductions in CBF that were coupled to hypometabolism. Alternatively, imaging of regional (rather than measurement of global) physiology may prove essential if we are to detect physiological derangements in spatially and physiologically resolved tissue compartments such as the ischemic and traumatic penumbra. The physiology in these tissue compartments represents targets for our therapeutic interventions. The use of global monitors allows the dilution of such pathophysiology by information from surrounding normal tissue, and decreases the sensitivity with which we can monitor the need for, and effectiveness of, therapy. It may also be important to develop new methods of data processing that provide clinically relevant summary measures of the burden of pathophysiology, since these may allow us to select patients for specific therapies.

Finally, we need to move away from simply monitoring the consequences of pathophysiology. The recognition of the importance of ischemia as a key pathophysiological mechanism in many forms of CNS insult has spawned a huge industry in monitoring ischemia and its consequences. However, we are increasingly aware that energy failure in the brain may arise from a range of pathophysiological processes, including derangements in systemic cardiorespiratory physiology, intracranial hypertension, microvascular ischemia, mitochondrial dysfunction, and abnormally increased energy demands associated with peri-infarct depolarizations or glutamate release. Not recognizing which of these mechanisms is operating in a given patient may lead to inappropriate and ineffective therapy. Further, access to the brain extracellular fluid (ECF), through microdialysis or CSF collection, allows us to measure the levels of various disease mediators. Such measurement on a routine basis is almost unique in critical care, and may be important for both the identification of pathophysiological targets, and the rational titration of treatment against these processes. For example, microvascular injury may be initiated by a large spectrum of oxidant and inflammatory processes; measurement of key cytokine levels may identify specific targets for anti-inflammatory therapy. Importantly, once effective therapies are developed, such monitoring will also guide the application of such therapy, both in terms of patient selection and the timing and duration of therapy.

It would also be extremely valuable to validate peripheral biomarkers of the type, progress and severity of brain injury. Thus, S-100B has been proposed as a prognostic marker in head injury, and its episodic release has been found in some settings to presage significant deterioration in physiology [62]. While no specific marker is available for intracranial hemorrhage, the development of a simple blood test that allowed separation of ischemic and hemorrhagic stroke would accelerate the delivery of thrombolytic therapy.

Better Imaging Will Improve Therapy Selection and Prognostication

The availability of MRI with DWI and PWI has rationalized the use of thrombolytic therapy in stroke. Some details of how these techniques should influence patient care algorithms require further assessment, but it is very likely that the paradigm of early physiological assessment developed for ischemic stroke will spread to other CNS insults. We already know that MRI provides better structural characterization of brain injury, with improved prognostic categorization, but its widespread use has been limited by the difficulties in continuing the full range of ICU interventions in MRI units. However, there are no longer technical barriers to using MRI to assess critically ill patients, and I am confident that MRI will become routine in the imaging of many patients with trauma and intracranial hemorrhage. There may be particular benefits with MRI in multiple trauma, since there is increasing disquiet regarding the long term risk of radiation exposure from abdominal and thoracic CT [63]. Within the brain, other functional imaging techniques, such as Xe-CT and PET, may provide more robust quantitative measures for the purist, but none can match MRI for the breadth of structural and functional data that it provides, or compete with it in the availability stakes. While magnetic resonance spectroscopy is attractive, I believe that its use will be limited to research and the assessment of selective neuronal loss in the chronic stage of disease.

Therapy Improvements: New Interventions and Better Use of Existing Ones

While both clinicians and the pharmaceutical industry would dearly love to find a magic neuroprotective silver bullet, past experience suggests that this goal may not be easy to achieve. After a substantial period of pessimism, there is now a burgeoning interest to evaluate novel therapeutic compounds, and I believe that we may soon be riding a new wave of clinical trials in stroke and acute brain injury. It would be inappropriate to discuss specific agents in this article, but it is important to ensure that these new studies do not make the mistakes that invalidated many of the first generation of clinical trials of neuroprotection.

First, we need to initiate therapy early enough to give it a chance to succeed. It seems clear that the recruitment windows for many previous trials were too lax. For example, the NABISH trial [14] used a cut off of eight hours, despite the fact that experimental studies suggested loss of neuroprotective efficacy when hypothermia was initiated more than three hours post injury [64]. There have been attempts to assess the benefit of early hypothermia in a subsequent study by randomizing only patients who are hypothermic at admission [65]. However, it has proven difficult to recruit patients into this study. The inference from this discussion is that any neuroprotective intervention will need to be initiated in the prehospital phase in many conditions. With non-drug interventions, such as hypothermia, the major problem may lie with initiating therapy. While 'high tech' solutions are an option, we may be able to achieve initial temperature targets (~ 35 °C; see below) in most patients by rapidly infusing one to two liters of cold intravenous fluid. Where the intervention is a drug, administration may only be limited by side effects. While systemic cardiorespiratory depression is the issue that has concerned most people, local cerebrovascular effects may be the limiting factor in some situations. Thus, prehospital thrombolysis has not been a viable option because it is clinically impossible for an ambulance paramedic to exclude intracranial hemorrhage. The availability of a robust peripheral biomarker of cerebral hemorrhage might allow this distinction to be made in the patient's home, or in the ambulance, and improve the risk benefit ratio to an extent that allowed prehospital thrombolysis.

Having initiated such therapies, it is important that we develop rational ways of titrating their intensity and duration. It is important to recognize that any intervention that we make may have significant side effects, and we need to consider different paradigms of intervention. There may be some agents that are given in fixed doses because we do not have effective means of monitoring therapy response. Other agents, or even the same agents in different doses, may need to be titrated to physiological response or evidence of activity in a pathophysiological process. For example, minimal hypothermia (35-36 °C) can be widely applied as a neuroprotective intervention in head injury, since it has limited side effects. However, more profound hypothermia (33–34 °C) is known to cause significant cardiovascular compromise, renal dysfunction and electrolyte abnormalities, all of which may adversely influence outcome. Restricting this intervention to patients with the most florid pathophysiology would shift the risk/benefit ratio in a favorable direction, and this goal can be achieved by restricting these levels of hypothermia to patients with refractory intracranial hypertension [66]. Importantly, ICP also provides a useful indicator of the duration for which hypothermia may be needed. Such an approach may allow better individualization of therapy than has been possible in the past.

This discussion also underlines the importance of minimizing and combating the side effects of such neuroprotective interventions through meticulous intensive care [45]. Both pharmacological and physical neuroprotection may result in significant cardiorespiratory compromise. While these complications may be a problem for diseases that have traditionally not been managed in critical care units (e.g., ischemic stroke), this should not preclude use of these approaches if we can provide the supportive intensive care that negates their dangers.

Novel interventions with cell based therapies and trophic factors are likely to come to clinical trial, and perhaps into clinical practice, by 2015. Indeed, acute brain injury, where the blood brain barrier is disrupted, may provide an excellent scenario to test the effectiveness of systemic delivery of such therapies. In contexts where intracerebral delivery of cells or cell-derived therapies is required, routine access to the ventricular system and cerebral parenchyma (through ventricular and microdialysis catheters, respectively) may make head injury and intracranial hemorrhage prime clinical settings for early evaluation.

Widening the Scope of Neurocritical Care and Improving Outcome Assessment

It is now being increasingly recognized that critical care in general needs to look beyond the walls of the ICU. This is particularly true of neurocritical care, since early physiological insults can profoundly affect outcome, and the airway and ventilatory problems are common beyond the acute phase, and may require repeated critical care readmission. Given these considerations it is vital that neurocritical care services develop outreach services, both to stabilize patients early, and to consolidate the gains made during the ICU stay during the post ICU period. It is also essential that neurocritical care services develop their own follow up of patients, so as to facilitate audit and enhance education of staff. Unlike illnesses that present to general intensive care, outcomes from acute neurological disease may require long periods of recovery and rehabilitation to maximize functional recovery. Assessing patient outcome at discharge from hospital may result in unduly pessimistic views of the benefit of neurocritical care amongst nursing and medical staff.

Such assessments will also improve our assessments of outcome, and allow us to test important hypotheses regarding the effect of intensive care on neurocognitive outcome. Crude estimates of mortality are not appropriate outcome measures for neurocritical care [8], which should ideally improve the quality of outcome rather than survival rates. At the other end of the outcome scale, advanced techniques of assessing neurocognitive function, such as functional imaging [67], may alter our perception of what currently seem to be hopeless outcomes.

Making Sure that Legislative Developments Do Not Upset the Applecart

The developments that have been discussed in this chapter can only be realized with continuing clinical research. Unfortunately, there has been a strong and irrational trend to make clinical research in incapacitated adults more and more difficult. New regulatory hurdles for research in these settings, ostensibly developed to improve ethical accountability, may mean that care of patients in such categories of disease can never benefit from rational scientific development. These trends have been most prominent in Europe [68], but have created difficulties in North America as well. We have an ethical imperative as critical care physicians to interact with legislators and the public and ensure that they are informed and educated about these issues, which are of vital importance for our specialty.

Conclusion

It seems likely that the next ten years will see substantial advances in diagnosis and monitoring of patients with acute CNS insults. While there will clearly be new therapies unveiled, my prejudice is that substantial benefits are also likely to be gained from using existing therapies more appropriately, with individualization of therapy based on genotype and monitoring of disease process activity. While current developments promise significant improvements in clinical care, we must insure that the appropriate and rational assessment of new developments is not hampered by ignorance and misinformation amongst legislators and the public.

References

1. Menon DK (1999) Cerebral protection in severe brain injury: physiological determinants of outcome and their optimisation. Br Med Bull 55:226–258
2. Kermer P, Klocker N, Bahr M (1999) Neuronal death after brain injury. Models, mechanisms, and therapeutic strategies in vivo. Cell Tissue Res 298:383–395
3. The Brain Trauma Foundation and the American Association of Neurological Surgeons. Management and prognosis of severe traumatic brain injury. Part I: Guidelines for the management of severe traumatic brain injury. Brain Trauma Foundation 2000, New York At: http://www2.braintrauma.org/guidelines/downloads/btf_guidelines_management.pdf Accessed July 2005
4. Wahlgren NG, Ahmed N (2004) Neuroprotection in cerebral ischaemia: facts and fancies–the need for new approaches. Cerebrovasc Dis 17 (Suppl 1):153–166
5. Narayan RK, Michel ME, Ansell B, et al (2002) Clinical trials in head injury. J Neurotrauma 19:503–557
6. Steiner LA, Coles JP, Johnston AJ, et al (2003) Responses of posttraumatic pericontusional cerebral blood flow and blood volume to an increase in cerebral perfusion pressure. J Cereb Blood Flow Metab 23:1371–1377
7. Zygun DA, Doig CJ, Gupta AK, et al (2003) Non-neurological organ dysfunction in neurocritical care. J Crit Care 18:238–244
8. Patel HC, Menon DK, Tebbs S, Hawker R, Hutchinson PJ, Kirkpatrick PJ (2002) Specialist neurocritical care and outcome from head injury. Intensive Care Med 28:547–553
9. Elf K, Nilsson P, Enblad P (2002) Outcome after traumatic brain injury improved by an organized secondary insult program and standardized neurointensive care. Crit Care Med 30:2129–2134
10. Diringer MN, Edwards DF (2001) Admission to a neurologic/neurosurgical intensive care unit is associated with reduced mortality after intracerebral haemorrhage. Crit Care Med 29:635–640
11. Varelas PN, Conti MM, Spanaki MV, et al (2004) The impact of a neurointensivist-led team on a semiclosed neurosciences intensive care unit. Crit Care Med 32:2191–2198
12. Suarez JI, Zaidat OO, Suri MF, et al (2004) Length of stay and mortality in neurocritically ill patients: impact of a specialized neurocritical care team. Crit Care Med 32:2311–2317
13. Bulger EM, Nathens AB, Rivara FP, Moore M, MacKenzie EJ, Jurkovich GJ (2002) Management of severe head injury: Institutional variations in care and effect on outcome. Crit Care Med 30:1870–1876
14. Clifton GL, Choi SC, Miller ER, et al (2001) Intercenter variance in clinical trials of head trauma–experience of the National Acute Brain Injury Study: Hypothermia. J Neurosurg 95:751–755

15. Kochanek PM, Snyder JV, Sirio CA, Saxena S, Bircher NG (2001) Specialty neurointensive care–Is it just a name or a way of life? Crit Care Med 29:692–693
16. Chesnut RM (2002) Should we be using evidence-based quality assurance benchmarks to choose brain injury management centers? Crit Care Med 30:1927–1929
17. Marshall LF (2001) Intercenter variance. J Neurosurg 95:733–734
18. Naredi S, Koskinen LO, Grande PO, et al (2003) Treatment of traumatic head injury–U.S./ European guidelines or the Lund concept. Crit Care Med 31:2713–2714
19. Cowan JA Jr, Dimick JB, Wainess RM, Upchurch GR Jr, Thompson BG (2003) Outcomes after cerebral aneurysm clip occlusion in the United States: the need for evidence-based hospital referral. J Neurosurg 99:947–952
20. Menon D (2004) Neurocritical care: turf label, organizational construct, or clinical asset? Curr Opin Crit Care 10:91–93
21. Bramlett HM, Dietrich WD (2004) Pathophysiology of cerebral ischemia and brain trauma: similarities and differences. J Cereb Blood Flow Metab 24:133–50
22. Roof RL, Hall ED (2000) Gender differences in acute CNS trauma and stroke: neuroprotective effects of estrogen and progesterone. J Neurotrauma 17:367–388
23. Nathoo N, Chetty R, van Dellen JR, Barnett GH (2003) Genetic vulnerability following traumatic brain injury: the role of apolipoprotein E. Mol Pathol 56:132–136
24. Millar K, Nicoll JA, Thornhill S, Murray GD, Teasdale GM (2003) Long term neuropsychological outcome after head injury: relation to APOE genotype. J Neurol Neurosurg Psychiatry 74:1047–1052
25. Kirkpatrick PJ, Czosnyka M, Pickard JD (1996) Multimodal monitoring in neurointensive care. J Neurol Neurosurg Psychiatry 60:131–139
26. Czosnyka M, Pickard JD (2004) Monitoring and interpretation of intracranial pressure. J Neurol Neurosurg Psychiatry 75:813–821
27. Springborg JB, Frederiksen HJ, Eskesen V, Olsen NV (2005) Trends in monitoring patients with aneurysmal subarachnoid haemorrhage. Br J Anaesth 94:259–270
28. Silva Y, Puigdemont M, Castellanos M, et al (2005) Semi-intensive monitoring in acute stroke and long-term outcome. Cerebrovasc Dis 19:23–30
29. Morganti-Kossmann MC, Rancan M, Stahel PF, Kossmann T (2002) Inflammatory response in acute traumatic brain injury: a double-edged sword. Curr Opin Crit Care 8:101–105
30. Hillered L, Vespa PM, Hovda DA (2005) Translational neurochemical research in acute human brain injury: the current status and potential future for cerebral microdialysis. J Neurotrauma 22:3–41
31. Kirkpatrick PJ, Smielewski P, Czosnyka M, Menon DK, Pickard JD (1995) Near-infrared spectroscopy use in patients with head injury. J Neurosurg 83:963–970
32. Gupta AK, Hutchinson PJ, Fryer T, et al (2002) Measurement of brain tissue oxygenation performed using positron emission tomography scanning to validate a novel monitoring method. J Neurosurg 96:263–268
33. Menon DK Coles JP, Gupta AK, et al (2004) Diffusion limited oxygen delivery following head injury. Crit Care Med 32:1384–1390
34. Huisman TA (2003) Diffusion-weighted imaging: basic concepts and application in cerebral stroke and head trauma. Eur Radiol 13:2283–2297
35. Coles JP (2004) Regional ischemia after head injury. Curr Opin Crit Care 10:120–125
36. Latchaw RE (2004) Cerebral perfusion imaging in acute stroke. J Vasc Interv Radiol 15: S29–46
37. Jager HR (2000) Diagnosis of stroke with advanced CT and MR imaging. Br Med Bull 56:318–333
38. Yonas H, Pindzola RP, Johnson DW (1996) Xenon/computed tomography cerebral blood flow and its use in clinical management. Neurosurg Clin N Am 7:605–616
39. Schellinger PD, Kaste M, Hacke W (2004) An update on thrombolytic therapy for acute stroke. Curr Opin Neurol 17:69–77

40. Rinkel GJ, Feigin VL, Algra A, Vermeulen M, van Gijn J (2002) Calcium antagonists for aneurysmal subarachnoid haemorrhage. Cochrane Database Syst Rev CD000277
41. Bernard SA, Gray TW, Buist MD, et al (2002) Treatment of comatose survivors of out-of-hospital cardiac arrest with induced hypothermia. N Engl J Med 346:557–563
42. Hypothermia after Cardiac Arrest Study Group (2002) Mild therapeutic hypothermia to improve the neurologic outcome after cardiac arrest. N Engl J Med 346:549–556
43. Clifton GL, Miller ER, Choi SC, et al (2001) Lack of effect of induction of hypothermia after acute brain injury. N Engl J Med 344:556–563
44. Langham J, Goldfrad C, Teasdale G, Shaw D, Rowan K (2003) Calcium channel blockers for acute traumatic brain injury. Cochrane Database Syst Rev CD000565.
45. Polderman KH (2004) Application of therapeutic hypothermia in the intensive care unit. Opportunities and pitfalls of a promising treatment modality–Part 2: Practical aspects and side effects. Intensive Care Med 30:757–769
46. Hoyte L, Kaur J, Buchan AM (2004) Lost in translation: taking neuroprotection from animal models to clinical trials. Exp Neurol 188:200–204
47. Kwan J, Hand P, Sandercock P (2004) A systematic review of barriers to delivery of thrombolysis for acute stroke. Age Ageing 33:116–121
48. Wirth A, Baethmann A, Schlesinger-Raab A, et al (2004) Prospective documentation and analysis of the pre- and early clinical management in severe head injury in southern Bavaria at a population based level. Acta Neurochir Suppl 89:119–123
49. Scott PA, Temovsky CJ, Lawrence K, Gudaitis E, Lowell MJ (1998) Analysis of Canadian population with potential geographic access to intravenous thrombolysis for acute ischemic stroke. Stroke 29:2304–2310
50. Martino G (2004) How the brain repairs itself: new therapeutic strategies in inflammatory and degenerative CNS disorders. Lancet Neurol 3:372–378
51. Peterson DA (2004) Umbilical cord blood cells and brain stroke injury: bringing in fresh blood to address an old problem. J Clin Invest 114:314–316
52. Chopp M, Li Y (2002) Treatment of neural injury with marrow stromal cells. Lancet Neurol 1:92–100
53. Alexander MP (1995) Mild traumatic brain injury: pathophysiology, natural history, and clinical management. Neurology 45:1253–1260
54. Rudd AG, Hoffman A, Irwin P, Lowe D, Pearson MG (2005) Stroke unit care and outcome: results from the 2001 National Sentinel Audit of Stroke (England, Wales, and Northern Ireland). Stroke 36:103–106
55. Douglas VC, Tong DC, Gillum LA, et al (2005) Do the Brain Attack Coalition's criteria for stroke centers improve care for ischemic stroke? Neurology 64:422–427
56. Molyneux A, Kerr R, Stratton I, et al (2002) International Subarachnoid Aneurysm Trial (ISAT) of neurosurgical clipping versus endovascular coiling in 2143 patients with ruptured intracranial aneurysms: a randomised trial. Lancet 360:1267–1274
57. Priestley G, Watson W, Rashidian A, et al (2004) Introducing Critical Care Outreach: a ward-randomised trial of phased introduction in a general hospital. Intensive Care Med 30:1398–1404
58. Pollack SJ, Lewis H (2005) Secretase inhibitors for Alzheimer's disease: challenges of a promiscuous protease. Curr Opin Investig Drugs 6:35–47
59. Imahara SD, O'Keefe GE (2004) Genetic determinants of the inflammatory response. Curr Opin Crit Care 10:318–324
60. Schmidt EA, Czosnyka M, Gooskens I, et al (2001) Preliminary experience of the estimation of cerebral perfusion pressure using transcranial Doppler ultrasonography. J Neurol Neurosurg Psychiatry 70:198–204
61. Czosnyka M, Piechnik S, Richards HK, Kirkpatrick P, Smielewski P, Pickard JD (1997) Contribution of mathematical modelling to the interpretation of bedside tests of cerebrovascular autoregulation. J Neurol Neurosurg Psychiatry 63:721–731

62. Raabe A, Kopetsch O, Woszczyk A, et al (2003) Serum S-100B protein as a molecular marker in severe traumatic brain injury. Restor Neurol Neurosci 21:159–169
63. Dawson P (2004) Patient dose in multislice CT: why is it increasing and does it matter? Br J Radiol 77:S10–S13
64. Markgraf CG, Clifton GL, Moody MR (2001) Treatment window for hypothermia in brain injury. J Neurosurg 95:979–983
65. Clifton GL, Miller ER, Choi SC, et al (2002) Hypothermia on admission in patients with severe brain injury. J Neurotrauma 19:293–301
66. Polderman KH, Tjong Tjin Joe R, Peerdeman SM, Vandertop WP, Girbes AR (2002) Effects of therapeutic hypothermia on intracranial pressure and outcome in patients with severe head injury. Intensive Care Med 28:1563–1573
67. Menon DK, Owen AM, Williams EJ, et al (1998) Cortical processing in persistent vegetative state. Wolfson Brain Imaging Centre Team. Lancet 352:200
68. Liddell K, Menon DK, Zimmern R (2004) The human tissue bill and the mental capacity bill. BMJ 328:1510–1511

Disaster Medicine

P. E. Pepe, K. J. Rinnert, and J. G. Wigginton

Introduction: The Nature of the Problem

Throughout history, disasters, primarily in the form of natural catastrophes, have plagued the human race. Today, however, the risk of multiple injuries and deaths from a given incident has increased dramatically [1–4]. Not only is the earth more heavily-populated with human life settled across many more regions of the planet, but there are also larger pockets of human inhabitants. Most of these population centers are concentrated in high-risk locales such as metropolitan cities where very frequent and multiple person-to-person contacts occur. In addition, the world now faces a broadened spectrum of disasters, ranging from unconventional wars, nuclear releases, transportational mishaps, terrorist bombings, infectious disease epidemics and chemical discharges to floods, famine, earthquakes, tornadoes, cyclones and fires [2, 4].

While epidemics, famine, war, earthquakes and the like have always played a role in human experience, the ever-increasing spiral of human populations, the rapid growth of technology, swift world-wide travel for millions of persons, and exponential expansion of at-risk industries and residences conspire to increase human exposure to disasters. Accordingly, the numbers of casualties resulting from each incident are more likely to be large [2]. The recent undersea earthquake in the Indian Ocean that sent towering, 700 kilometer per hour tsunamis across Southern Asia resulted in a tremendous number of deaths and morbidity because of the sheer volume of exposures. Expanding population bases living and working in vulnerable situations along the at-risk seashores provided a baseline set-up for disaster.

Also, although the recent tsunami disaster occurred in Southern Asia, it affected many other countries worldwide because their citizens and their businesses were involved. In this modern era, mass air travel, expanding technology and economic imperatives have all changed the nature of 'localized' disasters. Over the past 50 years, because of the rapid growth of technology and relatively affluent worldwide economies, travel and sightseeing have evolved from an occasional pastime of the very privileged and the odd adventurer into a prevailing norm of worldwide mass tourism. In many parts of the globe, a 1950s seacoast village of 5,000 inhabitants is very likely now a cosmopolitan resort with millions of annual visitors.

Likewise, industries have also become global, often seeking heavily-populated sites where labor may be more economical and local workforces readily available to work for lower wages. A large number of the victims of the Indian Ocean tsunamis were foreign nationals operating businesses and many, many tourists, including celebrities, were caught up in this Asian calamity as well. Thus, in many ways, disasters throughout the world have now become multi-national in nature, having global impact, an impact amplified by mass media coverage and internet streaming of the events.

Similarly, despite the relatively fewer number of deaths, the September 11, 2001 attack on the World Trade Center in New York could be considered a multi-national event because of the hundreds of persons from dozens of countries working there. It also pointed out the concepts of modern vulnerability. Not only were highly-concentrated populations in one building an easy target to induce multiple casualties, but because of modern technology (i.e., a large modern transportational device laden with explosive fuel), such a dramatic disaster can now take place, intentionally or otherwise.

Perhaps more worrisome, is the threat of worldwide spread of contagious disease, both naturally-occurring and malicious (bioterrorist) promulgation [5, 6]. Again, with more people on the planet who have the potential to become an infected vector and with more global concentrations of highly-mobile populations (and thus more opportunities for exposure), the risk for pandemics has clearly increased. And while overt threats of nuclear holocaust have seemingly dissipated following the fall of the former Soviet Union, the underlying devices of mass destruction still exist, causing great concern for those who must anticipate how to deal with the aftermath [2, 4].

Beyond the initial impact of injury and illness are the subsequent public health sequelae such as insufficient food supplies, contaminated water, lack of shelter, and the subsequent threat of associated diseases. Finally, the psychological impacts of disasters on populations is only just now beginning to be better appreciated, not just for those directly affected, but for the population as a whole [2]. For example, the economic down-turns in the United States, Europe and elsewhere after the events of fall 2001 are often considered one of the casualties of the terrorist attacks. It emphasizes the under-recognized widespread affects that disasters can have on the international public psyche. Even when loss of life and infrastructure are relatively minimal in the grand scheme of the particular nation involved, disasters can have significant and far-reaching psychological impact (e.g., the 2001 U.S. anthrax postal system attacks). The old adage, "all disasters are local", may be somewhat anachronistic in the 21st Century.

From a sociological point of view, it is logical that countries might stand a better chance of mitigating mortality and morbidity with robust health care systems, solid public infrastructures, substantial community resources and early detection-warning systems. This would occur not only through forewarned prevention of injury and illness, but also through rapid access to sustenance, medical and rescue assets. It could be emphasized that much of the loss of life and morbidity from the 2004 Indian Ocean tsunamis and their subsequent sequelae actually resulted from relative limitations in terms of such characteristics. Nevertheless, the events of the fall of 2001 in the United States and the subsequent Toronto experience with severe acute respiratory syndrome (SARS) also exposed the vulnerability of even relatively healthy and well-resourced nations.

From a medical point of view, even though the death and long-term morbidity toll was not as high as the staggering consequences of the Indian Ocean tsunamis, the public health risk management issues associated with the 2001 U.S. anthrax attacks and other identified *potential* threats were still enormous [2, 5, 6]. Facilitated by obsessive mass media mania, the potential threat of other public health crises (involving large populations) as a result of either terrorism or natural disease (e.g., small pox and avian flu pandemic scenarios) became more of a reality in terms of *public perception*. As a result, tremendous political pressure has developed for medical clinicians and public health officers alike to become better prepared to protect the public from all disasters, let alone doomsday scenarios. This response has played out in political venues such as the development of the Department of Homeland Security in the U.S. and improved worldwide intelligence-gathering cooperation both domestically and internationally. Nevertheless, while some improvements in surveillance and pharmacological resource allocations have evolved, the *medical aspects* of homeland security and public health emergency preparedness remain worrisome and under-developed relative to public expectations of the safety net, be they appropriate expectations or not.

More specifically, at the present time, the great majority of healthcare facilities and emergency medical systems (EMS), even in prosperous Western nations, are overwhelmed in terms of emergency care surge capacity, be they government-based or private entities. Many of the key trauma centers and EMS crews are deluged on a day-to-day basis, brimming with fully-occupied beds, sub-optimal nurse and ancillary personnel staffing, despite increasing demands for service and a higher acuity of illness and injury. One could argue that these existing health care services, including ambulances, emergency centers, operating rooms, and intensive care units (ICUs) are facing a disaster each day as available medical resources outstrip the daily demands for urgent and critical care. This tenuous situation causes the looming threat of additional surges from disasters to become an even deeper concern.

Summarizing these points, there is a spiraling risk for catastrophic events involving multiple casualties and population-based medical morbidity, including proximal injury and illness and subsequent psychological and public health concerns. Such events will likely be multi-national in nature, even when localized to a particular venue. Therefore, this will require international cooperation in terms of prevention, mitigation and relief. However, the medical care infrastructure, even in wealthy countries already seems to operate at capacity, making a major multiple injury event or an influenza pandemic a true challenge. One might, therefore, ask what our ICUs would need to be like in the year 2015 and, in this case, our ICUs would not only be those located in the traditional in-patient facilities, but also ambulances, emergency centers and even field hospitals. In the following discussion, the issues, concerns and respective potential solutions will be analyzed and proposed.

Where are we Now: Specific Vulnerabilities in Current Disaster Management

As multi-faceted as the threats of disasters have become, so are the medical sequelae [2, 4, 6]. Explosions carry the triple threat of thermal, penetrating and blunt trauma [2, 4]. Associated building collapses cause crush injury syndromes and fires induce carbon monoxide poisoning and respiratory tract impairment [2, 4]. Earthquakes cause all of the above. Hurricanes, floods and tidal waves result in drowning, snake bites, and contaminated water supplies [2]. Chemical releases can result in pulmonary injury, burns, nerve system dysfunction, liver damage, and cellular dissolution [2, 4]. Severe radiation exposures cause burns, immunological suppression and diffuse epithelial damage, internally and externally. Biological agents result in a myriad of physiological insults. From pneumonia, coagulopathies, and central nervous system compromise to cardiac suppression and liver failure, the viral and bacterial agents provide often-insidious challenges to clinicians and public health officers alike, regardless if the root source is a natural epidemic or a malicious dissemination.

In turn, there is a need for dealing with surge capacity, not only in terms of medical care equipment, but also the personnel that utilize them. Not only are additional ventilators, dialysis machines and antibiotics anticipated, but also additional nurses, technicians, therapists and specialists. While existing medical personnel would best be used, coordinated plans to incorporate them into a disaster plan (providing them with timely respite and staggered shifts) are the challenges. While additional personnel theoretically could be imported from nearby (unaffected) medical facilities or from other regions or countries, the local personnel best work in their own environments and still would need to provide coordinating leadership roles.

This concept is in keeping with the number one rule of multiple casualty incident management, namely to follow day-to-day routines as closely as possible or modify day-to-day routines as much as possible to meet the unique demands of a disaster [7–9]. The logic here is that unfamiliar activities or settings result in logistical and procedural learning curves for clinicians and that such medical care obstacles can be amplified in a strange venue with overwhelming patient care demands. Learning how the laboratory or pharmacy works or how to operate less familiar equipment or communications systems, can delay and impair the true focus of patient care.

Along this same line of thought, proposed plans to develop specialized turnkey facilities that could be made available for use primarily at the time of a public health emergency (such as a pandemic or smallpox attack) would seem to have its limitations. Even when well-designed with all of the proper accoutrements (negative pressure rooms, modified ventilation systems, appropriate security design, and fully-equipped with the most modern ICU equipment), learning curves for the imported staff could be significant. Also, such a free-standing facility would be less useful for acute injuries (because of delays), with the exception of some burns and focal injuries. Unless the facility operates on a day-to-day basis, its user-friendliness becomes less effective. In some nations, some specialty hospitals do exist, but if their utilization is not brisk, deterioration in medical skills competencies may occur.

In contrast, utilization of highly-experienced trauma centers and ICUs would optimize the medical care skills needed and the efficiency of the delivery of care assuming that they could be off-loaded from some of their day-to-day activities. For example, a busy emergency department could off-load sore throats, urinary tract infections, and broken arms to clinics (a place where surge and delays in care would have less concerning consequences). Likewise, through prospective, government-moderated agreements, ICUs at major receiving centers for disaster victims could transfer certain critical care patients to other community hospitals if necessary. This kind of arrangement has been worked out to a significant degree in venues like Miami, USA, a frequent target for major hurricanes in which certain hospitals themselves are at risk for damage.

In fact, this latter scenario is most likely the option that developed communities will choose for several reasons. Contrary to popular perception, *most* disastrous events do not create an immediate influx of critical patients [7–9]. Victims are either killed outright or they have generally survivable injuries. In most traditional situations, experience has shown that less than 10% of patients (those not killed outright) will require critical care or critical care monitoring [7–10].

For example, in the New York World Trade Center attack in September 2001, despite approximately 3,000 deaths, only about 1,400 patients were seen in area hospitals emergency centers by 0200 hours the next morning, more than 16 hours after the event. Less than a hundred were admitted to ICUs or monitoring beds. Most of these patients had chest pain or respiratory distress, presumably resulting from particulate matter and smoke. Despite being the largest terrorist disaster in US history, the local emergency care system was, in retrospect, able to handle all of these cases. Moreover, a large percentage of these patients were the rescuers sent into the incident such as firefighters and police. Previously, in the March 1993 New York City US Airways crash off the runway at La Guardia Airport, most of the passengers were killed outright and only four or five patients were deemed serious (and not necessarily critical). Again, dozens of the rescuers were injured from jet fuel-induced eye burns, sprains, and evolving hypothermia.

In addition to involving a small percentage of critical care cases, most conventional disasters can be handled by existing resources when those resources are not involved or currently overwhelmed [8]. In fact, the medical skills and experience of traditional, busy burn, trauma, and critical care centers offer more optimal care for patients. In many respects, such centers may see many critical patients in a given evening just on a day-to-day basis. As a result, they are already more familiar with some of the pressures and triage decisions imposed by disasters. Also, most conventional disasters, be they a tornado, explosion, chemical release or transportational mishap, are generally localized and acute medical care is needed only in proximity to the event, unless, of course, the local medical resources are themselves disabled or destroyed (such as the Yrevan earthquake in the late 1980s).

These concerns become further confounded by legal issues such as licensure and credentialing of medical professionals at hospitals. A physician coming to provide aid at another locale or hospital may not be authorized to do so if they are not licensed to practice medicine in that jurisdiction (i.e., country, state, province). Moreover, even if licensed, hospital accreditation, in most venues, requires prospective scrutiny of physicians with relevant background checks and certain administrative requirements. All of these procedures take time and are therefore essentially impossible to provide at the time of a catastrophic event. While some communities have set up mechanisms to cross-credential physicians, only a few have done so and this does not account for the issues of familiarity and skills utilization. Moreover, the key practitioners that might be needed to provide assistance at alternative locations in a disaster are skilled nurses, respiratory therapists, dialysis technicians, pharmacists and the like. While all of these practitioners could also be 'cross-credentialed', it still does not account for motivators to have any of those persons participate. Motivators are not just the dedication of an avid volunteer or the lure of a financial incentive, but they also include care for those practitioners' families in the midst of a disaster during which time the families may be vulnerable as well (no food or water, loss of electricity, trapped by flooding, possible exposure to contagious disease, etc). Furthermore, there are concerns about liability coverage and protection from malpractice lawsuits when providing services outside of one's routine location [5].

All of these concerns strengthen the argument that existing facilities, particularly major trauma centers and critical care hospitals, should all be fortified and better prepared for surge capacity. Not only are there issues of skills, experience, familiarity, learning curves, licensure, credentialing, motivation and liability protection with which to be concerned, but, again, this paradigm follows the basic disaster tenet to follow one's day-to-day routines as closely as possible [7–9]. It relies on the premise that one should prepare for such events by modifying day-to-day activities to accommodate requirements for a multi-casualty event. One of the major reasons why disaster scenarios, be they drills or actual events, often go awry is that they are encumbered by plans or procedures that fall outside normal routines. Therefore, working in environments that facilitate familiar clinical and procedural behaviors in a disaster is the most advisable strategy.

On the other hand, a major nuclear or biological event can pose a more regional-national threat, if not a global risk [4–6]. For example, even if only a fifth of a population becomes infected with a highly contagious disease over a several week period and only 5% of such patients require critical care, this can mean 10,000 critical care patients in a city of 1,000,000 residents. Assuming a week's stay for each patient whether they live or die, it still translates into the need for thousands of ICU beds at any given time. Also, under such circumstances, patients more than likely would not be transferred out to other communities because those other venues also may be experiencing similar, or even worse, surges in patient demands in such scenarios. Similarly, certain catastrophes may involve those 'routine facilities' and transport services themselves. They may be destroyed or inaccessible due to flood, earthquake, terrorist bombing or contamination. This scenario also entreats a plan for working outside one's normal routine or enormous surge at other facilities, either local or at a distance.

Ultimately, another problem with either building separate specialized facilities or modifying current resources for dealing with a major disaster is that it requires major economic resources to re-build or replace existing infrastructures. Obviously, the construction and operation of a free-standing facility in a stand-by mode for a low probability mega-event with mass casualties (i.e., a once or twice in a generation event somewhere in the world such as Bhopal, Chernobyl, or the Indian Ocean Tsunamis), especially considering the likely vulnerability of that facility in such catastrophes. In like manner, re-building or renovating current medical facilities to make them more secure and more appropriate for dealing with weapons of mass effect, bioterrorism and natural epidemics, would cost some nations billions of dollars. The re-working of water supplies, the renovation of ventilation systems, the creation of universal capabilities for negative pressure rooms, expansion of critical care units and operative capabilities, the installation of decontamination mechanisms, both internal and external, and the acquisition of many additional ventilators, pharmaceuticals, and antidotes (placed in storage) would entail costs that are almost incomprehensible for many governments and the administrators of most medical facilities.

Already strapped with budgetary challenges, such infrastructure changes would be unreasonable without full public support (government assistance) and the commitment that all other facilities would share in similar burdens. In fact, beyond the costs of constructing circumferential barricades (e.g., mitigating the effectiveness of car-bombs) and better controlling and minimizing hospital entrances, are the sociological conflicts. Such security measures defeat the purpose and current philosophy of hospitals, clinics and medical facilities which should strive to provide even easier, patient-friendly access to medical care, particularly for the elderly, sick and chronically-ill who need comfortable entrance.

Such financial concerns are one matter, but without appropriate education and training of healthcare personnel in these matters, all of this expense would be less meaningful. Up until the last few years, there were only pockets of international expertise, mostly military in nature, in terms of dealing with weapons of mass effect. In terms of training healthcare personnel as a whole, there was little interest and 'NBC' (nuclear, biological, chemical) training courses were often referred to as NBC meaning 'nobody cares' courses. Worse yet, the training offered by military might be different from governmental training efforts, even within the same country. In turn, these efforts were also independent of civilian medical care training initiatives as limited as they have been.

For example, in the US, this disconnect was epitomized by just the titular aspects of training. The military used 'CBRNE' (for Chemical, Biological, Radiological, Nuclear and Explosive) and the federal agencies used 'COBRA' (for Chemicals, Ordinance, Biologicals, RAdiation). Also, the focus was not always an 'all-hazards' approach to disaster management and it did not focus on other risks to the civilian populations such as hurricanes and pandemics. Moreover, just as a few examples, it did not always address the needs of all levels of healthcare workers in multiple disciplines (e.g., nursing, pharmacy, physicians, primary care providers, paramedics, veterinarians) nor did it focus on ancillary hospital staff (custodians, engineers, security) who need to know about decontamination procedures. As a result, there was a clear need to provide an all-hazards, multi-disciplinary, interoperable, standardized training initiative that provided uniformity and consistency in nomenclature, procedures and protocols for major disasters [2].

Such standardized, multi-disciplinary courses have been developed for the management of other major threats to life, namely cardiac arrest and trauma (e.g., the American Heart Association [AMA] Advanced Cardiac Life Support [ACLS] and the American College of Surgeons Advanced Trauma Life Support [ATLS]). They have even been demonstrated to be effective in increasing life-saving. However, unlike cardiac arrest and trauma cases that can present in certain facilities on a daily basis, disaster events are uncommon and infrequent events, even worldwide, making additional training and practice even more critical.

What Challenges Does the Future Hold?

It has been made clear that due to facilitated global travel, exponential growths of underserved populations and burgeoning technological advances, the risk for disasters is also accelerating. Added to those factors is the ever-evolving threat of terrorism, a problem that may even be further exacerbated by several nations' efforts to thwart such threats. Even in the post-Cold War era, the threat of nuclear bomb detonation and radioactive exposure still remains a concern, whether by rogue operatives or governments at war. This past year alone, the state of Florida in the United States experienced four major hurricanes over an expanding at-risk population base and many experts claim that major earthquakes along major fault lines are long overdue throughout the globe. The December 2004 Indian Ocean 9.0 Richter Scale event may have been a heralding event.

More likely, many infectious disease experts would predict that we are due for a clear 'shift' in the genetic make-up of influenza virus. Versus the typical drift that leads us to modify our influenza vaccines each year, most of the population will have little immunological memory and limited protection from any aspect of this new antigenic entity. It is feared that with the typical current processes for producing vaccines, an entirely new influenza virus could sweep through even healthy worldwide populations in a matter of months, long before a vaccine could be developed, processed, and distributed, not to mention the time it takes for inoculated persons, particularly children, to develop adequate protective antibodies.

A similar genetic jump from animal populations (e.g., 'avian flu') could proliferate with the same scenarios. In both cases, with more people to infect, more ways of rapidly transmitting the virus around the globe, and more persons with immunological suppression alive today, the risk for pandemic will become even more of a threat, not only for the population as a whole, but also for the ambulance crews, emergency department staff and ICU practitioners. If they become ill as well, there will be even fewer healthcare providers available to care for the throngs of ill persons, making the disaster scenario even worse.

Recently, there have been other evolving threats such as methicillin resistant *Staphylococcus aureus* (MRSA) found in untraditional sites. It is unknown what other new transmissible processes will occur. For example, the concept of SARS was unknown three years ago. Also, with tremendous advances in genetic engineering, it is feared that both malicious and unintentional contagion threats will become new realties. In the realm of chemical disasters, everyday there seems to be an ever-widening fleet of chemicals being transported by rail, highway and ships, increasing the likelihood of mishaps.

While threats for disaster are increasing, medical care resources are being spread thinner and thinner, from sociological factors (nursing shortages and increased re-focus on families in affluent societies) to financial constraints (decreasing reimbursements for medical practitioners and facilities or sparser resources from governments for healthcare). Ironically, with increased demands for protection from terrorism and other public health threats, financial resources have been diverted from healthcare to national defense and homeland security efforts. Unfortunately, most security efforts are overhead costs and not at all revenue-generating. Even within hospitals, dealing with disaster management is generally administrative in nature (training, equipment, procedures, personnel) and consumes and diverts medical care professionals' time and efforts from their day-to-day patient care activities.

To summarize these concerns about the future, it is predictable that, over the next ten years, there will be a substantial risk for more disasters, both natural and otherwise, and that these disasters will occur with dwindling healthcare funding and resources and more populations at risk. From the enhanced alerts for terrorism and pandemics to increased potentials for natural disasters in a more vulnerable world, there is a growing need to address solutions to these issues.

What Are the Possible Solutions?

It has become clear that many disasters are, in several respects, multi-national in nature. Also, with modern technology, every disaster can be brought into almost every home worldwide through television or the internet, sociologically affecting humans worldwide, even those not affected by involvement of loved ones or business colleagues. At the same time, most conventional disasters truly are local in terms of the medical response. Be it a chemical release, terrorist bombing, tornado touchdown or jumbo jet crash, it makes sense that existing local services still need to be fortified.

Structural Solutions

In a cyclone, tornado or hurricane belt, reinforced hospitals will have their ICUs secured within the center of the edifice, well above the level of potential storm surges and flood levels and far below the roof-top levels where spin-off tornadoes can rip off the top floors and blow out exterior windows. All hospitals, particularly those in recognized earthquake zones, should have 'earthquake-proof' designs with applicable structural integrity. When a hospital is a potential terrorist target such as any main receiving facility, trauma center, burn center, or children's hospital, security measures will dictate the need for barricades to bombs and specialized ventilation systems that detect and can control the spread of aerosolized poisons or biologicals. These hospitals will have a disproportionate number of negative pressure rooms and well-established decontamination zones around the potential entrance and receiving personnel (e.g., trained triage nurses and security personnel will be staged further out into the periphery and prepared with universal precautions and easy access to decontamination suits, including high level personal protective equipment (PPE).

Access to the hospital from more distant entry points may be facilitated by moving walkways or light rail systems (such as those used in many airports) to ease access from parking, drop-off points and mass transportation sites. However, entrances will be limited in terms of the number of access points with detection devices at all sites. Just as our airports are protected, so should our medical care facilities be.

Within the next ten years, spurred on by additional major terrorist events and further recognition of the vulnerability of the medical safety net, governmental resources will begin to make these changes and architects for new facilities will incorporate them into future design. But, economically-intensive, this aspect of preparation will lag being other efforts.

While the first approach to enhancing the structural aspects of disaster management would be to make improvements in existing facilities, this paradigm would be most value to handle the more likely conventional disasters. However, one might then return to entertaining the concept of a specialized facility to manage pandemics and disseminated bioterrorism incidents such as a mutated smallpox organism. In this case, to overcome the concepts of lack of familiarity with equipment and resources, credentialing, liability and medical skills utilization, a mitigating solution would be to dedicate a reserve team of medical personnel in the way a government entity deploys a fire service or army as a dedicated standing force. Currently, a hybrid for this type of concept is accomplished through the mobile medical teams and tent hospitals designed by the National Disaster Medical System (NDMS), an element of the Federal Emergency Management Agency (FEMA) in the United States Department of Homeland Security. Although it does not employ a round-the-clock standing team, it does utilize a 'stand-by' team of medical and allied health volunteers who are trained and routinely exercised to operate mobile hospitals. Currently, these teams would likely be inadequate for a mass casualty scenario with tens of thousands of victims, but still they are somewhat helpful in areas where the standing facilities have been destroyed, impaired or rendered inaccessible.

In the future, such mobile hospitals may have reasonable value in some circumstances, but community-wide plans to enhance existing facilities for surge capacity will supersede all other plans. Inter-hospital agreements to facilitate transfers of patients to balance out surges throughout the system will be in play in the best prepared communities. Such agreements will also include specialized storage facilities for antidotes and antibiotics, perhaps in a separate, undisclosed and protected storage facility, but close enough for easy access. The regional hospitals will purchase these items in bulk to leverage economies of scale (cheaper prices), but they will also coordinate receipt so that expiration dates on the drugs will be staggered and not all expiring at once. Such coordination would also include the use of healthcare and ancillary personnel in case of over-load at a given hospital or incapacity of another. Not only will prospective cross-credentialing be accomplished ahead of time using familiar mechanisms, but the process may even be facilitated by course completion in Advanced Disaster Life Support (ADLS) and Hospital Disaster Life Support (HDLS) types of courses [1, 2]. In all likelihood, arrangements will first focus intra-murally. For example, they may prioritize the use of nurses from the same hospital system (i.e., many hospital systems operate more than one hospital) because of the similarities in policies, procedures, liability coverage and payroll considerations. Such coordination of efforts would be a massive under-taking, but well-prepared communities will cooperate in such approaches.

Again, many disasters are multi-national and often occurr in under-resourced countries with relatively poor infrastructures. The creation of more than 100 disaster teams by the United Nations worldwide could be considered. Equipped with fast transport air-craft and mobile emergency units, these teams will be available on any site within less than 6 hours and will work closely with local organizations. Very likely, each disaster team will be staffed and operated by a multi-national force, and most likely a standing military team. As in any other military organization, teaching and training in disaster medicine will be part of military education in all countries and the teams will continuously drill and work together in coordination on a routine basis.

Training

Over the past two years, the AMA has begun to help develop a family of standardized, interoperable, multi-disciplinary, all-hazards courses to deal with the medical aspects of disaster medicine and counter-terrorism [1–3]. Working in close conjunction with several academic (university-based) trauma center leaders as well as multiple federal and military agencies and, more recently, other professional societies such as the American College of Emergency Physicians (ACEP) and the Society for Critical Care Medicine (SCCM), the AMA courses are beginning to lay the groundwork for standardized training and improved personnel preparations for disasters [1–3]. Like ACLS and ATLS courses, the ADLS course provides hands-on, multi-disciplinary scenarios in which participants learn to provide antidotes and other resuscitative skills in simulated austere, hazardous conditions requiring the donning and use of high-level PPE in insecure environments [1].

In addition to ADLS, a pre-requisite Basic Disaster Life Support (BDLS) course [2] provides intensive exposure to the didactic elements of disaster preparation from recognizing the main sequelae of explosions (tympanic membrane perforation, hollow viscus disruption, and contusions) to the elements of the Haddon matrix and other psychological aspects of disaster management as well as the main antidotes and therapies required in each scenario, be it chemical, biological, radiological, or traumatic in nature [2, 4].

Within the next ten years, it is predicted that, at the very least, within the United States, BDLS will be required for every medical student, paramedic student, nursing and other applicable allied health personnel [2]. ADLS will be provided to applicable trainees and nursing staff in critical care areas including advanced life support ambulances, emergency departments, and critical care areas. In addition, it is predicted that specialized in-hospital spin-off courses (e.g., HDLS) will address elements of decontamination tactics by custodians, engineers and others as well as the important and unique needs of caring for dozens of patients with highly-communicable diseases and strict need for nosocomial control.

Currently, many of these issues are already addressed in several excellent existing courses such as the SCCM's 'Fundamentals of Disaster Management' and other European counterparts [11]. However, it is predicted that these efforts will coalesce into a standardized set of courses that will be stewarded, in the future, by a team of consensus-building organizations and agencies worldwide. Such endeavors will become similar to the efforts conducted by the International Liaison Committee on Resuscitation (ILCOR) for cardiac resuscitation medicine. Although such training in itself will not fully prepare healthcare professionals for dealing with infrequent events such as disasters, it certainly will improve the chances of mitigation and improved outcomes, not to mention better safety for the healthcare providers themselves.

In addition, paramedics and emergency medical technicians will be trained to deliver prophylaxis in a public emergency preparedness situation such as a smallpox or yersinia outbreak or even a influenza pandemic. Prospective rules about who can be denied or provided vaccination or antibiotics and how one receives protection from liability will be arranged in the most prepared systems.

Equipment

In anticipation of a major event, facilities will develop a cadre of antidotes, antivirals and antibiotics for biological threats. More importantly, they will ratchet up ICU equipment, ventilators and respiratory care equipment as well as PPE and decontamination equipment. Ambulances and emergency departments and hospitals at large will be fortified by new computerized technology that enhances detection and discrimination of abnormal gases, chemicals, aerosolized biologicals and other threats in ventilation systems and ambient air, just as a carbon monoxide detector or Geiger counter would provide sentinel detection of carbon monoxide or radioactivity in one's home.

New ventilators will be impervious to chemical and biological agents and provide protected ventilation in such environments. In addition, artificial hemoglobin-based oxygen carriers that can be stored in ambulances or in far-forward military conditions will be placed in massive storage places as well and ready to use for mass casualties [12]. Some products now in early test stages can be stored without refrigeration for several years and are likely to be standard equipment in all critical care settings, be it pre-hospital, emergency center or ICU settings [12].

Inter-Governmental and International Cooperation

In the end, the new challenges will require a new level of international cooperation particularly because many natural disasters can be superimposed upon on-going complex emergencies, including on-going famines, civil wars or rebel insurgencies [13]. Such circumstances can further complicate rescue and restoration of normalcy [13]. At the same time, in the recent tsunami crisis, the World Health Organization (WHO) predicted the potential for many additional deaths from subsequent water-borne or mosquito-borne disease epidemics. However, it appears that such problems were apparently prevented by a prompt and well-funded response by both local and international communities.

Conclusion

Worldwide, there is a spiraling risk for catastrophic events involving multiple casualties and medical morbidity, not only in terms of acute injury and illness, but also subsequent psychological and public health concerns. Today, such events will likely be multi-national in nature, even when localized to a particular venue. Such events will require international cooperation in terms of prevention, mitigation and relief. Nevertheless, the best approach to preparing for disasters is to expand, modify and enhance current local infrastructures and capabilities for managing the multiple types of disaster scenarios and also to create a number of inter-facility cooperative agreements in advance. Aside from safer internal locations for ICUs and surgical theaters, certain structural changes will need to be installed such as modified ventilation systems, protected water supplies, decontamination mechanisms and security renovations. Another key action will be the proliferation of an international, interoperable, multi-disciplinary, all-hazards training initiative such as that being currently developed by the AMA and the NDLS family of courses. Specialized surveillance equipment that can detect and isolate poisons and infectious biological agents will be placed throughout medical facilities and cadres of antidotes, antibiotics and hemoglobin-based oxygen carriers will be stored in secure locations and made readily available for the applicable disaster scenario.

References

1. American Medical Association (2003) Advanced Disaster Life Support® Version 2.0. American Medical Association Press, Chicago
2. American Medical Association (2002) Basic Disaster Life Support® Version 2.0. American Medical Association Press, Chicago
3. American Medical Association (2004) Core Disaster Life Support® Version 2.0. American Medical Association Press, Chicago
4. Keyes DC, Burstein JL, Schwartz RB, Swienton RE (2004) Medical Response to Terrorism: Preparedness and Clinical Practice. Lippincott, Williams and Wilkins, Philadelphia, USA

5. Pepe PE, Rinnert KJ (2002) Bioterrorism and medical risk management. The International Lawyer 36: 9–20
6. Bartlett JG (2002) Bioterrorism and Public Health. Thomson Medical Economics, Montvale
7. Pepe PE, Stewart RD, Copass MK (1989) Ten golden rules for urban multiple casualty incident management. Prehosp Disaster Med 4:131-134
8. Pepe PE, Anderson E (2001) Multiple casualty incident plans: ten golden rules for prehospital management. Dallas Med Journal November:462–468
9. Pepe PE (1990) Responding to emergencies – review of the Phillips Petroleum explosion. Council of State Governments, March issue. Council of State Governments, Louisville, p 9
10. Pepe PE, Kvetan V (1991) Field management and critical care in mass disaster. Crit Care Clin 7:401-420
11. Farmer JC, Jiminez EJ, Rubinson L, Talmor DS, Markenson DS (2003) Fundamentals of Disaster Management, 2nd Edition. Society for Critical Care Medicine, Des Plaines
12. Manning JE, Katz LM. Brownstein MR, et al (2000) Bovine hemoglobin-based oxygen carrier (HBOC-201) for resuscitation of uncontrolled, exsanguinating liver injury in swine. Shock 13:152–159
13. Spiegel PH (2005) Differences in world responses to natural disasters and complex emergencies. JAMA 293:1915–1918

How Might Critical Care Medicine be Organized and Regulated?

Hospital and Medical School Organization of Critical Care Services

M. P. Fink

Introduction

The way departments and divisions are organized in hospitals and medical schools has evolved over time as a consequence of myriad influences. The evolution of these organizational structures is reminiscent of the way hospitals grow by adding new wings and remodeling old wards. But, any nurse or doctor, who has worked for a while in a 'modernized' but still old hospital and then has transferred to a brand new state-of-the-art facility, will tell you that one can go only so far by updating an obsolete structure. The workflow is far better in the newer facility, the quality of life is better for both patients and staff, and, in some instances, even quality of care is improved. Therefore, it is reasonable to ask: if we could start from scratch, would we still organize the specialties and subspecialties of medicine the way we do now, or would the 'org chart' look different?

Changing Physician Grouping

As the reader may have guessed by now, the author suspects that the most rational and efficient way to group physicians in hospitals and medical schools is quite different from current practice. Specifically, consider the case of emergency medicine physicians, hospitalists, and intensivists. Often, patients with an acute serious illness enter the health care system through the emergency department (ED). After being stabilized, many such patients are admitted to an intensive care unit (ICU), either directly or, if emergency surgery is required, via the operating room (OR). If the outcome in the ICU is favorable, then patients typically are transferred to a general medical or surgical ward to recuperate further before either going home or receiving additional rehabilitation at a facility specializing in this component of the continuum of care.

Thus, emergency medicine physicians, intensivists and hospitalists all 'touch' many patients requiring hospitalized care. The types of patients and the kinds of problems encountered by these three specialties are distinct. For example, many patients presenting to the ED can be discharged to home to be followed by a physician or surgeon on an out-patient basis. By the same token, many 'ward patients' are never so sick as to require care in an ICU, and much of the emphasis during hospitalization is (or should be) on discharge planning and education to minimize the likelihood of unnecessary repeat hospitalization for the same problem.

But, the similarities among these specialties are greater than the differences. Indeed, emergency medicine specialists, hospitalists and intensivists all must be broadly trained and capable of viewing patients in an integrated fashion rather than focusing only on one specific organ system or type of procedure. Furthermore, specialists in all three of these fields should be able to intervene in a timely fashion to deal with acute life-threatening problems, such as airway emergencies, hemorrhage, and derangements in electrolyte status. And, of course, all three groups of physicians focus on those patients that require care – even if only transiently – in a hospital.

Since the ED, the ICU, and the ward are all components of the continuum of care within the hospital environment, these three areas are all intimately co-dependent with respect to the allocation and availability of resources. Thus, when beds are unavailable on the wards, patients 'back up' in the ICUs, even when a lower intensity of monitoring and intervention is warranted. Lack of ICU beds leads to crowding and delay of services in the ED, compromising care and leaving patients and families dissatisfied.

Ideally, the practice of high quality critical care medicine does not begin when the patient arrives in the ICU, but rather begins as soon as critical illness is identified by health care workers, whether these individuals are emergency medical technicians, paramedics, nurses, emergency medicine specialists, surgeons or intensivists. Certainly, as pointed out recently by Cawdery and Burg, rapid stabilization and diagnosis are fundamental principals in both emergency medicine and critical care medicine [1]. These authors also point out that the demand for critical care services in the ED has increased over the past decade and continues to rise. For example, in California, the number of critically ill patients presenting to EDs increased by 57% from 1990 to 1999 [2]. In the United States, ED visits have increased by about 20% from 1992 to 2002 while the number of hospitals has decreased by 15% [3]. In 2002, 22% of patients were classified as true emergencies and 919,000 required "immediate medical attention" [3].

Most tertiary and quarternary care medical centers are large enough to support full-time staffing in the ED and the ICUs and many also incorporate hospitalist services to provide round-the-clock attending-level coverage for ward patients. But, few secondary community hospitals can support '7-by-24' staffing of the ED, ICUs and wards. In practice, the ED is staffed on a full-time basis and except for brief periods when daily rounds are being conducted or during extreme emergencies, patients in the ICUs and the wards are 'covered' from physicians' offices or homes by telephone. Emergency coverage for ward and ICU patients – to deal with airway crises or hypotension unresponsive to intravenous fluid administration – typically is provided by the emergency physician or, possibly, an in-house anesthesiologist.

Changing Training

Critical care medicine requires fellowship training, but currently it is not a 'primary specialty' in the United States or most European countries (Spain and Switzerland are notable exceptions). At least in the USA, critical care medicine is considered to be a subspecialty of one of four primary specialties: medicine, surgery, anesthesiology and pediatrics. The credentialing pathway requires board certification in one of these primary specialties then subspeciality fellowship training, ultimately leading to a 'certificate of added qualifications' in critical care medicine. It is noteworthy that there is no accredited pathway in the United States for emergency medicine physicians to obtain certification as experts in critical care medicine. Nevertheless, a sizeable number of emergency medicine physicians have received additional fellowship training in critical care medicine; many of these individuals are graduates of the Multidisciplinary Critical Care Training Program (MCCTP) at the University of Pittsburgh. Most of these physicians have obtained certification in critical care medicine by sitting for an examination offered by the European Society of Intensive Care Medicine. Many but not all hospitals in the United States regard the European Diploma in Intensive Care as an acceptable credential to permit practice critical care medicine. This view is the one taken by the University of Pittsburgh Medical Center.

Clearly, a far more rationale approach for providing the epoch of care that occurs in the hospital is to train a cadre of physicians, who are experts in emergency medicine, critical care medicine, and ward-based medicine. One way to achieve this goal is illustrated by the diagram shown in Figure 1. According to this concept, medical students could opt to obtain training in a Hospital-based Medicine (HBM) residency program. In contrast to conventional training in Internal Medicine, which appropriately emphasizes outpatient care, training in HBM would deal exclusively with the management of hospitalized patients.

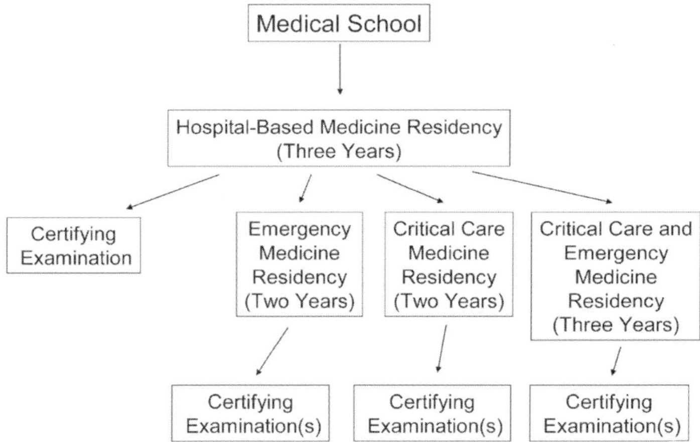

Fig. 1. Pathways to training as a hospitalist, emergency medicine physician and/or intensivist.

In addition to rotations on general medical and surgical wards, the three-year curriculum would include a substantial block of time in the OR, gaining experience with airway management skills. Additional rotations would include time in medical and various surgical ICUs as well as the ED.

After completing training in HBM, trainees would be qualified to sit for a certifying examination in this specialty. Many graduates of HBM programs might elect to obtain no further formal training, but rather start careers as hospitalists. However, other trainees might elect to complete two years of additional training in Emergency Medicine, two years of additional training in Critical Care Medicine, or three years of additional training, leading to added qualifications in both Emergency Medicine and Critical Care Medicine.

Currently, in most tertiary care medical centers in the United States, the ED is staffed by full-time emergency physicians under the auspices of a Department of Emergency Medicine. The hospitalist service – if it exists at all – is managed by the Department of Medicine or division of this department (e.g., General Medicine Division). Typically, critical care services are barely organized at all. Often, a general medical intensive care unit (MICU) is staffed by members of the Division of Pulmonary Medicine in the Department of Medicine. Some surgical units may be staffed by members of the Department of Surgery or the Department of Anesthesiology (or members from both Departments). Other units, such as neurosurgical ICUs, transplant ICUs or cardiothoracic ICUs, may be staffed by members of the relevant Departments or Divisions or, remarkably, not be staffed at all (at least by a cadre of geographical full-time experts in critical care medicine). It is well-known that the organization structure for critical care medicine in most North American community hospitals is even more problematic. Despite the availability of fairly convincing data to support the value – both in terms of lives and dollars saved – of 'high intensity' staffing of ICUs [4], the vast majority of ICUs in the United States adhere to a 'low intensity' model (i.e., open unit configuration, no geographical full-time physician staff).

Changing Organization

The new training pathways outlined above suggest a better way to organize emergency medicine, hospitalist and intensivist services within hospitals. According to this new model, the Department of Hospital-based Medicine would be responsible for staffing the ED and ICUs and would also provide hospitalist services for the wards. Large tertiary or quarternary centers might have multiple divisions in the Department (e.g., Emergency Medicine Division, Critical Care Medicine Division, Hospitalist Division), whereas smaller institutions might be better served by having a flatter organizational scheme and utilizing the same cadre of physicians to provide services on the wards, ICUs and ED. But, whether constructed with multiple divisions or not, hospitals and patients would be well-served by the existence of a Department of HBM. What would be the advantages of this approach?

First, except for very small hospitals, enough physicians would work under the umbrella of the Department of HBM to make providing full-time –

'7-by-24' – in-house coverage feasible without burdening any single doctor with an excessive number of nights on call per month. Full-time in-house coverage by well-trained intensivists or hospitalists is essential for the proper functioning of medical emergency teams (METs) that can respond at any time of the day or night to the deterioration of a patient on wards or in special care units.

At the University of Pittsburgh Medical Center we do not (yet) have a Department of Hospital-based Medicine. Nevertheless, we do have a fully independent Department of Critical Care Medicine that includes approximately 50 full-time faculty members. Departmental status for Critical Care Medicine has permitted us to effectively implement the MET concept at our institution. At the University of Pittsburgh Medical Center, the MET consists of a fully trained 'Resource Intensivist', a critical care medicine fellow, an ICU nurse and a respiratory therapist. The Resource Intensivist is not responsible for any particular ICU, but rather serves as the intensivist on call for the whole hospital, being available to respond to emergencies in the special care units, on the wards or in the ED. When a 'Condition C' (C stands for crisis) is called, the members of the MET coalesce together at the appropriate bedside. The critical care medicine fellow carries an 'Orange Bag' to the scene. The Orange Bag contains endotracheal tubes, laryngoscopes, and other intubation equipment (including tools for dealing with a difficult airway) plus a small assortment of emergency medications (e.g., etomidate, succinyl choline, and naloxone). Thus, the MET is capable of transiently bringing an ICU environment to the bedside of any patient in the hospital. Since the MET is empowered under the hospital by-laws to make whatever interventions are medically indicated to stabilize the patient, correctable problems are often identified and managed before the patient's status deteriorates further. Implementation of the MET concept has resulted in a substantial decrease in the incidence of cardiopulmonary arrests at the University of Pittsburgh Medical Center [5].

A second potential advantage of having a Department of HBM is the clear assignment of responsibility for the quality of HBM services. Under the organizational scheme that is common in most medical centers today, the seams between the ED and the ICU and the ICU and the ward are potential weak spots in the handling of care. Since no single Chair takes responsibility for patients in all three areas, the temptation to assign blame rather than fix problems is sometimes overwhelming.

A third advantage of having a Department of HBM is that it should be easier to lessen variations in practice across different settings in the hospital. For example, the approach used for resuscitating patients with severe sepsis ideally should be the same (or nearly so) for patients on the ward, in the ICU or in the ED. Although hard data regarding this issue are lacking, the author suspects that patients in many institutions are likely to be treated quite differently for the same problem, depending upon whether the care is delivered by hospitalists on a ward, emergency physicians in the ED, or intensivists in an ICU.

Conclusion

The author recognizes that each hospital has its own culture. Moreover, complex human organizations are rarely, if ever, designed from the ground up to optimize function and workflow. Thus, we almost always are confronted with making compromises between the traditional ways of doing our jobs and our notions of how we might do our work better. But, unless we try to envision a better model, we will be forever constrained by the imperfections in the current paradigm, or worse still, will change our practices only because of external factors beyond our control.

References

1. Cawdery M, Burg MD (2004) Emergency medicine career paths less traveled: cruise ship medicine, Indian health, and critical care medicine Ann Emerg Med 44:79–83
2. Lambe S, Washington DL, Fink A, Herbst K, Liu H, Fosse JS, Asch SM (2002) Trends in the use and capacity of California's emergency departments, 1990–1999 Ann Emerg Med 39:389–396
3. McCaig LF, Burk CW (2002) National Hospital Ambulatory Medical Care Survey: 2002 emergency department summary. Advance Data 340:1–36
4. Pronovost PJ, Angus DC, Dorman T, Robinson KA, Dremsizov TT, Young TL (2002) Physician staffing patterns and clinical outcomes in critically ill patients: a systematic review. JAMA 288:2151–2162
5. DeVita MA, Braithwaite RS, Mahidhara R, Stuart S, Foraida M, Simmons RL (2004) Medical Emergency Response Improvement Team (MERIT). Use of medical emergency team responses to reduce hospital cardiopulmonary arrests. Qual Saf Health Care 13:251–254

Physician Staffing in the ICU 10 Years from Now

J. A. Russell and A. Sutherland

Introduction

Physician staffing of intensive care units (ICUs) is a key element of the success of the clinical, teaching and research programs of an ICU. Indeed, recent studies show that the nature of physician staffing is highly associated with ICU and hospital mortality and length of stay [1]. Furthermore, regional and national shortages of resident physicians to cover ICUs have lead to the recruitment of full-time and part-time ICU hospitalists. It is likely that there will be further changes in the number and nature of physician staffing of ICUs over the next decade.

Physician staffing is already an issue in many ICUs for several reasons. First, ICU patient volume and complexity both continue to increase. Second, there is clear evidence that staffing an ICU with dedicated intensivists decreases mortality, morbidity and costs. Third, the quality improvement revolution in health care has entered the ICU and has impacted the skill sets and activities expected of ICU physicians. Fourth, training of residents and fellows in critical care medicine has been accredited in most countries and increases the rigor of training requirements, teaching and need for excellent clinical experience. Fifth, hospitals, health maintenance organizations (HMOs) and regional health districts have rationalized and re-organized hospital services (such as the volume and types of specific surgeries) that have impacted the size and nature of ICUs. Sixth, intensivists are entering into areas of clinical care outside the ICU such as medical emergency teams (METs), air transport, and other consultative services. Seventh, research in intensive care continues to be scientifically stronger, deeper and more widely appreciated, increasing the need for clinician-scientists in intensive/critical care medicine. Eighth, there are growing leadership needs in administrative, clinical, teaching and research arenas of intensive care. Ninth, the 'baby boomer' age of physicians will be entering retirement age and will be decreasing clinical activities and then fully retiring from clinical intensive care. Finally, changes in health care budgets have impacted the number and types of physician services in intensive care.

Because changes in physician status due to disability, retirement and death do not change the net number of full time equivalents (FTEs) in an ICU, I will focus on changes that will impact net FTEs of ICU physician services and will assume that disability, retirement and death will be dealt with by recruitment to those FTE slots of new intensivists.

What will the nature of ICU staffing be in 10 years from now? We will address this question by reviewing in more detail current physician staffing. Then, we will discuss in more detail the drivers that will influence physician staffing over the next decade. Then, we will present a model of future physician staffing that is a mix of projection, conjecture and a vision for future ICU physician staffing. The template that we will use for this discourse will be a case study of the ICU of St. Paul's Hospital in Vancouver, BC, Canada, where one of us (JR) has worked as an intensivist, as the ICU Director, and then as Chair of the Department of Medicine. We will use this case study to build the general case and draw on the literature to illustrate and support key observations and recommendations.

Current Physician Staffing of Intensive Care Units

The ICU of St. Paul's Hospital is a 14 bed multidisciplinary, closed Medical Surgical ICU closely affiliated with the University of British Columbia. There is a strong teaching program for medical students, rotating residents (from Medicine, Surgery, Anesthesia and Emergency Medicine), and Critical Care Medicine Fellows. There are about 700 admissions per year; about 85% of the patients require mechanical ventilation, and 40% of the patients are referred from other hospitals and the tertiary care programs of the hospital. There is a comprehensive research program ranging from molecular mechanisms of myocardial dysfunction and of epithelial injury, to genomics of sepsis and acute lung injury (ALI), to clinical trials in sepsis and ALI, to population research in critical care medicine. With that understanding of the ICU, how would one expect it to be staffed by physicians? At present, there are five full-time intensivists who rotate on call for one week at a time. The intensivist faculty member is the leader of the physician team (Fig. 1). There is almost always a first or second year critical care medicine Fellow on a 2-3 month rotation in the St. Paul's ICU. There are three to four residents from other services (Anesthesia, Medicine, Surgery and Emergency Medicine) who do a 2-3 month rotation in ICU. At all times there are one to three medical students doing an elective in intensive care medicine. The primary in-house call in the ICU is by the residents with a faculty intensivist on call each night. The critical care medicine Fellows take call every third or fourth night. Because of resident vacations and differences from month to month in resident numbers on ICU rotation, there is a cadre of intensive care Clinical Associates who provide clinical care on selected night and weekend day shifts.

How does this template compare to national guidelines for intensive care physician staffing? Recommendations from the Canadian Critical Care Society

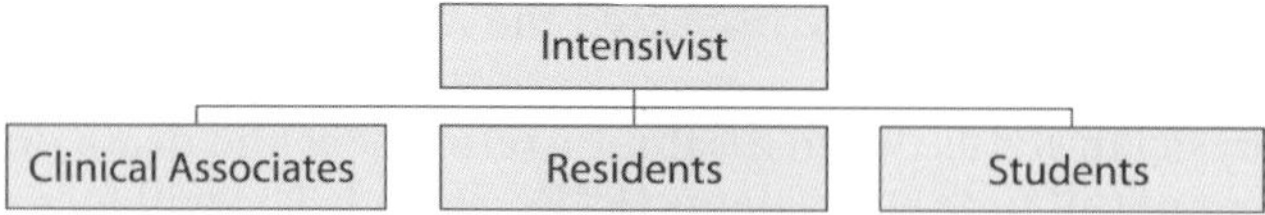

Fig. 1. Current ICU physician staffing at St. Paul's Hospital

have been updated and recommend one faculty intensivist for each ICU up to a maximum of about 14 beds. This recommendation is founded on the assumption that there is a separate in-house on-call physician such as a senior resident or a Clinical Associate.

How does this template compare to reports in the literature? Pronovost and colleagues did an extensive survey of ICU physician staffing in the USA [1]. They systematically reviewed 26 papers and abstracts representing 27 studies examining ICU attending physician staffing strategies in over 150 ICU in the United States, Europe and Asia. Study sample sizes varied from 177 to 5415 patients (mean: 1001, SD: 1190) and included ICU patients treated between 1979 and 2000. Study populations included medical ICUs (41%) surgical ICUs (9%), mixed medical-surgical ICUs (15%) and pediatric ICUs (11%) [2-27]. Eleven of the studies were from academic medical centers, six were from community teaching hospitals, four were from non-teaching community hospitals, and five included a variety of hospitals [1]. Pronovost and colleagues categorized ICU physician staffing in the studies as 'high intensity' (mandatory intensivist consultation or closed ICU [the intensivist is the patient's primary attending physician]) or 'low intensity' (no intensivist or elective intensivist consultation). The hospital mortality, ICU mortality, hospital length of stay and ICU length of stay were compared as outcome measures between patients treated in a high intensity staffing environment versus a low intensity staffing environment. Pronovost et al. calculated the random-effects, summary relative risk (RR) of mortality and the relative reduction for length of stay data from the studies for which the data was available.

Seventeen of the studies Pronovost and colleagues examined reported hospital mortality. Sixteen of the 17 studies showed a decrease in hospital mortality for ICU patients treated in a high intensity physician staffing environment, while one study reported a non-significant increase in hospital mortality with high intensity physician staffing. Fifteen studies reported ICU mortality according to ICU physician staffing. Fourteen of the 15 showed a decrease in ICU mortality for patients in a high intensity staffing environment. Thirteen of the studies that Pronovost et al. examined reported the hospital length of stay according to ICU physician staffing. Hospital length of stay was reduced for patients treated in a high intensity staffing environment (7-24 days for high intensity vs. 8-33 days for low intensity). Eighteen studies evaluated the ICU length of stay according to ICU physician staffing. ICU length of stay was reduced for patients treated in a high intensity staffing environment (2-10 days for high intensity vs. 2-13 days for low intensity). Overall, increased use of intensivists in the ICU led to significant reductions in hospital and ICU mortality and length of stay. In 1999, it was estimated that only one third of ICU patients in the United States were treated by intensivists as the primary physicians [28]. Since the greater use of intensivists in the ICU appears to be associated with reductions in ICU and hospital mortality and length of stay, increased intensivist staffing of ICUs may improve ICU patient outcomes.

All of the studies that Pronovost and colleagues examined were observational studies. There have been no randomized controlled trials to compare outcomes of patients in low versus high intensity staffing environments for practical and ethical reasons [1]. Three studies examined the impact of full time critical care physician staffing and other quality-of-care factors on mortality in pediatric ICUs [12, 20, 21]. The remaining 24 studies examined the impact of physician staffing strategies on outcomes in adult ICUs. While ICU and hospital mortality rates and length of stay were the primary outcomes, a number of the studies compared other clinically relevant outcome measures of patients treated in high- and low-intensity staffing environments. A number of studies compared the number of patients requiring mechanical ventilation and the duration of mechanical ventilation in low- and high-intensity staffing environments [6, 7, 18, 19, 23, 27]. Three of the studies examining post-surgical ICU patient care found that complications such as cardiac arrest, acute renal failure, septicemia, platelet transfusion, and reintubation were associated with low-intensity staffing strategies [11, 22, 25]. Interestingly, one of these studies found that using telemedicine as a means of achieving 24-hr intensivist oversight improved clinical outcomes, suggesting an alternate strategy to an around-the-clock, on-site intensivist care model [25].

In summary, the current St. Paul's Hospital ICU physician staffing is likely similar to physician staffing of other closed ICUs of similar size, patient complexity and with similar teaching and research responsibilities. What are the drivers that will impact physician staffing over the next decade at St. Paul's Hospital and at other hospitals?

Drivers of Changes in Physician Staffing in Intensive Care

Table 1 shows the major drivers that could impact physician staffing needs of a typical, tertiary care ICU over the next decade.

Patient volume in ICU is likely to increase over the next decade because of an aging population, because of increased complexity of surgery, because of increasing immuno-suppression from cancer chemotherapy, because of the increasing incidence and prevalence of septic shock [29] and because of evidence

Table 1. Drivers of changes in physician staffing in intensive care medicine

1. Patient volume – number of admissions per year
2. Patient complexity – source (e.g. Emergency, Medicine, Trauma, Surgery), severity of illness (e.g., APACHE II score), complexity of interventions (e.g., mechanical ventilation, vasopressor support, continuous renal replacement therapy [CRRT])
3. Quality improvement – clinical guidelines, clinical paths, quality improvement projects
4. Training requirements – medical students, residents, specialty fellows
5. Hospital and regional re-organization – impact on ICU beds
6. Other activities – research, teaching, administration, other clinical non-ICU programs
7. Budget – hospital, ICU, billing/fees/salaries
8. Leadership needs – administrative, research, teaching, clinical

of improved outcomes of intensive care medicine based on several randomized controlled trials. All of these factors are driving patient, family and referring physician demand for intensive care. At St. Paul's Hospital, population growth in the Vancouver downtown core as well growth in the Greater Vancouver Region are being used to project growth in the number of ICU beds in the Vancouver region and in particular at St. Paul's Hospital. Growth in specific programs (such as cardiovascular surgery) has been and will likely continue to be a factor driving demand for ICU beds at St. Paul's Hospital.

Complexity of patients and of the care that is delivered in the ICU is a second driver of ICU physician staffing. In the St. Paul's Hospital ICU, a comprehensive ICU database is used and captures all ICU admissions with data such as demographics, APACHE II scores, underlying diagnosis, interventions while in ICU and outcomes (ICU and hospital). This database is useful for tracking the ICU patient complexity and the impact on work-load and outcomes. Average APACHE II scores have risen over the last decade and will likely continue to increase. The growing evidence of the potential value of aggressive dialysis has lead to an increase in the proportion and numbers of patients on continuous renal replacement therapy (CRRT). In cardiovascular disease, the emergence of left and right ventricular assist devices, the use of early interventional cardiology and of intra-aortic balloon pumps have improved outcomes and therefore have also increased the numbers of patients on these complex modes of supportive care. The recent success of randomized controlled trials of therapies in intensive care medicine such as low (6 ml/kg) tidal volume [30], early cardiovascular resuscitation of sepsis and septic shock [31], activated protein C [32], intensive insulin therapy [33], and corticosteroids for septic shock, to name a few, while considered controversial by some, have generally increased recommendations for a comprehensive care approach to conditions such as sepsis and ALI. This complex care plan is likely best directed by full-time intensivists. It is likely that as even more therapies are 'proven', intensive care medicine will emerge as an even more independent evidence-based specialty which will increase demand for full-time intensivists to accurately and reliably apply best practice.

The Quality Improvement Initiative in health care lead by Donald Berwick [34] has had a substantial impact on virtually all fields of medicine including intensive care. There has been a parallel demand from groups such as Leapfrog for high quality intensive care under the direction of full-time intensivists. There will be a growing need for intensive care physicians to be aware of and indeed to lead quality improvement projects in the ICU to assure patients, peers, payers, and society that patients admitted to an ICU are receiving optimal care. Recent examples at St. Paul's Hospital of quality improvement projects are implementation of a sepsis care package developed by a Canadian Collaborative for Patient Safety with leadership from faculty at St. Paul's Hospital and citrate-based CRRT for patients who require CRRT but cannot tolerate heparin.

There are large jurisdictions (such as Canada) that have a physician shortage that is still not stable. As a result, the number of medical student places in Canada will increase over the next decade. The University of British Columbia medical school is doubling in size so that in a few years there will be double the number of residents requiring intensive care training. While there are other ICUs in community hospitals, it is likely that many of these residents will receive ICU training in the two major teaching hospital ICUs in Vancouver. This increase in resident numbers will likely increase the teaching load and have an impact on the number of intensivist teaching hours and thus overall physician staffing.

Regions and health maintenance organizations have re-organized in-patient services by rationalizing services such as trauma, cardiovascular surgery and neurosurgery. In Vancouver, St. Paul's Hospital took on major roles in the delivery of cardiovascular care, renal care and acquired immunodeficiency syndrome (AIDS) care in the mid 1990s. As a result, there were secondary effects on services such as the ICU, which provide part of these comprehensive tertiary care programs. In other jurisdictions, the ICU is impacted by other similar changes and there are 'ripple' effects of the physician staffing needs. There will likely be continued efforts to reorganize and rationalize care within regions and states in publicly-funded systems and these changes will indirectly influence numbers and types of ICU beds and so needs for ICU physician staffing.

There are several non-ICU clinical programs and important research, teaching and administrative responsibilities that drive intensive care physician staffing. At St. Paul's Hospital, the intensivists are responsible for a British Columbia Ambulance Service Air Transport Advisor program. This program provides 24/7 on-call intensivists for the paramedic-based air transport program which logs about 7,200 flights per year. The faculty intensivists provide emergent consultation by phone to the paramedics for all of the critical care transports. The faculty also provides a 24/7 Critical Care consultation service to a provincial maternity hospital in Vancouver for assessment and resuscitation of critically ill maternity cases. A recent example that will impact the St. Paul's ICU is the establishment of an ICU-based MET.

Obviously, a significant driver of changes in physician staffing is the overall ICU budget. Whether physicians bill fee-for–service, have overall service contracts or are salaried employees of an organization, there is usually a direct relationship between the overall magnitude of the ICU budget and the overall budget available for ICU physician staffing. Thus, changes in negotiations of fees and contracts can also drive change in ICU physician staffing. The ICU is often not a 'profit center' for for-profit hospitals and is a great consumer of costs in state or publicly-funded hospitals. Therefore, there may be a tension between needs of the hospital for clinical care as opposed to the reimbursement the hospital receives for critical care. Furthermore, hospitals in the private and in the public sectors often receive higher funding for specialized programs such as cardiovascular surgery and transplantation so that there may be a better case for ICU beds to support such programs. In contrast, ICU beds to support Emergency Department referrals of pneumonia and septic shock may not be as easily funded.

Leadership needs drive changes in ICU physician staffing. Virtually all ICUs have a Director/Department Head who is responsible for physician administrative aspects of the ICU. The skills that these individuals need are increasingly business skills such as preparing business cases, negotiation skills, conflict resolution skills, and organizational skills, none of which are in the medical school or residency curricula. The ICU Director is primarily responsible for issues such as budget, external relationships (e.g., hospital and university department heads, hospital administration (e.g., Vice-President of Medicine), other hospital

Table 2. Leadership skills of the ICU physician group

Leaders	Director/ Dept. Head	Clinical champion	Teaching leader	Research leader
Expertise & Portfolios	Budget	Outstanding clinician	Outstanding teacher	Outstanding researcher
	External relations	Implements quality improvement projects	Bedside teaching leader	Peer-reviewed grants
	Other Dept heads	Implements guidelines	Classroom teaching leader	Peer-reviewed manuscripts
	Hosp (VP Med)	Implements clinical paths	Focus on adult medical education	Mentors junior faculty
	University (dean)		Niche expertise (e.g. simulators)	Trains graduate students and fellows
	Nursing, RT			
	Divisional meetings			

RT: respiratory therapy

departments (such as Nursing and Respiratory Therapy) and coordinates the ICU group's divisional meetings. The other leadership skills that a teaching hospital ICU physician team must possess are a clinical champion, a teaching leader, and a research leader (Table 2). The clinical champion is the individual who is recognized as an outstanding clinician, who keeps abreast of the leading edge clinical and translational research literature, who is comfortable and can lead a quality improvement process, and can direct and lead implementation of clinical guidelines in the ICU. The teaching leader is the best teacher in the group, chosen for bedside teaching skills, for classroom teaching skills, and who has a special interest in the leading edge of adult education in medical care, such as in use of simulators for teaching or some other unique education niche. The research leader is an acknowledged strong scientist who has peer-reviewed grants and peer-reviewed manuscripts, mentors junior faculty, trains graduate students and critical care fellows, and is a resource for the group for research expertise.

Future Model of ICU Physician Staffing

Figure 2 shows a model of likely future physician staffing at St. Paul's Hospital that may be representative of other teaching hospitals that face similar drivers of change. The growth in patient volume, complexity, teaching, and other drivers will

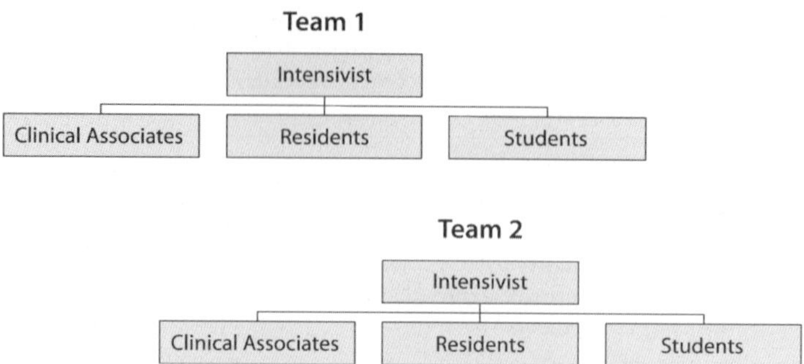

Fig. 2. Future ICU staffing

likely increase the number of ICU beds such that there are at least two ICU physician teams in the ICU and likely a third team responsible for other clinical non-ICU activities such as the MET, air transport and maternity critical care. Each team will still be lead by a faculty intensivist and the composition of teams will likely include a mixture of housestaff/residents and clinical associates (also known as hospitalists). There may be a need for further differentiation of the ICU-based teams such as Team 1 for more acute recent admissions and Team 2 for subacute cases in ICU. The third team will likely be responsible for all clinical non-ICU activities.

We foresee that there will be an even greater need for a strong foundation under each team of quality improvement, research, teaching, and a robust, real-time database of all ICU and non-ICU activities to aid future planning, research and quality improvement initiatives.

Processes For Planning Future ICU Physician Staffing

We have reviewed the current staffing of ICUs, drivers of changes in ICU physician staffing, and presented a model of a future ICU physician staffing example. However, there will be a great need for a much more robust process to get from now to 2015 and to optimize the ICU physician staffing in 2015. We suggest that there are (simplistically) three processes that most ICUs use to plan such changes in physician staffing (Table 3).

We suggest that the least likely to be successful and effective is simple lobbying and whining to authorities such as hospital administrators. There is no

Table 3. Processes for planning changes in ICU physician staffing

1. Business case proposals
2. Data-driven projections of ICU size and likely physician staffing requirements
3. Lobbying (also known as whining)

doubt that administrators will be overwhelmed by such lobbying and will more likely than not react negatively to emotional arguments without data and projections.

A common approach taken by many ICUs is to use a data-driven summary of current and future ICU volume and derive likely ICU physician staffing requirements. This is a step better than lobbying but does give the administrators the information they need to balance conflicting requests for funding and staffing. It is merely the ammunition but not delivered effectively.

The optimal and most likely successful process for planning physician staffing will be a well-written, well-documented business case that is carefully-prepared and can be read by several levels of the administration (e.g., Vice President Medicine, other Department Heads, Vice President Finance, Chief Executive Officer of the hospital and Dean of the medical school). The common sections of a business case include the 'business' of the ICU at present, the current ICU volume and complexity profiles, the drivers of change and likely impact on the specific ICU including patient volume and complexity and other anticipated drivers of change, the 5 (and even 10) year projections of physician staffing, the justification of the proposed staffing, the benefits to patients, the ICU, the hospital and the communities served, the budget projections and summary cost/benefit projections. The ability to articulate how altered physician staffing will enhance patient care and outcomes by activities such as QI and use of guidelines can be compelling for administrators. The needs for more and better teaching and research can be compelling for Deans and university department heads but are sometimes less compelling for those who hold the hospital purse strings.

Optimized ICU Physician Staffing

The optimal ICU physician staffing model has yet to be realized. There is convincing data now that a closed ICU or at least mandatory intensivist consultation model is associated with improved outcomes and length of ICU and hospital stay. As Pronovost et al. state in their discussion, it is not clear what components of the closed ICU or mandatory intensivist consultation process are the main cause(s) of improved outcomes. Is it knowledge and technical skills? Is it frequency of rounds and availability to respond knowledgeably to crises? Is it team leadership skills and optimizing the combined skill sets of all health care members of the ICU team? Is it application of most relevant care based on knowledge of the very specialized literature of critical care?

Figure 3 shows a model that we currently favor for future ICU physician staffing. The key elements are strong leadership in administrative, business, clinical care, teaching, and research, well-organized teams with clear responsibilities, and a foundation of quality improvement, clinical guidelines, research, teaching, and a comprehensive ICU and non-ICU (but critical care-related) clinical database.

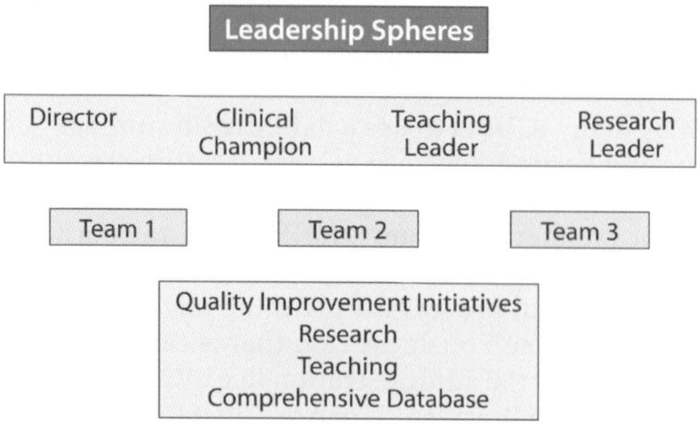

Leadership Spheres

Director	Clinical Champion	Teaching Leader	Research Leader

Team 1 Team 2 Team 3

Quality Improvement Initiatives
Research
Teaching
Comprehensive Database

Fig. 3. Optional ICU physician staffing

References

1. Pronovost PJ, Angus DC, Dorman T, Robinson KA, Dremsizov TT, Young TL (2002) Physician staffing patterns and clinical outcomes in critically ill patients: a systematic review. JAMA 288:2151-2162
2. Al-Asadi L, Dellinger RP, Deutch J, Nathan SS (1996) Clinical impact of closed versus open provider care in a medical intensive care unit. Am J Respir Crit Care Med 153:A360 (abst)
3. Baldock G, Foley P, Brett S (2001) The impact of organisational change on outcome in an intensive care unit in the United Kingdom. Intensive Care Med 27:865-872
4. Blunt MC, Burchett KR (2000) Out-of-hours consultant cover and case-mix-adjusted mortality in intensive care. Lancet 356:735-736
5. Brown JJ, Sullivan G (1989) Effect on ICU mortality of a full-time critical care specialist. Chest 96:127-129
6. Carson SS, Stocking C, Podsadecki T, et al (1996) Effects of organizational change in the medical intensive care unit of a teaching hospital: a comparison of 'open' and 'closed' formats. JAMA 276:322-328
7. DiCosmo BF (1999) Addition of an intensivist improves ICU outcomes in a non-teaching community hospital. Chest 116:238S (abst)
8. Dimick JB, Pronovost PJ, Lipsett PA (2000) The effect of ICU physician staffing and hospital volume on outcomes after hepatic resection. Crit Care Med 28:A77 (abst)
9. Dimick JB, Pronovost PJ, Heitmiller RF, Lipsett PA (2001) Intensive care unit physician staffing is associated with decreased length of stay, hospital cost, and complications after esophageal resection. Crit Care Med 29:753-758
10. Diringer MN, Edwards DF (2001) Admission to a neurologic/neurosurgical intensive care unit is associated with reduced mortality rate after intracerebral hemorrhage. Crit Care Med 29:635-640
11. Ghorra S, Reinert SE, Cioffi W, Buczko G, Simms HH (1999) Analysis of the effect of conversion from open to closed surgical intensive care unit. Ann Surg 229:163-171
12. Goh AY, Lum LC, Abdel-Latif ME (2001) Impact of 24 hour critical care physician staffing on case-mix adjusted mortality in paediatric intensive care. Lancet 357:445-446
13. Hanson CW, 3rd, Deutschman CS, Anderson HL 3rd, et al (1999) Effects of an organized critical care service on outcomes and resource utilization: a cohort study. Crit Care Med 27:270-274

14. Jacobs MC, Hussain E, Hanna A (1998) Improving the outcome and efficiency of surgical intensive care: the impact of full time medical intensivists. Chest 114:276S-277S
15. Kuo HS, Tang GJ, Chuang JH (2000) Changing ICU mortality in a decade: effect of full-time intensivist. Crit Care Shock 3:57-61
16. Li TC, Phillips MC, Shaw L, Cook EF, Natanson C, Goldman L (1984) On-site physician staffing in a community hospital intensive care unit. Impact on test and procedure use and on patient outcome. JAMA 252:2023-2027
17. Manthous CA, Amoateng-Adjepong Y, al-Kharrat T, et al (1997) Effects of a medical intensivist on patient care in a community teaching hospital. Mayo Clin Proc 72:391-399
18. Marini CP, Nathan IM, Ritter G, Rivera L, Jurkiewicz A, Cohen JR (1995) The impact of full-time surgical intensivists on ICU utilization and mortality. Crit Care Med 23:A235 (abst)
19. Multz AS, Chalfin DB, Samson IM, et al (1998) A «closed» medical intensive care unit (MICU) improves resource utilization when compared with an «open» MICU. Am J Respir Crit Care Med 157:1468-1473
20. Pollack MM, Katz RW, Ruttimann UE, Getson PR (1988) Improving the outcome and efficiency of intensive care: the impact of an intensivist. Crit Care Med 16:11-17
21. Pollack MM, Cuerdon TT, Patel KM, Ruttimann UE, Getson PR, Levetown M (1994) Impact of quality-of-care factors on pediatric intensive care unit mortality. JAMA 272:941-946
22. Pronovost PJ, Jenckes MW, Dorman T, et al (1999) Organizational characteristics of intensive care units related to outcomes of abdominal aortic surgery. JAMA 281:1310-1317
23. Reich HS, Buhler L, David M, Whitmer G (1998) Saving lives in the community: impact of intensive care leadership. Crit Care Med 25:A44 (abst)
24. Reynolds HN, Haupt MT, Thill-Baharozian MC, Carlson RW (1988) Impact of critical care physician staffing on patients with septic shock in a university hospital medical intensive care unit. JAMA 260:3446-3450
25. Rosenfeld BA, Dorman T, Breslow MJ, et al (2000) Intensive care unit telemedicine: alternate paradigm for providing continuous intensivist care. Crit Care Med 28:3925-3931
26. Tai DY, Goh SK, Eng PC, Wang YT (1998) Impact on quality of patient care and procedure use in the medical intensive care unit (MICU) following reorganisation. Ann Acad Med Singapore 27:309-313
27. Topeli A (2000) Effect of changing organization of intensive care unit from «open policy without critical care specialist» to «closed policy with critical care specialist». Am J Respir Crit Care Med 161:A397 (abst)
28. Schmitz R, Lantin M, White A (1999) Future Workforce Needs in Pulmonary and Critical Care Medicine. Abt Associates, Cambridge
29. Annane D, Aegerter P, Jars-Guincestre MC, Guidet B (2003) Current epidemiology of septic shock: the CUB-Rea Network. Am J Respir Crit Care Med 168:165-172
30. The Acute Respiratory Distress Syndrome Network (2000) Ventilation with lower tidal volumes as compared with traditional tidal volumes for acute lung injury and the acute respiratory distress syndrome. N Engl J Med 342:1301-1308
31. Rivers E, Nguyen B, Havstad S, et al (2001) Early goal-directed therapy in the treatment of severe sepsis and septic shock. N Engl J Med 345:1368-1377
32. Bernard GR, Vincent JL, Laterre PF, et al (2001) Efficacy and safety of recombinant human activated protein C for severe sepsis. N Engl J Med 344:699-709
33. van den Berghe G, Wouters P, Weekers F, et al (2001) Intensive insulin therapy in the critically ill patients. N Engl J Med 345:1359-1367
34. Berwick DM (1989) Continuous improvement as an ideal in health care. N Engl J Med 320:53-56

ICU Research – One Decade From Now

J. J. Marini and D. J. Dries

Introduction

Good planning requires insight and a clear vision of what lies ahead. But in a rapidly changing world, any attempt to make predictions over a long interval may be a fool's errand. ('Only two things are certain: Death and taxes'). Knowing this to be the assignment and perhaps our fate, our approach is to first describe the strong forces that appear currently to be shaping our intensive care unit (ICU) practice, to speculate on future opportunities and needs, and to extrapolate from this base to their implications for future conduct of research in critical care 10 years hence. Our collaboration in developing this projection blends the thoughts of two intensivists, who share clinical responsibilities and research interests, but who practice in different ICU venues (medical [JJM] and surgical [DJD]). The ideas expressed clearly represent our own perspective and stem from personal experience, gathered in the idiosyncratic environments in which we practice. Others undoubtedly hold radically different views of what lies ahead, shaped by their own experience and circumstances.

Categories of Research

Research in critical care – whether performed in a laboratory or in a patient care setting – can be broadly categorized into experimental and non-experimental work. Experimentation suggests a hypothesis-driven rationale that can be tested at the proverbial 'bench' or at the bedside. The intent is often to probe the mechanisms that underlie disease pathogenesis, evolution, resolution, or treatment response. *Clinical* research can be subdivided into qualitative and quantitative sectors (Fig. 1) [1, 2]. Observational studies – cohort, case control, and surveys – are focused on gathering information that adds to the useful database that informs clinical practice. Another branch of non-experimental clinical research is data synthesis, a category umbrella that includes meta-analysis, decision analysis, and cost-effectiveness evaluation. Quantitative clinical research in recent years has been dominated by its experimental branch – the conduct of clinical trials in which one or more treatments are compared. By their nature, clinical trials seldom provide information that elucidates mechanisms, but often provide a proof of principle, help settle issues regarding what works and what does not across a population, and yield results that may serve as a stimulus or

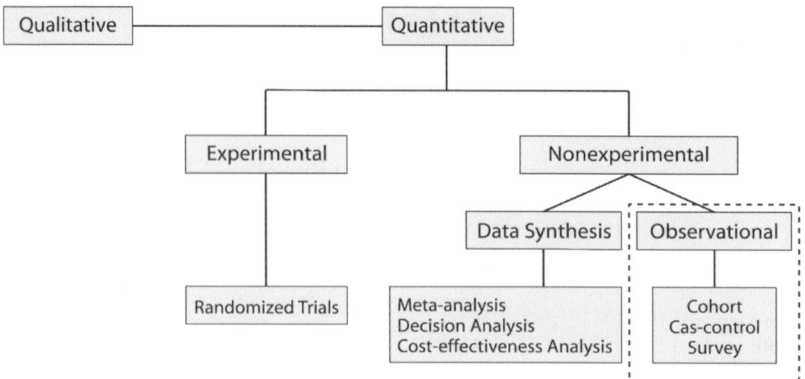

Fig. 1. Categories of clinical investigation (from [1] with permission)

point of focus for additional mechanism-defining experimental science. Health care delivery research also can be considered a form of clinical research, which is focused on the process of care execution. Here the emphasis may be to analyze how practice is currently conducted or to test alternative methods for providing care (e.g., protocol usage versus independent care giver decision-making).

Trend Drivers

From our perspective, six major forces are currently at work to shape the future of critical care research. These are:

- economic constraints
- escalating concern for patient safety
- constrained manpower for care delivery and academic activity
- technology advancement
- burgeoning complexity of patient problems and therapeutic options
- interconnections across disciplines and globalization across geographic boundaries

Each trend driver will be discussed in the following paragraphs.

Economic Constraints

Simply put, we would not be paying attention if we fail to feel or understand the dominance of this force upon our ability to conduct research. The cost of providing medical care has been escalating at an alarming rate that far out-strips the inflationary pressures within other major sectors of the economic activity [3]. Demographic shifts are also of concern. The aging populations of many economically advanced countries pose a rising demand for critical care services [4,

5]. Common sense dictates that increasingly disproportionate health expenditure cannot persist long into the future. As health-related economic pressures are brought to bear increasingly on the resources of government, business enterprise and individuals, standards of living will be threatened unacceptably. Attempts to contain costs by streamlining the organization of the health delivery system – to manage care – have met with only limited success, and the disappointing pace at which improved efficiency ('process') models have been implemented leaves little room for optimism [6]. Assuming that rationing will not be embraced without complaint and withering political 'push-back', the difficulty of resolving these economic issues threatens the 'optional' pool of health-related activity (i.e., education and research).

The difficulty of providing expected rates of service compensation to physicians has led to the increasing diversion of discretionary work time effort into 'dollar-productive' clinical activity, thereby minimizing their educational effort and research involvement. In the North American system, most academic faculty members are charged with covering their own salaries through research grants, administrative commitments, or clinical activity; relatively few perpetually funded 'chaired' positions are available, and virtually all of these are bestowed on well-published academicians with long-established reputations in medical science. A restricted number of salaried 'lines' designed to support a traditional academic career are available in governmental hospitals (state and military), but the compensation offered is generally less than that in the private community. Increasingly, even these dollars are being re-directed to encourage the care delivery mission for their constituents, leaving less discretionary time.

These same economic constraints also have given rise to a need for 'enhanced throughput' of patient encounters within the hospital system, leading to logistic difficulties in conducting clinical research that requires unbroken periods of observation time and/or a patient unaltered by a diagnostic or therapeutic interventions. The economic crunch also has impacted the private sector, which currently provides funding for the overwhelming majority of ICU research work. All too often, investigator-initiated work underwritten by industry has yielded to company-driven mandates that compensate the 'investigator' monetarily for enrolling patients and for data-collection services related to specific product/drug testing, rather than support him/her for intellectual endeavors with possible spin-offs for the company.

These economic pressures have given rise to 'bottom line thinking' directed toward finding out what works and what does not, rather than toward probing underlying mechanisms of action with less tangible long-term payoffs. Given the financial incentive/penalty structure that drives most administrators, this short-term orientation is certainly understandable. It may even be desirable *to some extent* in a highly volatile healthcare marketplace. Yet, over the long haul, devastating consequences associate with such an unrelenting preoccupation on near-term cash flow to hospital and physician; lack of investment has doomed many businesses to obsolescence and inefficiency as the general economic climate changes about them.

To us it appears no coincidence that the rise of 'evidence based' data quality rating systems and that of managed care were contemporaneous; both are consistent with principles of optimizing cost effectiveness [7]. The need for enhanced efficiency also has bolstered a movement towards research into standardization of care, a principle that has served in the manufacturing industries very well. By analogy, standardization of care to reduce variability makes good sense when there is uniformity of definitions of disease, similar levels of expertise among providers, similar behavior of diseases, uniformity of opinion regarding proper action, and perfection of the processes for the delivery of care. Unfortunately, in critical care, it can be argued that our definitions are too imprecise to broadly support such a standardization paradigm; there exist relatively few 'gold standard' indicators with which to certify and monitor disease. Moreover, standardization of process relies on unchanging, predictable conditions and uniform raw materials. But in fact, patients who carry the same disease labels are far from uniform in their co-morbidities and capacities to respond to treatment. Consequently, the ever-changing complex systems dealt with in the critical care setting often require timely feedback and continual readjustment of well-reasoned empirical management, and not scripted progression of care protocols.

Within the United States, the drive toward improved efficacy of inpatient care has given rise to the rapidly adopted 'hospitalist' career pathway [8, 9]. Hospitalist physicians, few of whom receive dedicated training beyond residencies in general medicine, now deliver increasing volumes of well remunerated *critical care* services, often without involving the intensivists trained specifically in their management. With their focus on cost-containment and care process streamlining, the priorities of the hospitalist are clearly not in the conduct of discovery-oriented research. Thus, this economics-driven trend is one that favors care delivery as opposed to research conduct but may be a logical necessity, given the relative dearth of critical care specialists (see below).

A lack of financial resources for discretionary use in research is a problem that has always been faced by struggling economies. Apart from the option not to participate at all in the development of new knowledge, some less well developed countries have opted to sponsor research only in designated government hospitals. Under the influence of the economic forces just outlined and of the constraints on academic manpower described below, tighter restriction of venues in which research is conducted may be a future consequence for investigator-initiated research in highly advanced countries, as well.

Escalating Concern for Patient Safety

Aligned tangentially with the economic trend driver of critical care research is the mounting concern for patient safety in the ICU environment [10, 11]. Almost by definition, critical care implies the application of advanced technologies and invasive treatments to patients who are unusually vulnerable to complications. Concern for patient safety in such an environment is entirely appropriate, and given the dangers inherent to ICU care, protection of the critically ill and preservation of their rights (and/or those of their surrogates) to autonomy of informed decision-making must be non-negotiable goals. Yet, against this background, recent studies have called to attention the unacceptable frequency of medical errors that continue to be made in all hospital settings [10, 11]. In the face of the rising costs of medical care, bill payers have exerted strident demands to lower their outlays for health benefits [12]. Some have banded together to bring real economic pressure to bear on the health care delivery systems to improve quality and reduce cost. The initiative of the 'Leapfrog' consortium prominently exemplifies the impatience of the business and community leaders to improve safety of their beneficiaries while reducing cost [11, 12]. These legitimate concerns for safety already influence the nature and quantity of ICU research and are likely to continue to do so well into the future.

In response to market forces that demand improved quality of service and safety of patients, the traditional complexion of the teaching hospital is in the throes of an impressive 'make-over'. The housestaff-driven care of yesteryear is increasingly considered a hazardous, outmoded model. Concern for errors arising from the lack of experience of trainees, sleep deprivation, and fatigue has mandated curtailment of working hours and pushed the more experienced academic staff into the caregiver roles formerly played by their trainees. Although this approach clearly has logical appeal, it has added pressure onto the academic physician to be primarily a doctor, not an investigator or even a teacher [13–15].

Awareness of patient vulnerability has led to ever-tightening restrictions imposed by institutional review boards concerning research conducted at the bedside. The clinical investigator is now severely limited in making observations and/or therapeutic interventions that place the patient at any significant risk, even if the interventions might be hugely informative and scientifically worthwhile. Indeed, most studies with negligible potential for benefit to the patient are discouraged or disallowed. Independent of ethical concerns, the economic and legal consequences of experimental misadventures restrain the conduct of hazardous research. When untoward consequences result from participation in a study, the expenses related to that care must be underwritten by the patient, the hospital, the research protocol, or the funding agency. Although infrequent, lawsuits resulting from adverse research outcomes have the potential to inflict enormous financial and public relations burdens on the hospital and care providers involved in their conduct. These practical liabilities may be as inhibitory to critical care research as any genuine concerns for patient safety.

Crisis in Education of Academic Physicians

The classical 'three-legged stool' of the academic clinical scientist has been threatened to be reduced to a single pillar [13–15]. In the not so distant past, the academic practitioner could undertake research, education, and patient care all within the scope of his/her daily practice. Currently, however, the academic physician must focus more sharply on only one of these elements; as the previous discussion suggests, it is the *clinical* leg that has overtaken the others, since time devoted to education or unfunded research cannot be spent on generating clinical revenue. Without question, early career salary grants have been helpful, and funding is available for research involvement *provided that* the work fits the template of the public or private funding agencies. Regrettably, the associated salary offset component is often insufficient, especially for more senior investigators. In the United States, the National Institutes of Health are charged with conducting research programs that meet certain political as well as scientific objectives. Consequently, targeted programs are generously supported and themes consistent with the prevailing forces within specific study sections garner the 'lion's share' of the available dollars. For at least the last two decades, the majority of funding has been directed toward sub-cellular and molecular biological work as well as toward epidemiologic studies and clinical trials. We do not contest that these topic areas are both exciting and beneficial, and it is entirely appropriate that they receive generous support. However, these overwhelming priorities have encouraged neglect of the study of practical problems occurring at the physician-patient interface, i.e., the areas that most physicians (and relatively few non-physician scientists) think of as 'translational research'. Too often, what is left in view of the student and resident physician is company-driven research almost devoid of intellectual appeal for either the site designated 'investigator' or for the potential academic recruit.

This lack of fundability of investigator-initiated projects focused at the bedside has had a devastating impact on the training milieu, as it has forced young trainees potentially interested in academic medicine to choose between laboratory science and clinical medicine. Quite understandably, these young physicians choose to be doctors first and see research as a diversion from that primary task. Complicating matters, these young physicians in the United States graduate from medical school seriously in debt and cannot forgo high rates of compensation [16]. Moreover, there has been attrition of the academic role models, who once served to attract students and residents into the academic community. Often, what the resident now encounters is not an accomplished physician dedicated to advancing the science and practice of medicine, but rather a time-hassled clinician with limited time to teach, considerable administrative responsibilities, and – if their supervisor is involved at all in science – crushing pressures to accomplish fundable research focused away from the bedside. Understandably, this mix of activities has limited appeal for the young physician with unprecedented financial obligations and a focus on starting a family and building a quality lifestyle.

There is another important factor to consider. Whether or not politically correct to call attention to it, the drastically altered gender demographics of medical practice also have fueled the push away from academic participation [17, 18]. Over the past 25 years, the percentage of women among physicians has increased several-fold. In reality, time priorities are shaped by factors outside of medicine, and for the highly trained woman facing the biological time clock, raising a family means limiting time for discretionary activities unrelated to generating income. Largely owing to their vital traditional roles in the family unit, women may be even less likely than men to enter the stressful, time consuming field of critical care medicine. Day care and domestic assistance alleviate some of these burdens, but neither addresses them all, nor are they always financially acceptable or logistically feasible options for the recent medical graduate. Perhaps as a consequence, women are seriously under-represented as academic contributors to our discipline of critical care medicine relative to their representation in physician workforce overall; this phenomenon is particularly evident at the more senior ranks. Critical care research and practice has been nurtured by a generation of great leaders, but the pool of such individuals is rapidly shrinking as they age and retire. Unless our gender-polarized field can attract and retain women investigators at a much greater clip, one can envision a steady attrition of research output as the aging generation of (predominantly male) intensivists retires [14, 15, 19].

Another repercussion of this sea change in gender demographics within medicine is that a much larger percentage of physicians now marry other professionals (often other physicians) than was true a quarter century ago. Both partners may have sizeable loans awaiting repayment. No longer is one spouse enabled to spend unlimited energy in climbing the hierarchy of academic professional prominence by a homebound spouse dedicated solely to family development. Given these domestic responsibilities, the prospect of pursuing an unfettered academic career and a balanced personal life appears unrealistic to many young physicians of both genders, and rightly so.

At present, there are very few young physicians, who see a secure upward path that makes optimal use of their skills and training for a career in research and allows adequate time for a rewarding personal life. In critical care, we confront a shrinking number of dedicated young investigators to fill in the ranks of those who have gone before them.

In contrast, the popularity of the hospitalist pathway within academic-affiliated hospitals may well be explained by several factors [20]. Despite the curriculum revisions of the past decades, the majority of internal medicine training still occurs within the hospital, a practice venue that offers familiarity to the graduating resident. Indeed, the rise of 'hospitalism' appears to validate the focus of traditional training on inpatient care. Those individuals, who have devoted their entire lives to their own education, see the academic medical center as an attractive place in which to continue that endeavor and to teach others, fearing the gradual attrition of their skills and not wishing to practice in the isolation from colleagues perceived to occur in traditional private practice. Increasingly, it is the hospitalists, not the specialists, who serve as the teachers in academic centers and role models. Because they are omnipresent and often perform their educational functions very well [20, 21], the student or resident may see this broad-based, non-research focused, administration-endorsed, and potentially *academic* career as a logical, familiar, 'do-able' extension of ongoing training. At least at present, hospitalism has the additional allure of offering full staff salaries (and scheduled hours) without requiring the additional economic and intellectual investments demanded of subspecialty fellowship training. This career path presents an attractive alternative at a time when most young doctors are sensitive to their financial condition and future lifestyle. Finally, it is not a field devoid of research potential, albeit one focused on health services delivery rather than on defining disease mechanisms and their correction.

Perhaps the most attractive aspect of the hospitalist choice involves the quality of lifestyle that it appears to offer. In most hospitalist assignments, there are predictable hours, no call assignments, competitive salaries and liberal amounts of 'off-time'. No subspecialty training is required to practice the full range of medical acuity. Once thrown, this 'toggle switch' choice to opt for lifestyle over subspecialty training all but precludes a research career in critical care medicine. Few seem to take account that the 'burnout' rate within this young field at this juncture already appears to be disturbingly high. As the hospitalist pathway matures, the composition of its scope of practice may also enrich sufficiently to stem this trend. Going forward, the increasing necessity of providing intensive care with these acute care oriented professionals, who lack subspecialty training in critical care and, as a rule, have responsibilities and interests focused outside the ICU, bodes poorly for future ICU research productivity, at least of the types traditionally and currently undertaken.

Complexity of Patients and Therapeutic Environments

At any single point in time, critically ill patients often have more than one dysfunctional organ system and carry more than one physiologically important diagnosis. The patient population receiving care in the ICU is inexorably ageing [4], and many patients reach old age with a variety of chronic debilitating diseases as the backdrop for their acute problems. As a consequence, the same disease labels often encompass patients with physiologically diverse characteristics and severity [22–24]. These co-morbidities and intersecting disorders of physiology often influence the response to interventions, perhaps in ways that are not well understood. Such complexity impairs the conduct and relevance of certain forms of ICU research that rely heavily on precise sample characterization. Moreover, the treatments brought to bear on these patients routinely include dozens of drugs and therapeutic devices. For just such reasons, attempts to standardize the care delivered to these patients that do not incorporate tight feedback loops are destined to fail in such a complex environment. The process of well-reasoned intervention, timely evaluation, and mid-course correction is fundamental to therapeutic success; other paradigms of one disease-one treatment approach serve us less well. When dealing with such complexity of co-morbidities and co-interventions, reductionist approaches of isolating a variable of interest are difficult or impossible to conduct and may be theoretically flawed when underlying mechanisms are incompletely understood [25–27]. Future research approaches that utilize techniques to more precisely define the sample population, e.g., by biochemical or genetic phenotyping [28], and probe the mechanistic hierarchy, e.g., by neural network analysis [29], promise to better inform the clinical trials that have preoccupied our attention over the past 15 years (Fig. 2). For many questions confounded by complexity, sophisticated animal models – especially those developed and conducted over lengthy periods in simulated ICU environments – may be the best that we can do.

Advanced Technology

In attempting to perfect the care delivery to critically ill patients and to make optimal use of an expanded range of therapeutic options, it is vital to have a high

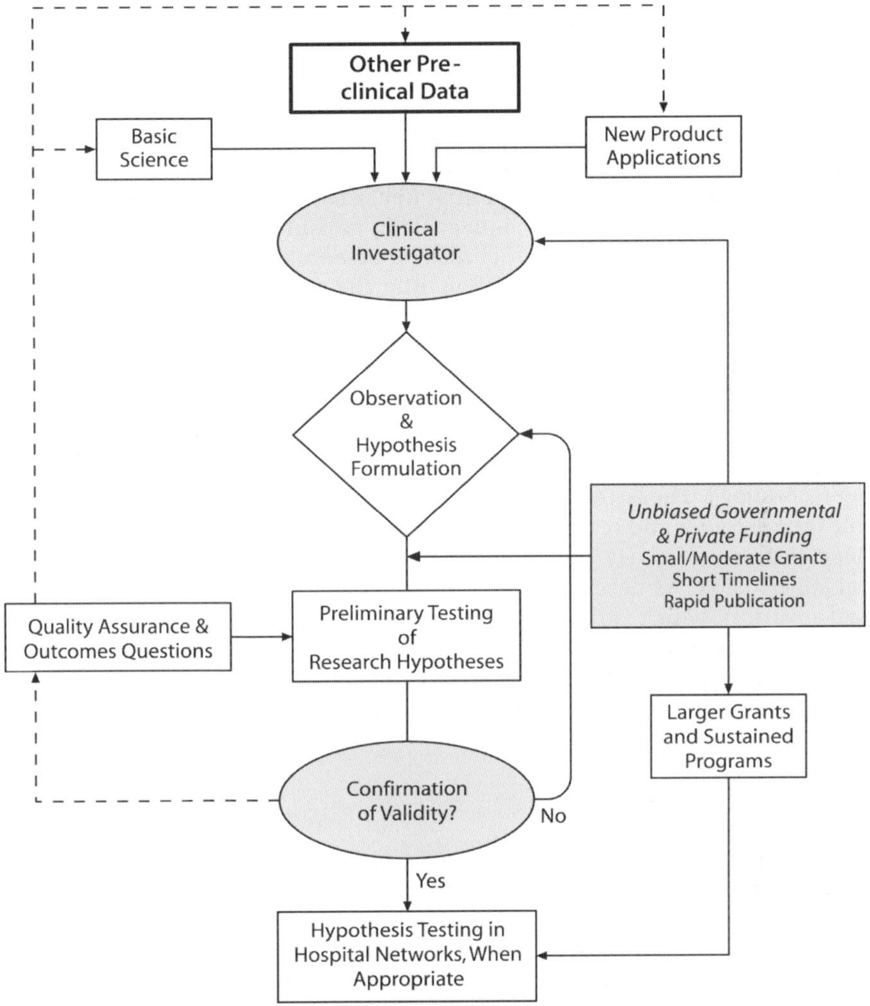

Fig. 2. Idealized clinical research paradigm circa 2015

quality, readily assessable information stream to draw from and sophisticated tools with which to accomplish our objectives. These tools should be non-invasive whenever possible. The explosive growth of molecular biology, telecommunication technology, and the medical applications of computer science has already begun to re-shape the clinical environment wherein we practice [28, 30, 31]. Retrieval of information from the literature or from the patient record is far easier in the electronic age, imaging methods are immeasurably more detailed, and minimally invasive procedures now effectively replace many surgical operations. With 'point-of care' testing and such accelerated laboratory methods as polymerase chain reaction (PCR), the turn-around time between measurement of key variables and intervention decision can be dramatically shortened [28, 31]. Recent advances, such as the mapping of the human genome, the development of microarrays, and the identification of disease-specific biochemical markers, are poised to initiate a torrent of research activity directed toward such important areas as bio-signature identification and drug discovery [28, 31–33]. The display of multiple computationally complex variables of monitoring interest can now occur in real time. Rapid transmission of key images and voluminous data offers the possibilities of 'off-site' management, consultation at a distance, and networked information sharing for clinical or research purposes. Miniaturized, wireless sensors and video transmission offer the promise of convenient, comprehensive monitoring at long distances, and perhaps the opportunity to reduce the need for continual human bedside surveillance [34, 35]. An extension of the telemetry concept, non-invasive, remote tele-monitoring could track vital physiologic parameters of patients at high risk for ICU admission (from other inpatient locations) or re-admission after ICU discharge. The latter is an important problem that has not been approached adequately for lack of an affordable facilitating technology. The latter appears to be at hand. Such technological advances enable the caregiver and researcher to manage otherwise overwhelming clinical problems more effectively or to undertake the care of more patients with less direct supervision. As described later under 'Opportunities', it is these technological advances, which appear to hold the greatest promise for mastery of a burgeoning number of very difficult clinical problems with fewer highly educated and trained personnel at the bedside. They hold equal potential for conducting certain kinds of informatics-aided research.

Globalization

Enhanced communication and data access as well as the ability to traverse great distances to attend conferences and observe behavior has tightened the cohesiveness of the scientific community and has helped to foster cross disciplinary interactions. This globalization now enables research to be conducted with appropriate collaborations from persons, who can contribute uniquely to the project at hand. The potential for information dissemination and telecommunication has had the effect of dramatically widening the pool of potential contributors of new information to our field. No longer is timely access to the latest scientific discoveries limited to the region wherein it occurs. Over the past 15 years, for example, scientific communications in critical care medicine, once overwhelmingly the responsibility of North America, have been fully internationalized. One reason is the sabbatical exchange of trainees; another is the transcendence of national boundaries for participation in scientific meetings. Even within the same geographic region, interdisciplinary information transfer ('cross-pollenation') and collaboration have become increasingly common, aided by rapid information transfer and accelerated 'Web' publishing. Information and techniques that are developed or used commonly in one non-medical field may be unknown to biomedical research, yet have dramatic applications. Rapid information transfer has aided such collaboration. There are numerous recent examples of medical applications from engineering and materials sciences.

Opportunities (Table 1)

Alongside the daunting problems for critical care science that may arise from the trend drivers just enumerated has been a parallel expansion of our ability to conduct research. Torrid expansion of the knowledge base has occurred not only in the specialties of medicine, but concurrently in every discipline, allowing unique research opportunities to emerge. The computerization of our society has worked with astounding rapidity within medicine to automate medical records and to dramatically improve our ability to mine our expanded database for valued insights. No present day academic practitioner needs to be reminded of how computerization has aided clinical, educational and increasingly research productivity by dramatically accelerated information retrieval and communication with peers. At present, it is possible to monitor physiological processes precisely and non-invasively, to have immediate access to scientific literature at the point of care, to perform direct order entry and to continuously record complex banks of data over extended periods. Once a research question is formulated, retrieval of the appropriate information is possible in many instances within a brief period of time. The availability of emerging techniques, such as microarray analysis of biological samples, allows us to ask detailed questions regarding gene expression, protein elaboration, and diagnostic identity. First described in 1995, microarrays utilize thousands of simultaneous DNA or oligonucleotide probes to determine levels of mRNA expression in a given specimen [32, 33]. The pattern of mRNA expression can be regarded as an expression 'fingerprint' of a cell or tissue. This newfound ability to probe at the micromolecular level has opened up exciting vistas for drug development and for targeting patients.

Table 1. Opportunities in critical care research

Advancing Telecommunication Technology
Long distance collaboration
Electronic libraries & remote data access
Electronic and portable medical records
Bedside Informatics
Anatomical & Physiological Imaging
Molecular Biological Applications
Microarray analyses
Rapid biochemical analyses
Non-Statistical Methods Geared to Complex Systems
Automation of Personnel Services

Roughly 5,000 genes of the approximately 35,000 genes in the human genome are believed to encode proteins with therapeutic potential; i.e, 90% of potential targets remain unexplored. Yet, as of 1996, successful drug treatments were directed toward only about 500 gene targets. Almost without question, future drug development for the problems of critical care will incorporate microarray technology [28, 32, 33].

Nowhere in the clinical setting has the influence of advanced computer technologies been more evident than in the field of anatomical and physiological imaging [36]. We now have imaging technologies that allow sophisticated surgeries and detailed anatomical and physiological investigations to be conducted with minimal invasiveness. Indeed, the same block of comprehensive data obtained non-invasively or semi-invasively at a single computer-enabled imaging session (e.g., helical 'spiral' CT) can be re-configured to ask questions that arise from the requested study and relate to detailed static anatomy or dynamic events (such as, regional ventilation). Functional imaging, using a variety of radiological, ultra-sonographic, acoustic, electrical conductivity and metabolic probes, is a currently blossoming area rich with opportunities for scientific investigation that were impossible to consider only a short time ago. Simultaneously, telecommunication advances have reduced the cost of transferring images and information sufficiently that long distance research collaboration, remote management of critically ill patients, and even long range specialty surgery can be undertaken [37, 38]. Such technologies have begun to move detailed monitoring from the ICU into the home setting, where they can track the progress of patients with high risk diseases or life threatening conditions or allow detailed follow-up of recently discharged individuals to ensure compliance with the intended treatment plan. In view of the scientific interest in the long-term impact of critical care, these technologies suggest unprecedented opportunity for longitudinal data collection.

Automation of services currently provided by highly trained and compensated personnel could help to free-up the financial resources needed to foster research in our field. Moreover, the expansion of wireless, non-invasive physiological monitoring and information processing promises to enable ancillary and technical personnel to gather and analyze sophisticated research data bases with only minimal guidance from the physician-investigator. The data intensive field of critical care medicine is highly likely to benefit from this technological leveraging of our research time.

Sophisticated monitoring may also enable more timely diagnosis and intervention. Although few examples of truly 'closed loop' systems that continuously monitor patients and intervene with appropriate goal-directed therapies can be enumerated at the present time, in many areas this ideal is closer to being realized [39]. For example, systems have been developed to monitor glucose and to meter out insulin in order to keep serum glucose concentration within desired range without the need for personnel to intervene. From a purely technical point of view, 'closed loop' mechanical ventilation has been close to implementation for at least a decade. Should such automation prove safe and effective, it could offload a large element of the service component of providing critical care, which currently consumes so many of the health care dollars allocated to intensive care. Research opportunities for addressing the benefits, dangers, and optimization of 'closed loop' therapy suggest an important new avenue for outcomes and physiology-oriented researchers alike.

Needs

The trend drivers and opportunities previously outlined suggest at least seven important unmet needs for the critical care research environment (Table 2).

Independent Funding Sources

If original investigation is to continue by the critical care practitioner at the bedside, there must be money to fund the investigator's time as well as the worthwhile projects they envision. Intensive care is extremely expensive. Limited funds from the public sector are now allocated to translational research *at the bedside*, and the tightly purpose-restricted funds available from the private sector beg for an independent funding source that would judge projects on the basis of their inherent worth and not on the basis of politics or economic potential.

De-Politicization of the Approval / Award Process

Project awards are made currently against a heavy background of academic and governmental politics. The absence of funds for work centered at the interface between patient and physician must be rectified, if we are to make timely progress in the common goal of achieving better results at lower costs. Currently, the interests of the clinician scientist are weakly represented in groups that judge the merits of research proposals. Securing stable funding for research conducted at the bedside has become a Herculean task.

Table 2. Needs for critical research

- Independent Funding Sources
- De-Politicization of the Grant Award Process
- Development of the Clinician-Scientist Pathway
- Restoration of Trust Between Patient and Physician
  - Legal tort reform
- Rejuvenation of the Educational Process for Critical Care Research
  - Applied respiratory physiology
  - Computer and communication skills
- Long Term, Realistic Animal Models of Critical Illness and ICU Care
- Long Range Vision & Planning By Policy Leaders

Development of the Clinician-Scientist Academic Pathway

We must nurture young physicians to encourage careers as clinicians actively engaged in critical care research [13, 14]. To facilitate this goal, it will be important to: prevent the accumulation of crushing debt burdens during the years of training; provide appropriate research training; define valid, durable mechanisms to free-up dedicated time to undertake meaningful research in all phases of the career cycle; make liberal use of care extenders, not only for execution of clinical duties, but also to facilitate the conduct of research. The clinical burdens and expectations for work hours and compensation are not likely to favor research participation unless means can be identified that facilitate and lighten the clinical workload.

Restoration of Trust Between Patient and Physician

The critical care unit is an alienating environment with an intimidating array of machines and procedures. Therapeutic decisions often carry the potential for harm as well as benefit. Patients and/or their families have very little opportunity to bond with the physician caring for the patient. Restoration of trust between patient and physician must be addressed for bedside research to flourish.

Rejuvenation of the Educational Process for Critical Care

Steady erosion of the role of physiology in the clinical aspects of critical care management has had adverse repercussions for the training of clinical investigators. When dealing with a complex system, a secure knowledge of physiology is vital for making reasoned judgments that integrate observations from the numerous channels in play and to respond appropriately to the feedback provided from the 'n =1' clinical trials we are forced to perform in when caring for individual patients. Univariate, population-based conclusions from clinical trials inform the decision making process, but do not and theoretically cannot provide a prescription for individual care at all points of decision. This concept is valid, even when all relevant questions have been adequately trialed and all answers are in.

Long Term Realistic Animal Models of Acute Illness

Virtually all animal models of critical care have been developed for completion over periods of minutes to hours, whereas critical illness evolves over days to weeks. Because of the complex physiological interactions extant in the clinical setting, appropriate and humane whole animal models of critical illness are sorely needed to perform experiments that integrate the numerous pathophysiologic and adaptive forces at work over the extended course of critical illness.

Long Range Vision / Planning By Policy Leaders

The crisis in critical care research conducted at the patient physician interface is genuine. Effectively addressing the issues will require considerably more far-sighted orientation and long range planning than has recently been exercised. Policies aimed at next year's bottom line or the prevailing political wind will encourage further erosion of our field's research health. Fundamental concerns regarding the fate of the clinician-scientist that began to surface more than 15 years ago have only intensified since. Our political and professional societal leaders must develop durable plans of action to preserve and renew our research and educational infrastructures.

Predictions

Ignoring the admonitions of the quotes given in the Introduction to this discourse, we two fools will now 'rush in' to make predictions 'where wiser men fear to tread' (Table 3). These are based on what we see as the primary trend drivers, opportunities, and needs for research in critical care medicine, as outlined above. Three sweeping predictions seem rather 'low risk' to make. First, we are confident that the funding crunch will threaten to stifle investigator-initiated research in the critical care setting. Investigator-initiated critical care research, already concentrated in the academic medical centers, will contract further into an even smaller number of academic centers of excellence, as it has been prudent to do in other economically stretched countries of the world. Second, technology will continue to advance very quickly, opening new opportunities to address the serious problems that confront us. Last, there will be continued trends for less invasive care that puts the patient at reduced risk for harm.

Table 3. Predictions for 2015

- Funding Crunch for Critical Care Research
- Contraction of Investigator-Initiated Investigation
- Less Invasive Testing and Intervention
  - Shift toward non-invasive/non-interventional research projects
- Increased Collaboration across Disciplines and Geographic Boundaries
- 'Outsourcing' of Patient Databases & Laboratory Analyses
- Computer Simulation & Facilitation of Data Collection
- Increased Volume of 'Process-Oriented'/ Outcomes Research
  - Hospitalist conducted and cost containment / safety oriented
- Improved Definitional Precision and Reduced Numbers of Clinical Trials
- Expanding Impact of Molecular Biology
- Investigations into Defining Appropriate Therapeutic Objectives for the Critically Ill

Certain other predications rest on less firm ground. Very briefly they are as follows:

Collaboration: There will be increasing efforts to collaborate in order to take advantage of the 'connecting' technologies afforded by technological and telecommunications advancements. Interdisciplinary collaborations will flourish to meet the needs for specialized expertise.

'Outsourcing': There will be even further 'outsourcing' of our investigational patient bases and of laboratory activities. As the depth at which research is conducted becomes more sophisticated, it becomes less likely that any single laboratory can perform all of the desired work in isolation of others. Enhanced telecommunications will facilitate such interchanges.

Noninvasive Investigation: In our risk-averse practice environment, investigation in critical care medicine will become increasingly noninvasive, especially for questions that require interventions unlikely to benefit individual subjects. Here, newer monitoring and imaging methods will assist in obtaining data without invasive interventions, and molecular probes will assist not only for more precise characterization of patient phenotypes, but also in the scientific exploitation of tissues and fluids removed for clinical purposes.

Computer Simulation and Facilitation of Research: Simulation technology, already making important inroads in the 'no-risk' training of physicians for technically demanding management skills, also will begin to be used to answer certain questions related to life support. Computerization will improve the detection, control, and feedback that are necessary for timely intervention. Linear, unidimensional statistical models of research design and analysis will be complemented by the numerically demanding, computer-dependent techniques that better take into account the multiple variables often at work to influence outcomes of interest in acutely ill patients. Integrative analytical techniques, both statistical and increasingly non-statistical (such as neural network analysis), will be applied to confront the complexities of critical care.

Process/Outcome Orientation: As demands for cost accountability intensify, so too will investigation into the processes of care delivery, ICU organization, and long-term outcomes. Research into the feasibility and efficacy of telecommunication-enabled remote ICU management will be conducted under the urgency to leverage scarce valuable personnel against the press of building populations needing expensive care.

This 'process/best practice/outcome' orientation toward care delivery will be pushed forward by the hospitalists as it is well aligned with their professional *raison d'etre*. Impetus for such information will only continue to strengthen as fewer personnel fully trained in critical care medicine are available at the bedside. As protocols are implemented to drive care in an environment of competence variation, they will accentuate the role of ancillary care givers such as nurse practitioners, respiratory therapists, and physiotherapists. It is reasonable to presume that these care extenders may be called upon increasingly to participate in clinical research conducted at the bedside.

Improved Clinical Trials and Definitional Precision: The rampant enthusiasm for clinical trials will moderate in the next decade unless more precise definitions and better identification of the patient bases can be accomplished, co-intervention controls are more tightly applied, and the questions addressed for trial rest on a solid pre-clinical research base. Attempts will be made to more precisely define the disease entities we now broadly classify. Such problems as the acute respiratory distress syndrome (ARDS), sepsis, and ventilator-associated pneumonia are too imprecisely classified at present to allow a build up of a solid database of proven observations and therapies. Increasingly, well conducted trials will be viewed as proof of principle, rather than as a prescription for care of the individual. The methodology is simply too expensive, too cumbersome, too time-anchored, and too unreliable to guide practice, particularly when external validity cannot be verified and funding remains within the private sector.

Expanding Impact of Molecular Biology in ICU Research: Molecular biology will penetrate effectively into intensive care practice and research. Patients will be better identified by nucleic acid and protein expression microarrays. Tracking of responses by detailed biomarkers will dramatically improve the insights gleaned from longitudinal research (see below). Drugs will be targeted towards promotion and inhibition of gene activity. The research field of drug development guided by molecular science will reach impressively into the ICU.

Identification of Appropriate Therapeutic Targets for the Critically Ill: Most of the current approach to critical care is based on the tacit assumption that aggressive attempts should be made to restore normal physiological parameters. Yet this underlying assumption must be questioned. In the ICU setting, therapeutic targets that lie outside of those that characterize health may be tolerable or even desirable. The lesson of permissive hypercapnia is an appropriate example. Moreover, given enough time, human beings are capable of impressive adaptive responses. Because examination of these questions is imperative, this research field will become more active as the decade progresses.

The development of long-term, large animal models of acute illness will provide essential insights to inform cautious forays of research into these important questions in the clinical arena.

Conclusion

Powerful trend drivers threaten to adversely transform the conduct of critical care research over the next decade. Despite an increased need, there will be continued erosion of the physician-scientist's role in critical care medicine, as movements away from specialized critical care training and toward both cost-effectiveness and hospitalist-based management intensify. Insecurity of the career pathway, disappearance of role models, and lifestyle issues will erode the attractiveness of academic appointments based in investigative pursuits. To preserve and enhance care delivery, we must confront these problems directly and urgently. We must embrace advances in technology and improve our educational environment to make optimal use of scarce resources and rejuvenate interest in the academic practice of critical care medicine.

References

1. Pronovost PJ. Kazandjian VA (1999) A new learning environment: combining clinical research with quality improvement. J Eval Clin Pract 5:33–40
2. Rubenfeld GD, Angus DC, Pinsky MR, Curtis JR, Conners AF Jr, Bernard GR (1999) Outcomes research in critical care: Results of the American Thoracic Society Critical Care Assembly Workshop on Outcomes Research. Am J Respir Crit Care Med 160:358–367
3. Halpern NA, Bettes L, Greenstein R (1994) Federal and nationwide intensive care units and healthcare costs: 1986–1992. Crit Care Med 22:2001–2007
4. Angus DC, Kelley MA, Schmitz RJ, et al (2000) Current and projected workforce requirements for care of the critically ill and patients with pulmonary disease: Can we meet the requirements of an aging population? JAMA 284:2762–2770
5. Kelley MA, Angus D, Chalfin DB, et al (2004) The critical care crisis in the United States: A report from the profession. Chest 125:1514–1517
6. Robinson JC (2001) The end of managed care. JAMA 285:2622–2688
7. Evidence-Based Medicine Working Group (1992) Evidence-based medicine: a new approach to teaching the practice of medicine. JAMA 268:2420–2425
8. Wachter RM, Goldman L (1996) The emerging role of "hospitalists" in the American health care system. N Engl J Med 335:514–517
9. Anonymous (2002) The who, what, when, where, whom, and how of hospitalist care. Ann Intern Med 137:930–931
10. Kohn LT, Corrigan JM, Donaldson MS (2000) To Err Is Human: Building A Safer Health Care System. National Academy Press, Washington
11. Milstein A, Galvin RS, Delbanco SF, Salber P, Buck CR Jr (2000) Improving the safety of health care: the Leapfrog Initiative. Eff Clin Pract 3:313–316
12. Galvin R, Milstein A (2002) Large employer's new strategies in health care. N Engl J Med 347:939–942
13. Khadaroo RG, Rotstein OD (2002) Are clinician-scientists an endangered species? Barriers to clinician-scientist training. Clin Investig Med 25:260–261
14. Schrier RW (1997) Ensuring the survival of the clinician-scientist. Acad Med 72:589–594
15. Phillipson EA (2002) Is it the clinician-scientist or clinical research that is the endangered species? Clin Investig Med 25:23–25
16. Naradzay JF (1998) Into the deep well: The evolution of medical school loan debt. JAMA 280:1881–1883
17. Nonnemaker L (2000) Women physicians in academic medicine: new insights from cohort studies. N Engl J Med 342:399–405
18. Tesch BJ, Wood HM, Helwig AL, Nattinger AB (1995) Promotion of women physicians in academic medicine: glass ceiling or sticky floor? JAMA 273:1022–1025
19. Levinson W, Lurie N (2004) When most doctors are women: What lies ahead? Ann Intern Med 141:471–474
20. Goldman L (1999) The impact of hospitalists on medical education and the academic health system. Ann Intern Med 130:364–367
21. Landrigan CP, Muret-Wagstaff S, Chiang VW, Nigrin DJ, Goldmann DA, Finkelstein JA (2002) Effect of a pediatric hospitalist system on housestaff education and experience. Arch Pediatr Adolesc Med 156:877–883.

22. Schuster DP (1997) Identifying patients with ARDS: time for a different approach. Intensive Care Med 23:1197–1203
23. Levy MM, Fink MP, Marshall JC, et al (2003) 2001 SCCM/ESICM/ACCP/ATS/SIS International Sepsis Definitions Conference. Crit Care Med 31:1250–1256
24. The ARDS Network (2000) Ventilation with lower tidal volumes for acute lung injury and the acute respiratory distress syndrome. N Engl J Med 342:1301–1308
25. Eichacker PQ, Gerstenberger EP, Banks SM, Cui X, Natanson C (2002) Meta-analysis of acute lung injury and acute respiratory distress syndrome trials testing low tidal volumes. Am J Respir Crit Care Med 166:1510–1514
26. Shanawani H (2004) Lessons from the ARDS network ventilator trial design controversy. Respir Care Clinics N Am 10:317–328
27. Eichacker PQ, Natanson C (2003) Recombinant activated protein C in sepsis: Inconsistent trial results, an unclear mechanism of action, and safety concerns resulted in labeling restrictions and the need for phase IV trials. Crit Care Med 31:S94–S96
28. Fink MP (2004) Research: Advances in cell biology relevant to critical illness. Curr Opin Crit Care 10:279–291
29. Hanson CW 3rd, Marshall BE (2001) Artificial intelligence applications in the intensive care unit. Crit Care Med 29:427–435
30. Celi LA, Hassan E, Marquardt C, Breslow M, Rosenfeld B (2001) The eICU: It's not just telemedicine. Crit Care Med 29:N183–N189
31. Villar J, Mendez S, Slutsky AS (2001) Critical Medicine in the 21st Century: From CPR to PCR. Crit Care 5:125–130
32. Napoli C, Lerman LO, Sica V, Lerman A, Tajana G, de Nigris F (2003) Microarray analysis: a novel research tool for cardiovascular scientists and physicians. Heart 89:597–604
33. Schena M, shalson D, Davis RW (1995) Quantitative monitoring of gene expression patterns with a complementary DNA microarray. Science 270:467–470
34. Rosenfeld BA, Dorman T, Breslow MJ, et al (2000) ICU telemedicine: Alternate paradigm for providing continuous intensivist care. Crit Care Med 28:1–7
35. Barie PS (1997) Advances in critical care monitoring. Archi Surgery 132:734–739
36. Trotman-Dickenson B (2003) Radiology in the intensive care unit. J Intensive Care Med 18:239–252
37. Schlag PM, Moesta KT, Rakovsky S, Graschew G (1999) Telemedicine: The new must for surgery. Arch Surg 134:1216–1221
38. Rassweiler J, Binder J, Frede T (2001) Robotic and telesurgery: Will they change our future? Curr Opin Urol 11:309–320
39. Branson R (2004) Understanding and implementing advances in ventilator capabilities. Curr Opin Crit Care 10:23–32

Organizing Clinical Critical Care Research and Implementing the Results

D. Cook and S. Finfer

Introduction

The overall goal of clinical research in the intensive care unit (ICU) is to increase our understanding of how critical illness can be prevented, diagnosed, treated or palliated, thereby improving outcomes for patients. The past ten years have seen great advances in critical care research with the advent of national and international consortia and the realization that research must focus on important patient-centered outcomes, and that collaborative multicenter research is the most efficient way to achieve this goal. These advances have been facilitated by the advent of the internet, email, and powerful but affordable personal computers. These advances from outside the field of medicine have revolutionized the way we access and process information, and have vastly improved the speed and efficiency of communication across research groups. Despite these advances, the future holds many challenges, both old and new. Some of these challenges are unique to critical care (e.g., multisystem disease, relatively small and heterogeneous population of patients), some are shared with other specialties (e.g., consent from unconscious patients, which is also a problem for neurosurgery, neurology and emergency medicine), and some are generic to medicine (e.g., making policy makers recognize the important role of research in improving outcomes, and ensuring efficient use of resources).

In this chapter, we identify five priorities that we believe should be actively pursued to take clinical research in critical care to the next level in the next 10 years.

Engage with Health Care Regulators and Funders

Although much has been achieved through the hard work and enthusiasm of individual researchers and research consortia, taking clinical research to its rightful place in 2015 will require more resources, and we will need the enthusiastic support of health care regulators and funders to achieve this. The clinical research community must convince funders and regulators that investing in clinical research is money well spent. Whilst the competition for funding is always fierce, and funders may shy away from diverting resources from clinical services to research, the value of investing in research has long been embraced by the pharmaceutical industry and should be self evident. Take for example the Saline versus Albumin Fluid Evaluation (SAFE) Study, the largest randomized trial in critical care to date [1]. The SAFE study was conducted on a cash budget of less than A$3million, although the true cost may have been closer to A$5million. Patients were enrolled over a 15-month period but from conception to publication the trial took 5 years to complete. During that time the Australian government spent close to A$100 million on albumin, and other healthcare systems will have spent many times that amount. Regardless of whether albumin is cost effective or not, an investment of A$3 million dollars seems worthwhile to define the role of an intervention costing many times that amount over the duration of the trial.

Many clinicians, educators, agencies and societies recognize the importance of evidence-based practice. To promote evidence based practice, governments have established bodies, such as the UK National Institute for Clinical Excellence (www.nice.org.uk). The Australian government has decided to purchase access to the Cochrane Library for the entire population of Australia. What governments have not done is systematically examine the many hurdles that obstruct the conduct of the clinical research on which evidence-based practice depends. Hurdles to conducting multicentered clinical research have been well documented. They include lack of standardized application forms, the need to submit protocols to many individual institutional ethics committees, individualized patient information and consent forms, the need to obtain funding from multiple sources to support a single trial, legislation designed to protect patient privacy that prohibits the collection of even anonymous aggregated data, failure to recognize that emergency research requires special provision to allow the participation of patients who are unable to give prior informed consent, and inability to understand that it may be unreasonable to expect surrogate decision makers to make informed decision within a few hours of a loved one becoming critically ill. Clinical researchers and the academic community at large are unlikely to solve these problems alone; to do so will require an alliance with health care funders and with governments.

We propose that the critical care community elicit the support of other specialties, and lobby health care funders and governments to achieve the following:

1. Standardized international grant application forms (or universal structured core content)
2. Standardized national (if not international) application forms for research ethics boards
3. Reciprocal recognition of research ethics board approvals both within and among countries (when research oversight standards are similar)
4. Standardized patient information and consent forms (with provision for minimal local adaptation as necessary)
5. Legislation allowing for delayed consent in emergency research (regardless of jurisdiction)
6. Appropriate national and international bodies to approve clinical trials to be conducted under emergency medicine provisions
7. National registries of approved emergency medicine trials into which participants may be enrolled without prior written informed consent

8. National 'opt out' registries of persons who do not wish to be included in emergency medical research projects in the event of sudden critical illness or injury
9. Financial support for the information technology needed to conduct large scale clinical trials cost-effectively within clinically relevant time frames
10. Government funded indemnity for clinicians conducting approved investigator-initiated and peer-review funded clinical trials

Improve the Quality and Quantity of Clinical ICU Researchers: A Physical and Virtual Network of Clinical Critical Care Research Training Centers

Critical care is a unique interdisciplinary specialty, and many fellowship training programs are small. Very few fellowship programs have a critical mass of trainees headed for careers as clinician-scientists. Accordingly, formal clinical research training in ICU programs is often underdeveloped [2], particularly in relation to basic science research training, which has led to calls for more organized educational initiatives [3]. To prepare intensivists to answer important questions of tomorrow, more formal opportunities for first class clinical research training are necessary.

Opportunities for research training cannot be considered in isolation, but must be seen against a backdrop of a shortage of critical care specialists and trainees in many countries. Clinical research can be an intrinsically rewarding and enjoyable activity. When taught by trained, experienced enthusiasts, and sustained by designated time and resources, it is possible to attract high quality clinician scientists to critical care.

We propose a global physical and virtual network of clinical critical care research training centers with several centers in each country. The goal of the Global Training Network will be to recruit, train and retain keen clinical ICU investigators by first attracting highly qualified critical care research trainees, graduate and post-graduate students, and junior faculty. Centers should partner with universities (e.g., Graduate Schools to identify Masters and PhD students) and existing critical care fellowship programs [4] to identify candidates who wish to pursue a career as a clinician scientist. Through these contacts, we will identify trainees with a variety of disciplinary and cultural backgrounds, who will contribute to, and benefit from, the Training Network. We will expand and formalize currently available programs for clinical research training around the world. Centers in the Training Network will offer at least one of the following: a) a range of core courses in clinical research, b) advanced methodology (e.g., factorial and cluster randomization), c) advanced biostatistics (e.g., survival analysis), or d) specialized research management (e.g., web-based data management platforms). Each trainee will have an individualized educational program, a lead project, a local mentor, and a small advisory panel. The mentor will provide personal advice, ideas, guidance and time management support to advance the trainee's projects and career [5]. The advisory panel will help to direct the trainee to specific resources, bridge funding, opportunities, and meetings that may advance the career of the trainee. The trainee will be required to establish a project under the supervision of the mentor and a few designated senior clinical investigators, who may be on the advisory panel.

Accepting that many talented individuals in both developed and developing countries may not be able to relocate to a Critical Care Research Training Center, we propose a Virtual Training Center be established at the same time as the physical centers. The Virtual Center will develop the same training opportunities as the physical centers but will deliver training using distance learning techniques, electronic communication and audio and video conferencing. Senior clinical researchers from Physical Training Centers will play a critical role in the Virtual Center and trainees from the Physical Training Centers will be encouraged to participate in exchange programs with Virtual Trainees.

Trainees will bring project proposals to annual Global Training Network protocol development meetings where more senior members will provide feedback using the community-mentoring model we have developed in the Canadian Critical Care Trials Group [6]. The venue will rotate around the cities of host institutions and will be available to virtual trainees by video linking. After presentations at these meetings, trainees will obtain crucial individual and community mentoring and receive valuable study-specific feedback, the combination of which will ensure the rigor, relevance and feasibility of their protocols. In addition, the Training Network will have a competitive Traveling Fellowship Program to allow structured, objective-specific training of candidates in several designated international Network Training Centers over 2–4 years. The Traveling Fellowship will allow trainees to create opportunities of greatest interest to their future, through exposure to different faculty supervisors and research groups around the world.

A Global Network of Clinical Critical Care Research Training Centers will provide dedicated junior clinician scientists with individualized training in clinical critical care research. Together, these centers will provide a transformational experience for future clinician scientists, helping to ensure their academic success and their future contributions to the optimal care of ICU patients.

Conduct More Large International Studies

To answer clinically relevant research questions with confidence, we need not only valid studies to minimize systematic error, but also large studies to minimize random error. Several landmark international epidemiologic studies and other observational studies in critical care medicine have been published. However, questions about prevention or therapy are best answered by rigorous multicenter interventional trials involving several thousand patients designed to detect small, but clinically relevant differences in heterogeneous groups of patients.

By 1995, approximately 1,300 randomized trials in critical care had been published [7]. Among 660 of these analyzed in two specialty journals, half randomized less than 100 patients, and 90% were single-center studies. In 2004, a new era in critical care research was heralded by the SAFE study [1], marked by the 'large simple randomized trial' first popularized in cardiology. The Australian and New Zealand Intensive Care Society (ANZICS) Clinical Trials Group tested the effect of 4% albumin versus 0.9% sodium chloride on 28-day mortality among 7,000 heterogeneous critically ill patients requiring fluid resuscitation. This sample size was chosen to provide 90% power for detecting a 3% difference in absolute mortality from an estimated baseline mortality rate of 15%. Traditionally, completion of such trials would take many years. However, 16 centers in two countries enrolled patients into SAFE at a rate of over 100 patients per week and the study was completed in 15 months rather than the scheduled 18 months. For countries conducting many ICU trials concurrently, completion of trials of this size would take even longer.

We propose to build on the existing relationships, and forge new ones, to increase formal international collaboration in both adult and pediatric clinical critical care research. The international critical care community is still relatively small, cooperative and cohesive. Currently, several national and international clinical research consortia exist, addressing pressing problems of the critically ill. Key features of these consortia include a cohesive spirit, a sense of mission to achieve shared goals, and acknowledgment that such networks are much more than the sum of their parts [8]. Investigator-initiated, peer-reviewed funded ICU trials have grown from a small cottage industry into a major academic enterprise, and many peer-reviewed funded international collaborations have already been completed [9, 10]. We still need to increase the number of ICUs involved in critical care research in each country, to enhance the capacity for rapid recruitment, while maintaining data quality. Involvement of suitable community ICUs (funding and infrastructure permitting) would also enhance the generalizability of subsequent trial results.

To achieve more international collaboration in peer-reviewed research, the following is necessary:

1. To change federal funding policies, explanatory documents should describe previous productive collaboration among national clinical research consortia, showing that this has been done before.
2. Formal mechanisms must be developed to leverage peer-reviewed sponsorship among agencies in different countries, which would help investigators to engage in international efforts (even those that might have started out originally as national efforts).
3. Peer review in different countries requires identifying expert reviewers outside that country, who are not already involved in these large trials.
4. Standardized web-based application forms for all major funding bodies would improve the logistics of concurrent trial applications in different countries (e.g., Canadian Institutes for Health Research and the National Health & Medical Research Council of Australia).
5. Contingency funding (one peer review agency only releases funds if the partnering agency in another country awards funds) results in asynchronous

decision making, which is a major inhibitor of multinational collaboration. Alignment of funding timelines is sorely needed.

6. Pediatric research should be a priority focus, since the community of pediatric ICU clinician scientists is smaller than adult ICU clinician scientists, and international collaboration is obligatory if clinical questions are to be answered efficiently.

Mandate Trial Registration

It is estimated that at least 41,000 randomized controlled trials (RCTs) are currently in progress in North America alone (www.centerwatch.com). How many RCTs are underway in the ICU setting internationally is unknown. Trials registration will help to answer this question.

Publication bias is the tendency for studies with positive results to be published in preference to studies with neutral or negative results. Traditionally, investigators are more likely to write up trials with positive than negative results [11]. Editors are also more likely to publish such trials [12]. However, more recent studies suggest that this may be less of a problem than in the past. Of 745 consecutive controlled clinical trials submitted to JAMA over three years, 51% had positive results, 46% had negative results, and 3% had results of unclear significance [13]. Publication was significantly more likely if trials were multicenter versus single-center (1.60, 95%CI 1.02-2.52, $p=0.04$), if patients were enrolled in United States versus elsewhere (2.06, 1.20-3.52, $p<0.01$), and if there was an *a priori* sample size calculation (1.90, 1.23-2.95, $p<0.01$). After adjusting for these covariates, the magnitude of the treatment effect was not an independent predictor of publication in JAMA (1.30, 0.87-1.96, $p=0.21$). Whether this is the case in other journals is not clear. Trial registries are a step in the right direction to avoid the problem of publication bias. Registries also minimize the possibility of duplicate publication, which gives the impression of a larger body of evidence than that which truly exists.

For clinicians, publication bias provides a more enthusiastic interpretation of an intervention's effectiveness than is warranted. Duplicate publications increase the chance that certain trials (usually with positive results) will be remembered. For reviewers, both publication bias and duplicate publications lead to biased meta-analyses. For researchers, both problems increase the risk of misinterpreting treatment effects cited in grant applications, and increase the risk of ceasing research prematurely on interventions erroneously perceived to be of established effectiveness. Trial registries may decrease the risk of these problems. For readers, trial registries may also have a positive influence on the quality of reporting. Although the advent of electronic communication and powerful but affordable personal computers has greatly enhanced our ability to conduct high quality research, the ability to perform complex statistical manipulation of both large and small datasets carries both great benefits and great risks. In particular, when a detailed analysis plan for important study is not published prior to the study results being known, there is the potential for investigators to perform multiple analyses with the attendant risk of reporting 'chance' positive findings.

A priori reporting of the study design and analytic plan is likely to result in more faithful descriptions of the methods than if the protocol had not been disclosed; this should be a requirement for publication in major general and critical care journals.

We propose obligatory trial registration for clinical critical care research. An example of a suitable registry is from the US National Library of Medicine (www.clinicaltrials.gov), which allows public access and electronic searching of contact information, study design, and funding source. The International Committee of Medical Journal Editors (ICMJE) recently has adopted a mandatory trials registration policy effective for any trials starting enrollment after July 1, 2005 [14]. This initiative will make the existence of every trial a public record, for free access by all research stakeholders. Moreover, registration will be a prerequisite to publication in the 11 journals represented by the ICMJE.

Improve Ethical Standards but Decrease Bureaucracy

In the ICU, just like outside the ICU, clinical research should fulfill seven ethical requirements [15]. These include: 1) social value, 2) scientific validity, 3) fair participant selection, 4) a favorable risk-benefit ratio, 5) independent review, 6) informed consent, and 7) respect for enrolled participants. We predict that these ethical requirements are unlikely to change substantially in the next decade, although the operationalization of some of them may evolve in some sectors.

Take informed consent, for example. Delayed or deferred consent has been used previously in emergency medicine trials when patients lack decisional capacity. Studies that do not involve emergency interventions have recently been conducted using deferred consent [1]. In an international trial called CRASH (Corticosteroid Randomization after Significant Head Injury), 20,000 patients were planned to be allocated to corticosteroids or placebo to detect a 2-week mortality reduction from 15% to 13% with 90% power [16]. The trial was stopped early after accrual of 10,008 patients due to a significant 20% relative risk increase in mortality. Participating hospitals set their own consent procedures; some allowed a complete consent waiver while others required consent from a legal representative. For most clinical research projects in the ICU, we suspect that family members or surrogates will continue to provide informed consent, whereas waived, deferred and/or delayed third party informed consent will be used more for emergency interventions in some jurisdictions. In North America, we predict that for most ICU studies, individual patient autonomy (choosing to participate or not, as expressed through the next of kin) will outweigh the default sense of social responsibility to answer research questions (waived, deferred and/or delayed third party informed consent, even if confirmed or refuted subsequently by the patient). A completely uniform approach in ICU research seems unlikely on this issue in the next decade.

We propose higher ethical standards but less bureaucracy in clinical ICU research. Although optimal research oversight is desirable, some developments and complexities are barriers rather than facilitators to sound ethical research. For example, in their effort to protect individual autonomy, the province of Québec in Canada passed legislation that required first person consent for all research. Québec's civil code began undergoing modifications to its original text in 1955 under the Duplessis government. The latest version was established in 1990 and passed as law in 1994, which provided new rules for research, but omitted consideration of the adult patient unable to provide consent. This resulted in immediate cessation of all clinical investigations involving acutely ill patients. The research community raised this as a serious problem and in 1998 it was resolved with the passing of Law 432, which modified Article 21 (which itself addresses consent for research experimentation). Since 1998, investigators in Québec have been able to obtain third-party consent. In some Québec hospitals, investigators are held by research ethics boards to confirm obtained consent from ICU patient surrogates or from the patients themselves. Deferred consent is not an option [Y Skrobik, Hopital Maissoneuve Rosemont, Montréal, Québec, personal communication].

Another problem is new federal privacy legislation, which has led to requests to obtain first or third party consents for registries and other large scale observational studies. A recent example of this ethics bureaucracy decreasing rather than increasing the validity of research is the attempt to create the Canadian Stroke Registry. Mandatory first-person informed consent before patients could be included in registries resulted in inclusion of only 39% of eligible patients, and subsequently 51% of eligible patients following a research nurse at each site [17]. This authorization bias [18] created a major selection bias; mortality was significantly lower in enrolled versus eligible patients (7% versus 22%, $p<0.001$). Unsuccessful attempts to obtain consent consumed an estimated C$500,000 over two years. Ultimately, the registry was abandoned. In 2004 in Canada, the Personal Information Protection and Electronics Documents Act took effect, which allows a waiver of informed consent when it is impracticable, prohibitively costly and/or when it threatens the validity of the research. Clinically sensible privacy legislation and policies such as this are needed to waive informed consent for low risk observational studies. This would allow unbiased disease surveillance and data acquisition about epidemiology and quality of care.

More focus on the ongoing implementation and monitoring of the ethics of clinical critical care research was also suggested at the recent American Thoracic Society (ATS) Conference on the Ethical Conduct of Clinical Research Involving the Critically Ill [19]. A proposed checklist includes these questions:

1. Do new data or hypotheses undermine the social or scientific value of the ongoing study?
2. Do new results from this or other studies unfavorably alter the risk-benefit ratio?
3. Is the participant selection process working as intended and designed?
4. Are investigators carrying out the study as intended and designed?
5. Are the data and safety monitoring procedures, including the detection and reporting of adverse events, working as intended and designed?

International standards are required to outline, optimize and standardize the reporting relationship, responsibilities, roles and disciplinary representation of Data Safety Monitoring Boards (DSMBs) for ICU studies. This is particularly true for observational studies in which adverse outcomes are expected due to the baseline critical illness, whether or not a control group exists. A consensus conference on which types of clinical ICU studies require a DSMB would be useful. For example, should criteria involve sample size, risk:benefit ratio, number of centers involved, or the types of interventions being investigated? In additional, national or international research ethics boards for some simple multicenter studies would potentially reduce redundancy, and allow local research ethics boards to evaluate protocols that had already been evaluated by national experts [20].

Finally, everyone involved in clinical research should recognize conflicts of interest and comply with existing mechanisms to deal with them [19]. Conflicts of interest exist when researchers, research ethics board committee members, DSMB members, institutions, reviewers, or editors have financial or other relationships with persons or organizations that influence their actions, whether or not these individuals believe that these relationships affect their scientific judgment [21]. Financial conflicts include acceptance of gifts, consultancy, honoraria, stock ownership, options, grants, patents, and royalties. Non-financial conflicts include academic competition, ghost and gift authorship, and personal, professional or political relationships. Dual commitments, competing interests or competing loyalties are alternative terms reflecting relationships that are less likely to bias judgment. Conflicts of interest can influence research at any stage. For example, overstatement of benefit or understatement of risk in the consent process challenges the ethical integrity of a study. Non-disclosure of conflicts to the research ethics board may undermine the scientific integrity of a study, and, thus, public and professional trust. Institutions themselves may have conflicts of interest because much of their prestige and financial support stems from their involvement in research. As proposed in the ATS Conference on the Ethical Conduct of Clinical Research Involving the Critically Ill, institutions and research ethics boards should develop guidelines to monitor, clarify, and manage personal and institutional conflicts of interest [19].

A Vision for 2015: Using Information Technology Collaboratively to Improve the Global Conduct of Clinical Research and to Implement Research Results

If we work on the foregoing five priorities, we could get close to the events described below in 10 years. Imagine this:

Today, in 2015, coordinated action by far-sighted governments, the alliance of healthcare funders, the internet, and the advent of electronic communication in medicine has revolutionized the conduct of clinical research. Just how far we have come is illustrated by the following account:

In the early hours of Thursday morning, January 1 2015 Janet Smith is admitted to Orange Base Hospital in central New South Wales, Australia. Janet is a 19-year old tourist from Worthing in southern England who is spending a year backpacking around Australia, New Zealand and Asia before taking up her university place to read law. Janet was leaving a New Year's Eve party when she was hit by a 4-wheel drive sports utility vehicle. She has suffered multiple long bone fractures, multiple rib fractures with underlying lung injury and a significant traumatic brain injury with subarachnoid and intracranial hemorrhage. On arrival in the emergency department, while Janet is being attended by the trauma team, the admitting clerk finds Janet's UK National Health Service photo card in her purse. As both the National Health Service and Australia's Medicare System have adopted the standardized international health care card, Janet's card is read by the hospital's clinical information system (CIS). As Janet is unconscious, her security and privacy code cannot be entered, but on accessing her advanced directives file, the clerk verifies that she has authorized emergency access to her electronic medical record in the event that she is critically ill or injured. The clerk enters his personal access code, which identifies him as the person who has been authorized under emergency provisions to access patient records without the security and privacy codes. Janet's medical record is downloaded into the hospital's CIS. As Janet is resuscitated and details of her injuries and vital signs enter the CIS, the system scans her permissions files and notes that she has authorized the use of her anonymized healthcare data for epidemiological studies. In addition to Janet's anonymized data, information on the mechanism of her injury, the vehicle type and speed, deployment of airbags and the fact that the vehicle was fitted with a bullbar are automatically sent to the Australian National Trauma Research Center in Melbourne, the Cochrane Injuries Group in London, and the Canadian Trauma Registry in Hamilton.

As more data enter the CIS, automated evidence-based treatment prompts are generated to encourage the trauma team to implement research findings in their treatment of Janet. The CIS recommends crystalloid-based resuscitation, it notes that blood gas data generated from the intra-arterial electrodes and the automated radiology reports are consistent with acute respiratory distress syndrome (ARDS); the CIS uses Janet's height and weight to reset the ventilator to a tidal volume of 6 ml/kg of ideal body weight, at the same time the respiratory rate is adjusted to maintain normocarbia. Noting the positive finding of the CRASH II trial and the studies recommending activated factor VII in patients with trauma and intra-cranial hemorrhage, the CIS recommends treatment with aprotinin and activated Factor VII and the use of sequential calf compression for thromboembolic prophylaxis. The CIS also orders enteral nutrition, stress ulcer prophylaxis with a histamine-2-receptor antagonist, and once cardiovascular stability is achieved the head of the bed adjusts to the semi-recumbent position.

After stabilization in the emergency department, Janet is transferred to the operating room, has an intracranial pressure monitor placed and undergoes surgery for her long bone fractures. Whilst she is undergoing surgery, her hospital location code is altered to indicate she will be admitted to the ICU. As the ICU at Orange Base Hospital is part of the Global Research Initiative in Critical Care, her permissions file is again accessed and indicates that she has not registered to opt out of research projects approved by the International Emergency Research Ethics Committee. At 03.00 in Eastern Australia, the CIS generates a list of projects for which she appears eligible. The list includes three RCTs and her details are automatically emailed to the on-call Global Research Initiative Coordinator. As it is 03.00 in Eastern Australia, the CIS selects the coordinator in Hamilton, Ontario, Canada where it is 11 AM. The research coordinator also receives an automated SMS message to alert her to a potential trial participant. The research coordinator acknowledges the alerts and that the estimated time of admission to the ICU is 06.00. She checks eligibility criteria and then allows the Research Initiative Database to assign a random order for the trials for which Janet is eligible. The database then randomly assigns Janet to a treatment arm of the first trial which is a trial of different cerebral perfusion pressure targets in patients with traumatic brain injury coordinated from Paris on behalf of the European Society of Intensive Care Medicine. The database informs the ICU at Orange Base Hospital of Janet's inclusion in the trial. The CIS at Orange Base hospital automatically generates a standard English language information and consent form for Janet and for her surrogate decision maker. Baseline clinical and demographic data are transferred from the CIS to the trial database in Paris, and trial-related treatment protocols are generated for the nursing staff at Orange Base Hospital. Janet's inclusion in the trial is also registered with the Medicare Database in Canberra and generates credits towards Orange Base Hospital's accreditation with the Australian Hospitals Accreditation Board. At 07.00, Janet enters the ICU where treatment continues and is guided by further evidence-based prompts from the CIS and according to the trial protocol. At 08.00 the local research coordinator arrives in her office, checks her automated SMS messaging service and notes Janet's inclusion in the trial. She makes contact with the ICU nursing staff and is informed that all trial-related procedures are progressing well and that Janet's parents will be arriving from the UK the following day. Janet's parents were aware that Janet had chosen not to opt out of clinical research trials and had consented to the use of her health data in epidemiological research. They are understandably very concerned for their daughter but are also pleased that she appeared to be receiving excellent care in a hospital dedicated to evidence-based practice and clinical research. They accept the offer of a meeting with the ICU research staff after they have spoken with the clinical staff caring for their daughter.

Over the next two weeks, Janet remained in the ICU; the majority of her research data was automatically captured from the CIS and clinical records. A Global Research Initiative Monitor based in Sydney conducted a monitoring visit to Orange Base Hospital and checked Janet's data against source documentation. Janet's progress through the hospital, transfer back to the UK and recovery in rehabilitation was similarly tracked and monitored with outcome data including vital status and extended Glasgow Outcome Scores being recorded at three, six, and 12 months. Outcome data are submitted to the RCT database in Paris and to the three centers in Melbourne, London and Hamilton tracking Janet's progress as part of epidemiological studies of road trauma victims. Janet and her parents receive email reports of all the RCT results and their interpretation at the same time as the investigators, and before the results are made public.

Conclusion

In summary, we have proposed five priority activities to take clinical critical care research to the next level in 2015: Engage with health care regulators and funders; improve the quality and quantity of clinical ICU researchers; conduct more large international studies; mandate trial registration; and improve ethical standards but decrease bureaucracy. We hope that achieving these five priorities will result in a reality in which we use information technology collaboratively to improve the global conduct of clinical research and to implement research results.

References

1. The SAFE Study Investigators (2004) A comparison of albumin and saline for fluid resuscitation in the intensive care unit. N Engl J Med 350: 2247–2256
2. Curtis JR, Rubenfeld GD, Hudson LD (1998) Training pulmonary and critical care physicians in outcomes research: Should we take the challenge? Am J Respir Crit Care Med 157:1012–1015
3. Pinsky MR (1998) Research training in critical care medicine. New Horiz 6:293–299
4. Barrett H, Bion JF (2005) An international survey of training in adult intensive care medicine. Intensive Care Med 31:553–561
5. Sackett DL (2001) On the determinants of academic success. Clin Invest Med 24:94–100
6. Cook DJ, Todd TRJ (1997) The Canadian Critical Care Trials Group: A collaborative educational organization for the advancement of adult clinical ICU research. Intensive Care World 14:68–70
7. Langham J, Thompson E, Rowan K (2002) Randomized controlled trials from the critical care literature: identifcation and assessment of quality. Clin Intensive Care 13:73–83
8. Cook DJ, Brower R, Cooper J, et al Multicenter clinical research in critical care. Crit Care Med 30:1636–1643
9. Esteban A, Anzueto A, Frutos F, et al (2002) Characteristics and outcomes in adult patients receiving mechanical ventilation: A 28-day international study. JAMA 387:345–355
10. Cook DJ, Rocker G, Marshall J, et al (2003) Withdrawal of mechanical ventilation in anticipation of death in the intensive care unit. N Engl J Med 349:1123–1132
11. Dickerson K, Min YI (1993) NIH clinical trials and publication bias. Online J Curr Clin Trials: Doc No 50
12. Dickerson K, Min YI, Meinert CL (1992) Factors influencing publication of research results: follow-up of applications submitted to 2 institutional review boards. JAMA 267:374–378
13. Olson CM, Rennie D, Cook DJ, et al (2002) Publication bias in editorial decision making. JAMA 287:2825–2828
14. DeAngelis CD, Drazen JM, Frizelle FA, et al (2004) Clinical trial registration: A statement for the International Committee of Medical Journal Editors. JAMA 292:1363–1364
15. Emanuel EJ, Wendler D, Grady C (2000) What makes clinical research ethical? JAMA 283:2701–2711
16. CRASH Trial Collaborators. Effect of intravenous corticosteroid on the death within 14 days in 10,008 adults with clinically significant head injury (MRC CRASH): randomized placebo controlled trial. Lancet 364:1321–1328
17. Tu JV, Willison JD, Silver FL for the Investigators in the Registry of the Canadian Stroke Network (2004) Impracticability of informed consent in the registry of the Canadian Stroke Network. N Engl J Med 350:1414–1421

18. Al Shahi R, Warlow C (2000) Using patient-identifiable data for observational research and audit. BMJ 321:1031–1032
19. Luce J, Cook DJ, Martin TR, et al (2004) The ethical conduct of clinical research involving critically ill patients in the United States and Canada: Principles and recommendations. Am J Resp Crit Care Med 170:1375–1384
20. Christian MC, Goldberg JL, Killen J, et al (2002) A central institutional review board for multi-institutional trials. N Engl J Med 346:1405–1408
21. Korn D (2002) Industry, academia, investigator: managing the relationships. Acad Med 77:1089–1095

Funding and Accounting Systems

P. M. Suter

Introduction

Health care will continue to get better and better in Europe and the United States, but its costs will increase. In parallel, the expectations of both the individual and society are changing clearly concerning the profile of physicians and the desired results of the system.

While the last 20 years have seen a steeper increase in health care costs worldwide than ever before, this has also resulted in marked improvements of outcome variables such as longevity and quality of life in patients with frequent diseases, such as cardiac problems or cancer. To limit the steadily increasing expenses for the health system, efforts have been made to improve the efficiency of the expenses, for instance by decreasing length of hospital stay and shifting management and care of many diseases to 'outpatient' systems. As a consequence, the following questions must be asked:

- How should we adapt the training of health professionals, funding and accounting systems to meet the expectations of the population?
- How can societal demands be satisfied in a consumer-driven system?

In the present chapter, some elements enabling us to meet the new objectives are presented

Training the Physician for a New Role in Tomorrow's Health Care: Reforming the Medical Curriculum and Introducing the Bologna System

Why?

During the late eighties and early nineties, a wind of change blew through a number of medical schools in the US and in Europe. The main reasons for the desperate need for a profound reform are summarized in the Robert Wood Johnson Foundation National Program Project report [1]:

- "Traditional medical school curricula required students to absorb impracticable amounts of scientific information in lecture format for the first two years, in preparation for standardized tests that grade their abilities in basic science. They received little practical experience in working with patients and were so busy with classes and tests that they had little time to think and proc-

ess what they were learning. Only in the third and fourth years did medical students have a chance to meet patients and apply what they had learned to clinical situations.
- Similarly, once students were into the third and fourth years of medical school, their experience was almost exclusively on the clinical side. Therefore, much of the basic science they learned in the first two years was forgotten, lost in the whirl of clinical rotations.
- The relevance of teaching basic sciences needed re-examination. At issue was the following question: Is it necessary for medical students to absorb the entire range of basic scientific knowledge, which is expanding exponentially year after year? Or would it be more productive to have them learn how to access such information easily when necessary in the course of clinical practice?
- Reorganization of basic sciences to take account of entirely new sciences, such as molecular biology and medical informatics, was long overdue. For many years, basic science education had been broken down into discipline-based departments such as cell biology or pharmacology. Innovations like problem-based learning and organ-based teaching, which integrate basic science with patient problems, had been largely stymied by the power of department heads.
- As medical schools started becoming major sites for biomedical research, and as their associated teaching hospitals have become the locus for cutting-edge medical care, teaching took a back seat to the research and clinical missions."

In addition to the necessary changes in organization of the curriculum, more autonomy of the students and newer pedagogic methods, a major shift in favor of expanded time for human and social science, the so-called soft sciences [2] became necessary.

How?

Recognizing these shortcomings and new demands, including for instance the scientific evidence linking biological, behavioral, psychological and social variables to health, illness and disease, the ongoing reforms have focused on the following:
- enforcement of human psychological and social sciences during the whole curriculum [2, 3];
- enhanced responsibility for students to organize their training and knowledge acquisition, by the problem-based-learning system;
- increased attention paid to clinical skills;
- earlier clinical contact and student-patient interaction;
- training for efficient communication;
- teaching of physician role and behavior
- more attention given to health policy and economics;
- learning practice skills and 'savoir-être'.

The Introduction of the Bologna System in all European Universities: An Additional Opportunity?

In 1988, the Ministers of Education of 29 European countries edited the "Bologna Magna Charta Universitatum". In this framework, the major objectives and changes needed to improve the university system of the continent were defined, including:

- a call for independence and autonomy of the universities
- a definition of the curriculum for:
- better compatibility, and
- increased comparability, for a
- greater student mobility between universities.

  To achieve these goals, the Charta proposed the introduction of a
- quality insurance for teaching, research and management
- uniform 3-level system:
  - first level: Bachelor 3 years
  - second level: Master 2 – 3 years
  - third level: Doctorate 2 – 3 years
- definition of the workload for the student by the introduction of a common 'European Credit Transfer System' (ECTS), whereby 1 ECTS corresponds to 30 hours, one full year of university study to 1800 hours and hence 60 ECTS; therefore the Bachelor degree corresponds to 180 ECTS, and the Master to 120–180 ECTS.

For the medical curriculum, the Bologna system adds an interesting opportunity to include the essential elements of the reform, to increase comparability between different countries and systems, and to ensure and improve quality aspects of formation and training.

In essence, the Bologna system is an occasion to improve training of tomorrows' physicians, which cannot be missed (Fig. 1).

How to Adapt Funding and Medical Education?

To define a good model for tomorrow's medical education funding system, we will have to consider the essential changes planned for the next decade (Table 1). These include the following:

- a reshaped curriculum of medical education (Bologna system) to select and train doctors;
- a reorganized postgraduate training system, to provide professional competence preferentially in domains where this is most needed;
- a quality-based pre- and post-graduate teaching system, with transparent financing, controlling and examination basis, leading to better international comparability, exchange and recognition;
- a performance controlled research promotion and improvement system - including national and European institutional coordination and financing agencies.

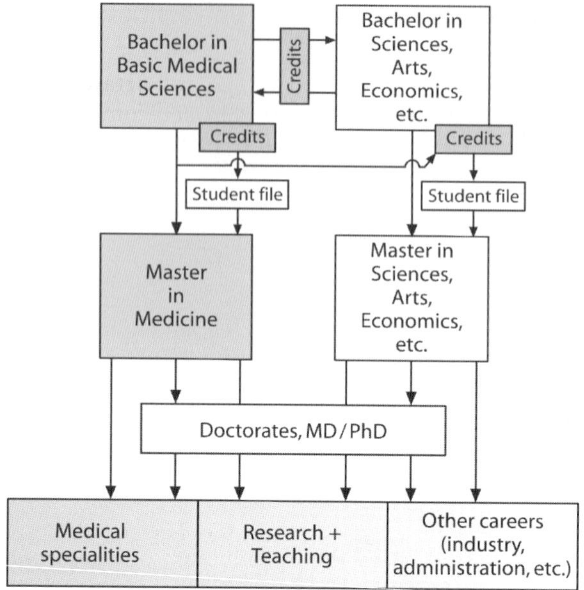

Fig. 1. Schematic representation of the Bologna system applied to the medical curriculum. Changes from and to the Bachelor and Master in Medicine are possible also during the studies, provided that the necessary credits are obtained and documented in the student file. Duration and ECTS: Bachelor 3 years / 180 ECTS, Master 2-3 years / 120-180 ECTS, Doctorate 2-3 years.

Table 1. Funding of teaching and research

Funding	Today – costs supported by	2015
Medical School	Federal + state, tuition	Federal + state, tuition + grants according to need + results
Postgraduate	Trainee (working hours) + teacher + institutions	Trainees + state according to specific needs for domains + results
Continuous education	Trainee, institution, industry - ± recognized	Idem - but also recognition for accreditation Quality control Incentives for quality
Research	Institutions (University, hospital, foundations, industry) based on expert evaluation or standards of institution	Idem - but more specific short / long term support according to quality control + performance indicators Basis for academic career

New Funding and Accountability for Health Care

When a system for an expensive area has to be reinvented, all important stakeholders must be involved to find a possible consensus or at least a compromise. Today, health spending *per capita* or in % of gross domestic product varies widely among developed countries (Table 2) [4].

The level of these expenses is not necessarily related to results or outcome. However, looking at a larger number of countries, including developing and poorer areas, a certain association between health expenditures and life expectancy at birth can be seen (Fig. 2) [5].

In countries where there is less than 1000 US$ of total health expenditure per head, life expectancy seems lower. On the other hand, no significant difference for life expectancy is evident for expenditures between 1500 and 3700 US$. This could suggest that in the latter, richer countries, efficiency of health expenditures are variable in terms of their effect on longevity.

Although longevity is frequently used as a simple variable to assess the effects of a health care system and its costs, this is not very satisfactory overall if we want to compare the most developed areas of the world, offering high standard care (Fig. 2). A better definition of health care outcome must include in addition infant and maternal mortality and potential years of life lost to common diseases below the age of 70. Such an approach was explored by Herzlinger ınd

Table 2. Health spending in 2002. From [4] with permission

Country	Health spending per capita PPP $*	% of gross – Domestic product
USA	5267	146
Switzerland	3445	112
Canada	2931	96
Germany	2817	10.9 ×
France	2736	97
Netherlands	2643	91
Sweden	2517	92
Australia+	2504	91
Italy	2166	85
United Kingdom	2160	77
Japan+	2077	78

PPP $ * indicates purchasing power parity international dollars
\+ Data are for 2001
× Nr high because the former East Germany contributed proportionally less gross domestic product to the unified Germany than added health expenditure

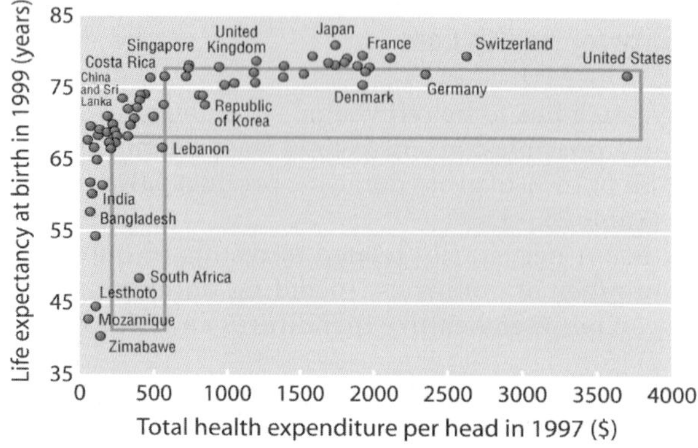

Fig. 2. Relation between total health expenditure per head and longevity for a number of developing and rich countries. It seems that health-expenditure above 1000 dollars per head (1997 figures) does not result in substantial further benefit in terms of longevity. From [5] with permission

Parsa-Parsi [6]. These authors noted that the most favorable outcomes resulted from a consumer-driven program. This could suggest that an appropriate sharing of responsibilities and financial efforts between patient public funds (= taxes), insurer and health care providers is important for a favorable cost/efficiency relationship [4].

As indicated in Table 3, this type of more precise analysis seems to indicate an advantage for a consumer-driven system [6].

Consequences for Intensive Care Medicine

Intensive care medicine is a complex area in terms of clinical tasks and constraints, collaboration with other health professionals and caregivers, interaction with hospital administrative, technical and other support services, and also concerning its relation with academic institutions. These institutions are responsible for the pregraduate and (in part) postgraduate teaching, but also for basic medical as well as clinical research. The multiple interactions of all partners and stakeholders in this field are not unique; these can be found in similar but not identical forms for other medical specialities.

Three main areas can be considered relevant for designing new models in funding and accountability (Table 4). Such new models should be built on the following conditions:

- the existence of a general service agreement, for the department/division of intensive care medicine, established with the partners and stakeholder most involved;
- a job description for the intensivist, cosigned by the main actors and revised regularly, including the tasks in clinical work, teaching, research and administrative duties;
- definition of budgets, distinguishing clinical and academic parts.

Table 3. Potential years of life lost to diabetes and myocardial infarction, life expectancy, and infant and maternal mortality – Canada, Switzerland, United Kingdom, and Germany. From [6] with permission

	Canada	Switzerland	United Kingdom	Germany
Potential years of life lost per 100 000 population aged < 70 y, 1997				
All causes	3803.3	3619.3	3951.5	4164.4
Diabetes	50.8	27.7	28.9	42.9
Acute myocardial infarction	184.9	122.6	248.4	239.5
Malignant neoplasm of colon	76.0	63.0	79.5	90.6
Malignant neoplasm of breast (among women only)	211.2			
Malignant neoplasm of prostate (among men only)	27.0	25,7	28.9	27.9
Infant mortality per 1000 live births, 1999	5.3	4.6	5.8	4.5
Maternal mortality per 100 000 live births, 1998	3.8	3.8	7.0	5.6
Life expectancy, y				
Total population at birth, 1999	79.9	79,7	77.4	77.7
Disability-adjusted total population at birth, 1997/1999	72.0	72.5	71.7	70.4
Men at age 65 y, 1997	16.3	16.5	15.1	15.2

The funding system of the future should be based on future possibilities and needs for specific training and more precisely defined tasks for the ICU physician. Dynamic career construction based on enlarged formation possibilities will open promising developments for intensivists, and provide better coverage of the main needs of hospital, ICU and university (Table 4).

The specific challenges of intensive care medicine may in part vary from one country to the other. Special consideration has to be given to an efficient handling of procedures and specific needs of other departments [7]. For staffing and career planning, the presence of the 'hospitalist' track [8] may play an important role.

The ICU as many other domains has felt increased competition with other units for income, increased costs, and a demand for a more business-like approach to operation. Its role in the hospital and the health care system in general is not always well defined, nor are its academic missions. Again, a 'general service agreement' ('convention d'objectifs') can help to define better tasks and duties, and the means required to do this.

Bekes et al. have recently described a real business model for critical care medicine as a product line [7]. They present a plan in the context of a specific hospital context and its board of trustees, based on the concept of a product line. It is shown that such a product line can be profitable for the hospital.

Table 4. Critical care activities relevant for funding and accountability

Today	General mixture of	– clinical tasks – management – teaching – research
Tomorrow	Clarification of main activities, early identification of different career possibilities and specific training	
	Medical school	Options (opportunity = Bologna), e.g. – clinical track – research track – MPH, MBA, etc
	Postgraduate	– enlarged possibilities for more than 1 medical specialty board – MD/PhD ± clinical training – PhD ± medical horizon – MBA / management
	Continuous education:	– according to activities in the ICU defined by curriculum, specific capacities and service needs – management, economics in health care, etc

Unlike other parts of the health system, the approach by Bekes et al. brings the ICU (and other sectors such as the emergency department) into focus as an essential part of the hospital. This can also mean that expansion of this line can only be achieved by increasing referrals from other hospitals, or offering new services requiring ICU beds, such as cardiology or liver transplantation.

Accountability of ICU services has to go primarily through hospital structure and university requirements of teaching and research. General health system discussions and funding models are therefore not applicable separately. From the patient's standpoint however, emergency and ICU services are typically part of the duties which should be taken care of by the state, its government and thereby the tax payer.

References

1. National Program Report. Preparing physicians for the future (PPF): A program in medical education. At: http://www.rwjf.org/reports/npreports/prephysicians.htm Accessed July 2005
2. Anonymous (2004) The soft science of medicine. Lancet 363:1247
3. Cuff PA, Vanselow NA (2004) Enhancing the Behavioral and Social Science Content of Medical School Curricula. US Institute of Medicine. At: http://www.nap.edu/books/030909142X/html Accessed July 2005

4. Reinhart UE (2004) The Swiss health system. Regulated competition without managed care. JAMA 292:1227–1232
5. Richards T, Tumwine J (2004) Poor countries make the best teachers. BMJ 329:1113–1114
6. Herzlinger RE, Parsa-Parsi R (2004) Consumer-driven health care. Lessons from Switzerland. JAMA 292:1213–1220
7. Bekes CE, Dellinger RP, Brooks D, Edmondson R, Olivier CT, Parrillo JE (2004) Critical care medicine as a distinct product line with substantial financial profitability: The role of business planning. Crit Care Med 32:1207–1214
8. Wachter RM (2004) Hospitalists in the United States – Mission accomplished or work in progress? N Engl J Med 350:1935–1936

Measuring Performance

G. D. Rubenfeld

Introduction: Performance = Quality

Measuring the performance of a complex service like critical care that combines the highest technology with the most intimate caring is a challenge. Performance is an elusive concept and I will use it interchangeably with another, equally elusive term, quality. Recently, consumers, clinicians, and payers have requested more formal assessments and comparisons of the quality and costs of medical care [1]. Donabedian proposed a framework for thinking about the quality of medical care that separates quality into 3 components: structure, process, and outcome [2]. An instructive analogy for understanding this framework is to imagine a food critic evaluating the quality of a restaurant. The critic might comment on the decoration and lighting of the restaurant, how close the tables are to each other, the breadth of the wine list and where the chef trained. These are all evaluations of the restaurant *structure*. In addition, the critic might comment on whether the service was courteous and timely – measures of *process*. Finally, the critic might comment on *outcomes* like eater satisfaction or food poisoning. Similarly, to a health care critic, structure is the physical and human resources used to deliver medical care. Processes are the actual treatments offered to patients. Finally, outcomes are what happens to patients, for example, mortality, quality of life, and satisfaction with care. It is also crucial to remember that while intensivists care deeply about the performance of intensive care units (ICUs), they are probably the only ones who do. Patients, their families, payers, and governments are much more likely to care about the performance of the hospital or the outcomes of a disease or procedure than the specific performance of one part of the hospital. It is irrelevant how superb the ICU care is if the patient is discharged to a ward that delivers poor care.

There is a debate about which of these measurements is the most important measure of quality. A compelling argument, and, in fact, one source of the growing 'outcomes research' movement, is that, ultimately, what happens to patients is the most important measure of medical care quality. To live up to the definition, better quality medical care must improve patient outcomes. Several attempts have been made at judging the quality of intensive care based on an important outcome, mortality adjusted for severity of illness [3–5]. Nevertheless, there are two good reasons to consider measurements of structure and process as measures of quality of care.

First, the only aspects of medical care that clinicians can directly influence are its structure and process. Therefore, to effect change in outcome, studies of medical care must be operationalized in terms of structure or process. A randomized controlled trial of the effect of a new drug for sepsis on mortality is an example of a study of the effect of a process on outcome. An observational cohort study of the effect on family satisfaction of increasing nursing continuity in the ICU is a study of the effect of structure on outcome. Studies that evaluate structure and process are important precisely because they are the factors that can be changed at the bedside. To link structure causally to outcomes and processes, clinicians draw on the tools of evidence based medicine. The extent to which the science will justify a claim between a given structure or process and improved outcome is the strength of evidence supporting that claim. Of course, some structures and processes are important even in the absence of empiric evidence that they change outcome. For example, one can decide that having oxygen available at the bedside in an ICU is a measure of quality without a randomized controlled trial showing that it reduces mortality.

The second advantage of structure and process as markers of quality is that they are more efficient to study than outcomes [6]. Because of the modest effect many medical processes have on outcome, it is easier to demonstrate the improvement in a process measure in a small sample size than an improvement in the outcome. For example, if the goal is to reduce the outcome of deep venous thrombosis (DVT) in the ICU, it is easier and less expensive to show that a given intervention has increased the number of patients receiving DVT prophylaxis than to show a reduction in the number of DVTs.

Measuring the Structure of Intensive Care

Studies of ICU structure are complicated by the variable nature and elusive definition of critical care. One must decide whether one is studying the structure of the ICU as a geographic location (as all existing studies have done) or of critical care as a service to a particular patient population. Are patients on prolonged ventilatory support in a nursing home in an ICU? Are patients being weaned in a post-anesthesia care area after cardiac bypass surgery receiving intensive care? Is the emergency department an 'ICU' because critically ill patients are cared for there for various periods of time? The answers to these questions will determine which special care areas and which processes of care constitute critical care.

In thinking about measuring ICU structure it is important to consider the instruments used to study structure. Some aspects of ICU structure are simple to identify and measure objectively, for example, the number of ICU beds, availability of bedside electrocardiographic (EKG) monitoring, or presence of respiratory therapists. Other aspects of ICU structure are more difficult to measure and require special qualitative or quantitative assessment [7, 8]. This would include how well the multidisciplinary providers in the ICU work as a team, the extent to which the ICU is managed by a core group of intensivists, and whether the ICU incorporates concepts of continuous quality improvement. Several investigators have developed explicit survey tools to measure these variables [8–10].

There is a limited number of studies describing ICU structure and its relationship to outcome. Four large studies deserve special mention because they compose most of the available data. Shortell, Zimmerman and their colleagues were involved with a number of studies using the APACHE database [8, 10, 11]. Three descriptive studies describe, in varying degrees of detail, the structure of ICUs in the US and Europe. In 1991, Groeger and colleagues surveyed ICU medical directors and used American Hospital Association data to describe ICUs in the US [12]. Recently, the COMPACCS (Committee on Manpower for Pulmonary and Critical Care Societies) produced a report that relied on a survey of critical care physicians and ICU directors to generate data on ICU structure in the US [13]. Finally, Vincent et al., used survey data from European ICUs participating in the European Prevalence of Infection in Intensive Care (EPIC) study to produce a picture of ICU structure in Europe [14].

While the best data available, these studies are difficult to summarize and compare because they did not use identical data elements or comparable definitions. Models for organizing critical care services are extremely variable and even the definition of which beds constitute 'intensive care' beds varies. Distinctions are subtle in separating a 'step-down' or 'intermediate care' bed from other beds and many hospitals use flexible staffing and moveable technology to convert emergency room and post-anesthesia care areas into critical care beds. Finally, these descriptive studies of ICU structure were based on the results of surveys filled out by ICU directors with varying response rates and incomplete attempts to verify the reported data.

Information about ICU structure can be gleaned from published recommendations. The Society of Critical Care Medicine has published a number of guidelines on these topics [15, 16]. The American College of Surgery's criteria for trauma center designation contains very explicit recommendation for the organization of critical services [17]. This detailed document lists criteria for four levels of trauma center designation. It includes specific structural criteria for human and material resources as well as their organization. Recognizing the significance of the physical layout, this document even recommends where individuals should stand during evaluation of the trauma patient and where instruments should be placed in a resuscitation bay. Of note, this document also recommends that Level I trauma centers use a dedicated ICU team run by an appropriately credentialed critical care surgeon. Because of the lack of data to guide the optimal structure for critical care, published guidelines and recommendations are, for the most part, based on expert opinion and common sense.

It is not surprising that the issue of structure is very important to intensivists. At its core, the ICU is a structural creation [18]. The ICU was born when the material and human resources devoted to caring for severely ill patients were focused in one part of the hospital. Two important themes emerge from a review of the literature on ICU structure. With one or two important exceptions, there is little evidence on which to base structural recommendations, and there is enormous variability in the structure and organization of ICUs around the world. Many important questions remain about the optimal structure for the ICU and the relationship between structure and process and structure and outcome.

Measuring the Process of Intensive Care

There are three primary challenges to using processes of care as measures of performance in the ICU. The first is that there is a relative lack of evidence and lack of agreement on the existing evidence for many processes of care in the ICU [19]. In the Surviving Sepsis Guidelines, there are only five 'Grade A' recommendations and none of these are specific positive recommendations for septic patients; two are recommendations to avoid treatments (high dose corticosteroids and increasing oxygen delivery to supranormal levels by use of dobutamine) and three relate to treatments that are not specific to sepsis [20]. Of the 10 'Grade B' recommendations for sepsis, only two – early goal directed therapy for initial resuscitation and recombinant human activated protein C - are specific positive recommendations for sepsis. For acute lung injury (ALI), only one intervention, a low tidal volume-low pressure ventilator has been shown to reduce mortality and there is considerable debate about the interpretation and application of this treatment [21].

The second challenge to using process measures in the ICU is that critical illness syndromes are much more difficult to identify than patients with acute myocardial infarction. For example, to ensure that everyone with an acute myocardial infarction has been treated in a specific way, one can screen troponin results from the clinical laboratory. To reliably identify patients with ALI or sepsis for process assessment requires a review of laboratory data, chest radiographs, and some clinical judgment about 'clinical assessment of left atrial hypertension' or 'clinical suspicion of infection'. Alternatively, a process assessment can rely solely on physician identified cases. This is limited as physician recognition and documentation of critical illness syndromes may be an important explanation of poor performance [22]. Therefore, evaluation of process variables in recognized cases will always overestimate performance. Finally, many of the processes that are of documented benefit and of greatest interest are difficult to measure. For example, many process benchmarks in managing acute coronary syndromes relate to timing of administration of specific medications or procedures. These are relatively easily identified in medical, billing, or pharmacy records. Compare this to the challenges of assessing the use of early goal directed therapy which requires assessing whether specific interventions were provided in response to specific physiologic cues.

Measuring the Outcomes of Intensive Care

In the context of the Donabedian model of measuring quality and with respect to the field of outcomes research, outcomes refer to a variety of variables that measure factors that are important to patients including: symptoms, quality of life, duration of life, quality of dying, the effect of their health care on their loved ones, and the cost of medical care. Patient-centered outcomes are distinct from any number of chemical, physiologic, and radiographic variables that may be measured in clinical research. Because of the importance of these outcomes to patients they are referred to as 'patient-centered' outcomes. Ideally, clinicians will offer, insurers will pay for, and patients will have the opportunity to use treatments that have been shown to improve patient-centered outcomes. High quality medical care is more likely to result in improved patient outcomes.

Mortality, or the probability of death measured at a fixed point, is the most common outcome variable in critical care. Usually, this is measured at ICU discharge, hospital discharge, or at a fixed number of days after ICU admission. There is always a tradeoff in selecting endpoint timing between sensitivity to treatment effect and clinical significance. Endpoints close to ICU admission (7-day mortality, for example) are most likely to detect the effect of critical care but are not clinically significant [1]. Measuring mortality 5 years after critical illness would arguably be more clinically relevant, but is expensive to collect and might miss important effects of critical care that would be washed out by 5 years. Mortality after hospital discharge is rarely captured in either administrative or electronic medical record databases. When unique patient identifiers are available, these databases can be linked to public death records to determine long-term survival. Recent evidence has focused on the effects of critical illness on long-term survival and quality of life; however, there is scanty evidence linking specific therapies in the ICU with these outcomes [23]. Although economists view it as an input to medical care, the other patient-centered outcome variable that is frequently available in computerized medical databases is cost and proxies for cost [24]. Actual costs, particularly the specific costs of critical care, are difficult to measure in health care. When using computerized medical databases, investigators frequently infer costs from lengthofstay or total charges [25].

There are several limitations to using outcomes to measure the performance of intensive care. The use of risk adjusted mortality remains a key component in attempts to define, report, and improve quality of care [26, 27]. Risk adjustment is designed to address the problem of confounding, that is, centers with sicker patients will have worse outcomes and appear to deliver worse care. By adjusting for severity of illness in a multivariate model, the baseline risk of death is mathematically equalized between institutions. The remaining differences in outcome are attributed to differences in structure and process of care. This is often expressed as a standardized mortality ratio (SMR) – the ratio of observed deaths to the number of deaths predicted by the risk adjustment model.

Unfortunately, there is now an extensive body of literature that demonstrates that risk adjusted outcome is neither a reliable nor a valid technique for identifying high or poor quality hospitals because of residual confounding, bias due to referral, upcoding of severity, and chance [28–32]. These limitations are poorly recognized as evidenced by a recent, widely publicized attempt to identify the "100 Top Hospitals" and their ICUs using risk adjusted outcomes based on administrative (non-physiologic) data from Medicare Provider Analysis and Review database [33] and from the Joint Commission on Accreditation of Healthcare Organizations' (JCAHO) recent decision to add risk adjusted length of stay and mortality to the ICU core measures of quality of care.

Another limitation to outcome measures is that they are usually limited to mortality and, perhaps, length of stay. There are, of course, many other outcomes that matter to patients, their families, and clinicians. Although instruments exist to assess a variety of other outcomes, they are not measured routinely, are not captured by standard electronic databases, and are more difficult to assess than simple measures like mortality and length of stay. These include medical error rates, nosocomial infections, patient and family satisfaction, provider burnout, quality of dying and death, and long-term health related quality of life [23, 34–36].

Although there are clear benefits to feeding back process and outcome data to individually motivated institutions, the promise of using this information as a tool to improve health care quality by informing marketplace decisions has not been fully realized [37]. Between 1991 and 1997, all 30 non-federal hospitals in greater metropolitan Cleveland participated in the Cleveland Health Quality Choice (CHQC) program. Every 6 months, models were used to analyze whether observed in-hospital mortality rates of participating hospitals were greater or less than expected and these results were distributed in a public report. While there was a trend over a 7 year period for hospitals with poor risk adjusted outcomes to lose market share, this effect was not statistically or clinically significant [38]. Therefore, the benefit of feeding back outcome data to hospitals does not seem to be mediated by changes in market share. In addition to pointing out the lack of evidence supporting the claim that public distribution of quality data improves care, a recent review raised the possibility of unintended negative consequences from reporting quality measures [39]. These included shifting of high-risk patients to adjacent healthcare systems that are not being assessed and denial of care to patients perceived at high risk for bad outcomes. An important question remains unresolved: if risk adjusted quality measures are useful to catalyze local quality improvement measures, is their effectiveness in this role linked to making the quality data public?

Measuring Performance: The Future

The future of measuring performance in critical care will require universal access to high quality data. This includes reliable and accurate coding of comorbid conditions, diagnoses, and risk factors for critical illness syndromes. Converting the clinically rich minute-to-minute data of the ICU electronic medical record into a meaningful tool for performance evaluation is a nontrivial exercise [40–42]. There have been multiple attempts to create a standardized ICU dataset for benchmarking and research including: Project IMPACT, an initiative launched by the Society of Critical Care Medicine [43], AORTIC (Australasian Outcomes Research Tool for Intensive Care) developed by ANZICS (Australia and New Zealand Intensive Care Society) [44], ICNARC (Intensive Care National Audit & Research) developed by the United Kingdom Intensive Care Society [45], and CCR-NET (Critical Care Research Network) developed by the Ontario Working Group in Critical Care [46].

In the future, documentation for clinical care and billing and documentation for performance evaluation and research will be simultaneous events [47, 48]. Direct data from the bedside will be filtered for these purposes to exclude the venous blood gas that is recorded as an arterial blood gas or the spurious oximeter reading that is captured when the sensor falls off the patient. While systems biology and bioinformatics including genomics, proteomics, transcriptomics, and metabolomics may provide novel insights into drug development and treatment selection for individual patients, their contributions to the field of performance evaluation are unlikely to be large. The primary role of these fields in performance evaluation would be better prognostication and risk adjustment, however, there is little evidence that the key to better performance evaluation and improvement is increasing the C statistic (a measure of predictive accuracy for risk adjustment tools) from 0.85 to 0.95. I suspect we in critical care may have more to learn about providing high quality care to patients from a careful observation of highly performing bioinformatics companies than we do from their products.

In the future there will be a relative de-emphasis of simple risk-adjusted mortality and the 'SMR' as the sole measures of performance. ICU performance will be viewed across multiple axes. These are likely to include the extent to which ICUs show improvement in their process and outcome measures over time rather than their fixed performance at a time compared to others. There will be an attempt to incorporate a variety of measures including medical error, family satisfaction, quality of dying and death, and complications into measures of performance. Individual clinicians' performance will be fed back to them so that, for example, an individual nurse will have an idea of what percentage of his or her patients received a daily interruption of sedation. An individual physician can see exactly how his or her patients with ALI are ventilated.

In the future, the focus will be on critical illness and not on critical care units. The structure, process, and outcomes of care will be tracked from emergency department to operating room to recovery room to ward to ICU to ward and perhaps even to home. There will be particular focus on the transitions of care between providers.

The hard question is not simply how to measure performance but how to report this information so that it is useful and how to use it to provide incentives to deliver high quality care. Measuring performance and feeding it back to providers can improve care [37]. Making benchmarks available to the public in the hope of driving care to high quality providers does not seem to be successful [38]. There have been calls in the United States to reimburse high-quality providers at a higher rate or to shift care to those providers who meet certain minimal standards, however, this is not uniformly accepted or effective [49].

Conclusion

One must be particularly circumspect in making predictions about the future of anything, particularly medicine. In 1973, in an article titled "Dollar and human costs of intensive care", the authors raised concerns about the enormous costs and poor survival of many patients in the newly organized ICU. However, they were optimistic about the future:

"[The] more promising approaches to cost reduction are all in an early stage of development now. Both deprofessionalization of the ICU by wider use of allied health personnel, and the automation of therapeutic functions are just beginning to be applied" [50].

Their optimistic predictions about increased use of advance practice nurses, physicians' assistants, respiratory therapists, and computerized monitoring all came true. Unfortunately, these have yielded quite the opposite of cost reduction.

References

1. Rubenfeld GD, Angus DC, Pinsky MR, Curtis JR, Connors AF Jr, Bernard GR (1999) Outcomes research in critical care: results of the American Thoracic Society Critical Care Assembly Workshop on Outcomes Research. The Members of the Outcomes Research Workshop. Am J Respir Crit Care Med 160:358–367
2. Donabedian A (1988) The quality of care. How can it be assessed? JAMA. 260:1743–1748
3. Sirio CA, Angus DC, Rosenthal GE (1994) Cleveland Health Quality Choice (CHQC)–an ongoing collaborative, community-based outcomes assessment program. New Horiz 2:321–325
4. Teres D, Lemeshow S (1993) Using severity measures to describe high performance intensive care units. Crit Care Clin 9:543–554
5. Knaus WA, Draper EA, Wagner DP (1983) Toward quality review in intensive care: the APACHE system. Qrb Qual Rev Bull 9:196–204
6. Mant J, Hicks N (1995) Detecting differences in quality of care: the sensitivity of measures of process and outcome in treating acute myocardial infarction. BMJ 311:793–796
7. Baggs JG, Ryan SA, Phelps CE, Richeson JF, Johnson JE (1992) The association between interdisciplinary collaboration and patient outcomes in a medical intensive care unit. Heart Lung 21:18–24
8. Shortell SM, Zimmerman JE, Rousseau DM, et al (1994) The performance of intensive care units: does good management make a difference? Med Care 32:508–525
9. Mitchell PH, Shannon SE, Cain KC, Hegyvary ST (1996) Critical care outcomes: linking structures, processes, and organizational and clinical outcomes. Am J Crit Care 5:353–363
10. Zimmerman JE, Shortell SM, Rousseau DM, et al (1993) Improving intensive care: observations based on organizational case studies in nine intensive care units: a prospective, multicenter study. Crit Care Med 21:1443–1451
11. Zimmerman JE, Rousseau DM, Duffy J, et al (1994) Intensive care at two teaching hospitals: an organizational case study. Am J Crit Care 3:129–138
12. Groeger JS, Strosberg MA, Halpern NA, et al (1992) Descriptive analysis of critical care units in the United States. Crit Care Med 20:846–863
13. Schmitz R, Landin M, White A (1998) Future Workforce Needs in Pulmonary and Critical Care Medicine. Abt Associates, Cambridge
14. Vincent JL, Suter P, Bihari D, Bruining H (1997) Organization of intensive care units in Europe: lessons from the EPIC study. Intensive Care Med 23:1181–1184
15. American College of Critical Care Medicine of the Society of Critical Care Medicine (1999) Critical care services and personnel: recommendations based on a system of categorization into two levels of care. Crit Care Med 27:422–426
16. Coalition for Critical Care Excellence: Consensus Conference on Physiologic Monitoring Devices (1995) Standards of evidence for the safety and effectiveness of critical care monitoring devices and related interventions. Crit Care Med. 23:1756–1763
17. American College of Surgeons Committee on Trauma (1998) Resources for Optimal Care of the Injured Patient: 1999. The American College of Surgeons, Chicago
18. Calvin JE, Habet K, Parrillo JE (1997) Critical care in the United States. Who are we and how did we get here? Crit Care Clin 13:363–376

19. Rubenfeld GD (2001) Understanding why we agree on the evidence but disagree on the medicine. Respir Care 46:1442–1449
20. Dellinger RP, Carlet JM, Masur H, et al (2004) Surviving Sepsis Campaign guidelines for management of severe sepsis and septic shock. Crit Care Med 32:858–873
21. Eichacker PQ, Gerstenberger EP, Banks SM, Cui X, Natanson C (2002) Meta-analysis of acute lung injury and acute respiratory distress syndrome trials testing low tidal volumes. Am J Respir Crit Care Med 166:1510–1514
22. Mahoney AM, Caldwell E, Hudson LD, Rubenfeld GD (2003) Barriers to physician recognition of acute lung injury. Am J Respir Crit Care Med 167:A738 (abst)
23. Angus DC, Carlet J (2002) Surviving Intensive Care. Update in Intensive Care and Emergency Medicine. Springer, Heidelberg
24. American Thoracic Society workshop on outcomes research (2002) Understanding costs and cost-effectiveness in critical care: report from the second. Am J Respir Crit Care Med 165:540–550
25. Rapoport J, Teres D, Lemeshow S, Gehlbach S (1994) A method for assessing the clinical performance and cost-effectiveness of intensive care units: a multicenter inception cohort study. Crit Care Med 22:1385–1391
26. Hadorn D, Keeler E, Rogers W, Brook R (1993) Assessing the Performance of Mortality Prediction Models. Rand, Santa Monica
27. Iezzoni LI (1994) Risk adjustment for measuring health care outcomes. Health Administration Press, Ann Arbor
28. Chassin MR, Hannan EL, DeBuono BA (1996) Benefits and hazards of reporting medical outcomes publicly. N Engl J Med 334:394–398
29. Escarce JJ, Kelley MA (1990) Admission source to the medical intensive care unit predicts hospital death independent of APACHE II score. JAMA 264:2389–2394
30. Park RE, Brook RH, Kosecoff J, et al (1990) Explaining variations in hospital death rates. Randomness, severity of illness, quality of care. JAMA 264:484–490
31. Hofer TP, Hayward RA (1996) Identifying poor-quality hospitals. Can hospital mortality rates detect quality problems for medical diagnoses? Med Care 34:737–753
32. Thomas JW, Hofer TP (1998) Research evidence on the validity of risk-adjusted mortality rate as a measure of hospital quality of care. Med Care Res Rev 55:371–404
33. Solucient (2000) 100 Top Hospitals: ICU Benchmarks for Success — 2000. Available at: http://www.100tophospitals.com/studies/icu00/introduction.htm Accessed July 2005
34. Heyland DK, Rocker GM, Dodek PM, et al (2002) Family satisfaction with care in the intensive care unit: results of a multiple center study. Crit Care Med 30:1413–1418
35. Curtis JR, Patrick DL, Engelberg RA, Norris K, Asp C, Byock I (2002) A measure of the quality of dying and death. Initial validation using after-death interviews with family members. J Pain Symptom Manage 24:17–31
36. Chen SM, McMurray A (2001) "Burnout" in intensive care nurses. J Nurs Res 9:152–164
37. Hannan EL, Kilburn H, Jr., Racz M, Shields E, Chassin MR (1994) Improving the outcomes of coronary artery bypass surgery in New York State. JAMA 271:761–766
38. Baker DW, Einstadter D, Thomas C, Husak S, Gordon NH, Cebul RD (2003) The effect of publicly reporting hospital performance on market share and risk-adjusted mortality at high-mortality hospitals. Med Care 41:729–740
39. Werner RM, Asch DA (2005) The unintended consequences of publicly reporting quality information. JAMA 293:1239–1244
40. Polderman KH, Jorna EM, Girbes AR (2001) Inter-observer variability in APACHE II scoring: effect of strict guidelines and training. Intensive Care Med 27:1365–1369
41. Fery-Lemonnier E, Landais P, Loirat P, Kleinknecht D, Brivet F (1995) Evaluation of severity scoring systems in ICUs–translation, conversion and definition ambiguities as a source of inter-observer variability in Apache II, SAPS and OSF. Intensive Care Med 21:356-360

42. Damiano AM, Bergner M, Draper EA, Knaus WA, Wagner DP (1992) Reliability of a measure of severity of illness: acute physiology of chronic health evaluation–II. J Clin Epidemiol 45:93–101
43. Cook SF, Visscher WA, Hobbs CL, Williams RL (2002) Project IMPACT: results from a pilot validity study of a new observational database. Crit Care Med 30:2765–2770
44. AORTIC. Available at: http://www.anzics.com.au/admc/software_aortic.htm. Accessed July 2005
45. Intensive Care National Audit & Research Centre. Available at: http://www.icnarc.org/. Accessed July 2005.
46. Critical Care Research Network. Available at: http://www.criticalcareresearch.net/. Accessed July 2005
47. Render ML, Kim HM, Welsh DE, et al (2003) Automated intensive care unit risk adjustment: results from a National Veterans Affairs study. Crit Care Med 31:1638–1646
48. Junger A, Bottger S, Engel J, et al (2002) Automatic calculation of a modified APACHE II score using a patient data management system (PDMS). Int J Med Inform 65:145–157
49. Corrigan J, Eden J, Smith BM (2003) Leadership by Example: Coordinating Government Roles in Improving Health Care Quality. Institute of Medicine. Committee on Enhancing Federal Healthcare Quality Programs. National Academies Press, Washington
50. Morgan A, Daly C, Murawski BJ (1973) Dollar and human costs of intensive care. J Surg Res 14 :441–448

Ethics and End-of-life Care

J. R. Curtis

Introduction: Statement of the Problem

Because of the severity of illness of patients in the intensive care unit (ICU), the ICU is a setting where death is common. Approximately 20% of all deaths in the U.S. occur in the ICU [1]. Although this proportion varies greatly in different countries, death is relatively common in most ICUs because of the severity of illness of these patients. Optimal palliative care of outpatients and patients in the acute care and long-term care settings and judicious use of the ICU for those with terminal or life-limiting illness may prevent many terminal ICU admissions. Nonetheless, the ICU will likely remain an important setting for end-of-life care both because of the severity of illness of critically ill patients and because many patients with chronic, life-limiting diseases and their families opt for a trial of intensive care if there is a reasonable chance that patients may have an extension of their life with a reasonable quality of life [2]. This chapter addresses the ethical issues and challenges that arise in providing high quality care to patients who ultimately die in the ICU.

Several studies have documented important shortcomings to end-of-life care in the ICU. For example, one study of six hospitals in the US showed that many patients die with moderate or severe pain [3], physicians are unaware of patients' preferences regarding end-of-life care [4] and the care patients receive is often not consistent with their treatment preferences [3]. Another US study demonstrated significant burden of symptoms among patients with cancer in the ICU [5]. Studies from the U.S. and Europe show that ICU clinicians frequently do not communicate adequately with family members [6–8]. For all these reasons, improving the quality of end-of-life care in the ICU is an ethical imperative.

Perhaps one of the best ways to improve quality of end-of-life care in the ICU is to clarify the goals of care in advance of critical illness and avoid the ICU altogether when ICU-based life-sustaining therapies are unwanted or unlikely to provide benefit. In the 1980s, many U.S. experts believed advance directives would allow patients to inform their physicians about the care they want at the end of life and to avoid technologic life-sustaining therapies at the end of life [9, 10]. Unfortunately, advance directives have not significantly affected the aggressiveness or costs of ICU care [11, 12] nor have they changed end-of-life decision-making [13, 14]. Nonetheless, advance care planning prior to hospitalization is likely to be an important component for improving end-of-life care in the ICU [15]. However, even with excellent communication, improved prognostication, and ideal advance care planning, many patients and their physicians and families will choose a trial of intensive care that may ultimately fail [2]. With an aging population and advances in the management of many chronic, life-limiting diseases, it seems likely that the shift from sustaining life to maximizing comfort after a trial of unsuccessful intensive care will continue to occur frequently in the ICU.

This chapter will review some of the important ethical issues regarding end-of-life care in the ICU identifying those for which there is consensus and those for which there is not. The chapter will also review some important components of end-of-life care in the ICU, including communication with patients and families, a focus on the interdisciplinary team, and striving for quality of care regarding withholding and withdrawing life-sustaining treatments. Finally, the chapter will review some recent studies of interventions that have been shown to improve end-of-life care in the ICU and finally will summarize some of the challenges to measuring quality of end-of-life care in the ICU.

Ethical Issues Regarding End-of-life Care

Intensive care practitioners have, from the earliest days of the specialty, recognized that many patients admitted to the ICU cannot benefit from, or do not wish to endure, the burdens of life-sustaining treatments [16, 17]. Accompanying, and in many situations leading this discussion, has been a rich literature concerning the *ethics* of end-of-life decision-making in the ICU [18]. The ethical principles of autonomy and beneficence are generally well accepted as guiding principles of ethical intensive care. However, challenges arise in trying to balance these principles in settings where they may conflict. Furthermore, there are additional ethical principles that are more controversial, playing a key role in end-of-life decision-making in some ICUs and not in others. For example, the principle of medical futility plays a central role in the decision-making to provide or limit intensive care in some hospitals [19, 20], while it has been decried by some authors as an unacceptable ethical principle because it conflicts with patient autonomy [21, 22]. The principle of 'double effect' has been cited as an ethical rationale for use of medication to relieve pain even when it may unintentionally hastens death, provided that the intent of the clinician is to relieve pain or other symptoms. However, this principle is also controversial [23]. Finally, the role of family in surrogate decision-making varies greatly in different countries. For example, in the U.S., family members of decisionally-incapacitated patients are provided with all the same rights for autonomy as the decisionally-capacitated patient, while in countries such as France this is not the case [24].

It is often said to be a general consensus among medical ethicists that withholding and withdrawing life-sustaining treatments are morally and ethically equivalent [25, 26]; several critical care societies have produced statements endorsing this view [27, 28]. However, it should also be noted that while this may be the predominant view in Western medical ethics, it is not the only view [29, 30]. Opposition to this view is strongest among some religious groups. In particular, many Jewish medical ethicists teach that there is an important moral distinction between withholding and withdrawing life-sustaining treatments [31]. There is also evidence that some clinicians believe that there is a difference between withholding and withdrawing life-sustaining therapies [30, 32]. Many of the empirical studies examining withdrawal of life-sustaining treatments in the ICU setting also examine withholding life-sustaining treatments. In the ICU setting, this distinction may be difficult to assess, especially in the case of intermittent life-sustaining therapies such as dialysis. Furthermore, decisions to withhold therapies are often subtle and more difficult to accurately assess by survey or medical record review than decisions to withdraw life-sustaining therapies.

Surveys and observational studies showing large variability in approaches to end-of-life care in the ICU suggest that application of these ethical principles vary greatly among different critical care clinicians [33–37]. Some have argued that there are no global ethics [38], meaning the ethical principles cannot be viewed outside of the culture of the medical systems and the patients and families while others have argued for the same set of ethical principles being applicable throughout the world. However, through international forums it seems likely that *some* global ethical principles can be identified [39] and then implemented in a way that allows for cultural competence both in the health care systems setting standards for clinicians that acknowledge the culture of clinicians and also in clinicians working with patients and families from other cultures. Figure 1 provides a conceptualization of the debate between global ethics and local ethics and a schematic proposal for balancing these two approaches. Much work is needed if we are to achieve such a balanced approach. Further work is also needed to identify those ethical principles that should be viewed as universal or global and those that should vary in different countries, regions, or cultures.

Conceptualization of global ethics in 2005: Tension between global ethics and local ethics

Tyranny of Global Ethics "One size fits all" Universal ethics regardless of local culture	VS.	All ethics are local "Ethical relativism" No global ethics

Conceptualization of global ethics in 2015: Balancing global ethical principles and using cultural competence in their implementation

A balanced approach to global ethics Consensus on global ethics principles Consensus on principles that vary by region or culture Implemented of all principles with cultural competence and sensitivity

Fig. 1. Moving toward a balanced approach to the issue of global ethics.

Since it seems likely that there are some components of end-of-life care in the ICU that should be universal and transcend cultural differences, the following sections attempt to identify some of these components.

Some Important Components of High Quality End-of-life Care in the ICU

Communication with Patients and Families

Several studies have shown that family members with loved ones in the ICU rate communication with the critical care clinicians as one of the most important skills for these clinicians [40]. Furthermore, observational studies suggest that ICU clinicians frequently do not meet families' needs for communication [6–8]. A study from France suggests that 50% of family members of critically ill patients have important misunderstandings of diagnosis, prognosis, or treatment after a meeting with physicians [6].

The ICU setting frequently involves complicated, confusing, and even discordant data that can be overwhelming to family members and make the family highly dependent on the health care team for assistance. A cross-sectional survey in France suggests that family members have a significant burden of symptoms of depression and anxiety [41] and a qualitative study in the US showed that families are also working through diverse processes such as reviewing the patient's life and understanding the effect of the loss of the patient on family relationships [42].

There has been little research on the content of clinician-family communication in the ICU. A recent observational study examined audiotapes of ICU family conferences about end-of-life care to develop a framework for understanding the content of these discussions and the techniques used by clinicians to provide support to family members [43]. Researchers found that critical care clinicians spent 70% of the time talking and only 30% of the time listening to family members [44]. In addition, the higher the proportion of time that family members spent speaking, the more satisfied they were with the family conference and yet there was no relationship with the duration of the conference and family satisfaction [44]. This study suggests that critical care clinicians may increase family satisfaction with communication about end-of-life care if they spend more time listening and less time talking. Another analysis from this study identified missed opportunities during family conferences about end-of-life care and found that common missed opportunities could be conceptualized in three categories: opportunities to listen and respond to family; opportunities to acknowledge and address emotions; and opportunities to pursue key principles of medical ethics and palliative care, including exploration of patient preferences, explanation of surrogate decision-making, and affirmation of non-abandonment [45]. Awareness of these commonly missed opportunities may provide critical care clinicians with some guidance for improving communication with families.

Inclusion of the Interdisciplinary Team

As the ICU team is made up of a number of health care professionals from many disciplines, it is important that all team members who are directly involved in patient care and in communication with patients and families be included in the process of end-of-life care in the ICU. Conflict is common in ICU decision-making and this conflict often occurs between members of the clinical team [46, 47]. One prospective cohort study of ICU patients for whom withdrawal of life support was considered found that conflict occurred between staff and family in 48% of cases and conflict among staff occurred in the same proportion of cases (48%) [47]. Furthermore, family members report that hearing different messages from different team members is a major source of distress for family members [48]. Therefore, communication and consensus within the ICU team is an important step in the process of high quality care for patients and families. Although consensus within the team may not always be achieved, it should be a goal of high quality care. Oftentimes, nurses come to the decision that life-sustaining treatments should be limited or stopped earlier than physicians, which several studies have demonstrated can be a source of frustration for some critical care nurses and a source of inter-disciplinary conflict for physicians and nurses [49, 50]. The best way to avoid and address such conflict is to ensure that lines of communication are open between team members .

Quality of Care Regarding Withholding and Withdrawing Life-sustaining Treatments

Many observational studies have examined the proportion of deaths in the ICU that are preceded by withholding or withdrawing life-sustaining therapies [51–55]. The proportion of deaths occurring in the ICU that are preceded by withholding or withdrawing life-sustaining treatments varies across the different studies, but most studies found that the majority of ICU deaths are preceded by either withholding or withdrawing life-sustaining therapies. This finding is generally true regardless of the time period or the country or continent in which the study was conducted, although most studies have been conducted in the U.S., Canada, and Europe. Nonetheless, several studies have documented significant differences across different institutions and across different countries. Prendergast and colleagues surveyed training program directors to determine the proportion of ICU deaths preceded by withholding or withdrawing life-sustaining treatments in 131 ICUs in 110 hospitals in 38 states in the US [34]. These authors showed dramatic variation ranging from 0 to 67% of deaths preceded by withholding life-sustaining therapies and 0 to 79% preceded by withdrawing life-sustaining treatments. Similarly, Sprung and colleagues and Vincent conducted studies of ICU deaths across Europe and showed geographic variation in the proportion of deaths preceded by withdrawing life support with higher proportions in Northern Europe, intermediate proportions in Central Europe, and lower proportions in Southern Europe [35, 36]. There was less variation in the proportion of deaths preceded by withholding life-sustaining therapy. However, in a more recent study of withdrawal of mechanical ventilation in 15 ICUs located in four countries, Cook and colleagues did not find variation by site [56]. This latter study raises the question of whether there was something different about these 15 ICUs or whether geographic variation may be decreasing in some areas as there is more attention paid to the issue of end-of-life care in the ICU. Nonetheless, geographic variation in withdrawing and withholding of life-sustaining treatments has been shown to be considerable and it remains unclear whether this variation is decreasing over time.

The reasons for the variations in the proportion of ICU deaths preceded by withholding or withdrawing life sustaining therapies are not entirely clear. Another study by Cook and colleagues examined the patient determinants of withdrawal of life support using a series of patient scenarios presented to critical care physicians and nurses across Canada [33]. These authors found that the most important predictors were the likelihood of long-term survival, pre-morbid cognitive function, and the age of the patient. There were also a number of clinician characteristics that were associated with an increased willingness to withdraw life-sustaining therapies including increased number of years since graduation, geographic location, and fewer number of beds in their ICU. Surveys of physicians' attitudes toward withdrawal of life-sustaining therapies have also identified a number of physician factors that influence physician willingness to withdraw life-sustaining therapies. A survey by Christakis and Asch showed that physicians who were younger, less religious, specialists, and had more time in clinical practice were all more willing to withdraw life support [57]. These studies suggest that some of the variation may be determined by clinician attitudes and biases regarding withdrawal of life-sustaining therapies.

Interventions to Improve End-of-life Care in the ICU

There have been a number of interventions that have attempted to improve end-of-life care in the ICU. One landmark study that attempted to improve the quality of end-of-life care for hospitalized patients and decrease the use of unwanted life-sustaining therapies at the end of life was the Study to Understand Prognoses and Preferences for Outcomes and Risks of Treatment (SUPPORT) [3]. SUPPORT randomized hospitalized, seriously ill adults to an intervention including feedback of prognostic data to physicians, patients, and families, feedback of patient preferences for end-of-life care to physicians, and facilitation of patient-physician communication about end-of-life care. SUPPORT was conducted by many experienced and talented health services researchers in the field of end-of-life care and yet the intervention did not improve quality of care. There have been a number of suggestions as to why this intervention was unsuccessful [58]. Some potential explanations include the fact that the intervention focused on individual physicians and patients and did not incorporate the systems of care and that the outcome measures may not have been sensitive to small but important changes. An intervention designed to improve the quality of care regarding withdrawal of life-sustaining therapies must incorporate the lessons from SUPPORT.

There have been seven studies published more recently that have suggested that an intervention focused on improving end-of-life care in the ICU setting can improve the quality of care. Table 1 summarizes these studies. The interventions include routine ethics consultation, routine palliative care consultation, a standardized order form for withdrawing life-sustaining therapies, a communication intervention in the form of mandated family conferences, and a quality improvement project. Only one of these interventions has been evaluated using the randomized controlled trial: routine ethics consultation. Each of the other interventions have only been assessed with before-after study designs.

Routine Ethics Consultation

In the first of two randomized trials, Schneiderman and colleagues assessed routine ethics consultation in a single center study [59]. Eligible patients were those for whom study nurses determined that "value-based treatment conflicts" arose. The goal of the ethics consultations was to identify, analyze, and resolve the ethical issues, to educate about ethical issues, and to help present personal views. They found that, among patients who went on to die, those randomized to receive a routine ethics consultation had a shorter length of stay in the ICU and fewer life-sustaining treatments. More recently, Schneiderman and colleagues performed a similar study as a multicenter, randomized trial in seven hospitals around the US [60]. Eligible patients were those in whom a study nurse and site principal investigator determined that "value-based treatment conflicts" arose. In this study, the intervention was described as a process that included assessing the ethical issues, making an ethical diagnosis, making recommendations for next step including meetings to improve communication, documentation of the consultation in the medical record, follow-up by the ethics consultant to provide ongoing support, and evaluation of the process for quality improvement of ethics consultation. They found that routine ethics consultations reduced the number of days that patients spent in the ICU and hospital, again suggesting that these consultations reduced the prolongation of dying. In addition, families and clinicians reported a high level of satisfaction with ethics consultation, although satisfaction was not compared with the group that was randomized to not receive routine ethics consultation.

Routine Palliative Care Consultation

There have been two studies of routine palliative care consultation in selected ICU patients. In a before-after study design, Campbell and Guzman [61] studied the effect of routine palliative care consultation on duration of life-sustaining therapies for patients with anoxic encephalopathy after cardiopulmonary resuscitation and also in patients with multiple organ dysfunction syndrome (MODS) with more than three organs affected for three or more days. The intervention conducted by the palliative care consultants included early communication with the family about prognosis, identifying advance directives or patient preferenc-

Table 1. Studies showing interventions that improve the care of patients undergoing withdrawal of life-sustaining therapies.

Reference	Study design	Population	Intervention	Number of patients	Outcome
Routine Ethics Consultation					
Schneiderman et al, 2000 [59]	Randomized trial	Patients in medical and pediatric ICUs in one hospital for whom "value-laden conflicts" arose	Routine ethics consultation	Treatment n=35 Control n=35	Intervention associated with decreased hospital and ICU days. Satisfaction with intervention high, but not compared to satisfaction in the control group.
Schneiderman et al, 2003 [60]	Randomized trial	Patients in adult ICU in 7 U.S. hospitals for whom "value-laden conflicts" arose	Routine ethics consultation	Treatment n=278 Control n=273	Intervention associated with decreased hospital and ICU days. Satisfaction with intervention high, but not compared to satisfaction in the control group.
Routine Palliative Care Consultation					
Campbell and Guzman, 2003 [61]	Before-after study	Patients in one medical ICU with anoxic encephalopathy after CPR or with multiple organ dysfunction syndrome (MODS)	Routine palliative care consultation	Before n=40 After n= 41	Intervention associated with decreased hospital days and decreased TISS score after developing MODS among patients with MODS; intervention associated with decreased hospital days for patients with anoxic encephalopathy

Table 1. *Continued.*

Reference	Study design	Population	Intervention	Number of patients	Outcome
Campbell and Guzman, 2004 [62]	Before-after study	Patients in one medical ICU with severe dementia	Routine palliative care consultation	Before n=26 After n=26	Intervention associated with decreased hospital and ICU days and decreased TISS score after DNR order
Standardized Orders to Withdraw Life-sustaining Therapies					
Treece et al, 2004 [63]	Before-after study	Patients in one of 6 ICU's in one hospital who died in the ICU	Implementation of a standardized order form with withdrawal of life support	Before n=41 After n=76	Intervention associated with: 1. high levels of physician and nurse satisfaction with form; 2. increase in average dose of narcotics and benzo-diazepines; 3. increased standard deviation of doses used; 4. no decrease in time from ventilator withdrawal to death
Routine Family Conferences					
Lilly et al, 2000 [66, 67]	Before-after study	Patient in one medical ICU for whom attending physician predicts ICU length of stay greater than 5 days or risk of mortality greater than 25%	Multidisciplinary family conference within 72 hours of admission	Before n=134 After n=396	Intervention associated with decreased ICU days

Table 1. *Continued.*

Reference	Study design	Population	Intervention	Number of patients	Outcome
Quality Improvement Project					
Hall et al, 2004 [68]	Before-after study	Patients who died in the ICU at two medical-surgical ICUs in one hospital	Quality improvement project with 3 components: 1) eliciting nurses concerns regarding end-of-life care, 2) altering nurses' progress notes regarding symptom assessment and treatment, 3) altering prescription policy for narcotics and sedatives	Before n=138 After n=168	Intervention associated with fewer patients receiving CPR in 12 hours prior to death; fewer numbers of narcotics and benzodiazepine drugs used and on average lower doses of benzodiazepines; high levels of satisfaction among nurses.

es, discussion of prognosis and treatment options, implementation of palliative care strategies when goals changed to "comfort measures only", and education of the primary team regarding palliative care strategies. These authors showed that routine palliative care consultation reduced the number of ICU days for the patients with anoxic encephalopathy and also reduced the number of ICU days after onset of MODS for patients with MODS. In a follow up study, these same authors applied the same routine palliative care consultation intervention to patients admitted to the medical ICU with severe dementia and again found that after implementation of routine palliative care consultation, patients who received the consultation had fewer ICU days and also had fewer life-sustaining treatments after initiation of a Do Not Resuscitate (DNR) order [62].

Standardized Order Form for Withdrawal of Life-Sustaining Treatments

There has been one before-after study of a standardized order form for withdrawal of life-sustaining therapies [63]. This study used a before-after design to evaluate the order form among patients who died in the ICU. The order form contained four sections: 1) preparation for withdrawal of life support (which included documentation of family conference; discontinuing routine labs and radiographic tests; discontinuing prior medications; completion of a DNR order); 2) a sedation and analgesia protocol that provided for continuous narcotic and benzodiazepine infusion if needed and provided nurses with wide latitude on doses and no maximum dose, but required documentation of the signs of discomfort that prompted increased doses; 3) a protocol for withdrawing mechanical ventilation that focuses on maximizing patient comfort; and 4) a set of principles that guide withdrawal of life-sustaining therapies. The intervention included development of the order form with input from multiple disciplines including nursing, physicians, pharmacists, and respiratory therapists as well as unit-based education on use of the order form prior to implementation. These authors showed that the order form was found helpful by the vast majority of physicians and nurses and resulted in an increased average dose of opioids and benzodiazepines used during the one hour prior to ventilator withdrawal and the one hour after ventilator withdrawal. However, the intervention was not associated with any change in the time from ventilator withdrawal to death. This study suggests that there was an increase in medication used for pain and sedation among some patients without evidence that these medications were used in a way that hastened death. The authors also examined a nurse-assessment of the quality of dying and death, using a validated questionnaire [64, 65], but this intervention did not show any significant change in the nurses assessment of the quality of dying and death.

Routine Family Conferences

Another intervention assessed in a before-after study was the implementation of a policy regarding routine family conferences in the ICU setting. Lilly and colleagues assessed this intervention among critically ill patients for whom the attending physician predicted a risk of mortality greater than 25% or anticipated an ICU length of stay of more than 5 days [66]. The intervention was a mandated family conference for these patients within 72 hours of admission to the ICU. The conferences were to be conducted by the attending physician and to cover four topics including: 1) review medical facts and treatment options; 2) discuss patient's perspectives on death and dying; 3) agree on a care plan; and 4) agree on criteria by which success or failure of the plan would be judged. This intervention was associated with a reduction in ICU days and the reduction was most prominent among the patients with the highest severity of illness who went on to die. These results were sustained in a four-year follow-up report from this group [67].

Quality Improvement Project

There has also been a published quality improvement project designed to improve quality of end-of-life care in the ICU [68]. This project was undertaken in response to legal actions taken against a critical care physician after withdrawal of life-sustaining treatments. In response, the quality improvement intervention was designed with three steps: 1) identify nurses and family concerns about end-of-life care in the ICU, 2) alter nursing progress notes entries to increase documentation of the withdrawal process, and 3) change orders to be used for analgesic and sedative medications to require a fixed upper limit to the amount of drug administered. Among those patients that died, the intervention was associated with reduction in the use of cardiopulmonary rseuscitation in the last 12 hours of life, fewer number of analgesic and sedative medications used, and lower cumulative doses of diazepam.

Summary of Interventions to Improve End-Of-Life Care in the ICU

The evidence described above, based on two randomized trials [59, 60], suggests that routine ethics consultation can reduce ICU days and decrease prolongation of dying for a subset of critically ill patients. These data also suggest that the ethics consultations are well received by family members and ICU clinicians. Although the process of the consultations are described, it is difficult to know what aspects of these consultations reduced ICU days and whether, as ICU clinician experience with ethics consultation increases, the benefit of consultation will persist. Before-after studies suggest that palliative care consultation may also have a similar effect on ICU length of stay for selected patients [61, 62]. Whether these two interventions have a similar mechanism is hard to assess based on existing data. A recent review article describes some of the models that can be used for ethics and palliative care consultation in the ICU and the settings in which either ethics consultation or palliative care consultation may be more useful [69]. The study by Lilly and colleagues also suggests that ICU clinicians may be able to have a similar effect by implementing routine family conferences in the sickest patients [66, 67].

One study suggested that a standardized order form for withdrawal of life-sustaining treatments in the ICU is associated with high levels of clinician satisfaction and can increase use of opioids and benzodiazepines, on average, for these patients without hastening death [63]. There are also some data to suggest that quality improvement projects targeting end-of-life care in the ICU setting can affect quality measures [68]. Interestingly, the former of these two studies had the goal of increasing critical care nurses' ability to give analgesic and sedative medications when needed while the latter had the goal of decreasing the variability in use of sedating medications in setting without standardized orders. Each study had its intended effect, although the intended effects were oppositional. Both studies attempted to increase nurses' documentation of the reasons for giving analgesic and sedative medications in the setting of withdrawal of life-sustaining treatment and one study showed that this documentation did increase [68].

Measuring the Quality of End-of-life Care in the ICU

Studies of interventions to improve the quality of end-of-life care in the ICU must address the issue of identifying the appropriate outcomes for such interventions. Several studies have used ICU length of stay among all patients or among patients that die as the outcome measure. The rationale for this outcome measure is that if ICU days are decreased for those patients that ultimately die and without an increase in overall mortality, the intervention has reduced the 'prolongation of dying'. This outcome assumes that prolongation of dying is a marker of poor quality care. There are some important potential limitations to ICU days as an outcome measure for such interventions. For example, an intervention that 'rushed' families might be associated with decreased family satisfaction with care and increased family depression and anxiety. There may also come a point in time when the prolongation of dying has been sufficiently minimized so that further improvements in the quality of care regarding withdrawal of life-sustaining treatments may not necessarily result in further reductions in ICU days. Nonetheless, in the current environment, reducing ICU length of stay, particularly if it is associated with high levels of family satisfaction, seems like an appropriate surrogate marker for improved quality of care.

Another similar outcome measure used in some studies is reduction in technologic life-sustaining therapies after a decision is made to limit life-sustaining therapies. Campbell and Guzman conducted two studies using a measure called Therapeutic Intervention Scoring System (TISS). TISS quantifies standard ICU and hospital interventions through the assignment of weighted points. These authors argue that TISS points after a DNR order are a surrogate marker of quality of care in the process of withdrawing life-sustaining treatments since the use of non-beneficial interventions that do not increase patient comfort are reduced [61, 62].

Another potential assessment of the quality of end-of-life care in the ICU is family or clinician satisfaction with care. Patient satisfaction is not a practical outcome measure for end-of-life care in the ICU since the vast majority of patients are not able respond to questions at the time that a decision is made to withdraw life-sustaining therapies [51]. Family and clinician satisfaction has been used in randomized trials by Schneiderman and colleagues, although in these studies the authors assessed satisfaction with the intervention and therefore did not survey family members of patients in the control arm [59, 60]. Treece and colleagues used a measure called the Quality of Dying and Death (QODD), a survey completed by nurses (in this study) to assess quality of withdrawal of life support [63]. The family-assessed QODD was validated in a study of 204 deaths in Missoula County and was shown to have good internal consistency (Cronbach's alpha 0.86) and construct validity, correlating significantly with measures of symptom burden, patient-clinician communication about treatment preferences, and several measures of quality of care [70]. The family-assessed QODD was also shown to correlate with other markers of quality of care in a study of patients in hospice [71]. The QODD has been used to evaluate the quality of ICU deaths in several studies. Levy and colleagues showed that this instrument could be completed by family members, nurses, resident physicians, and attending physicians. They reported that nurses and resident physicians gave more negative ratings than family members or attending physicians [64]. Hodde and colleagues showed that the ICU nurse-assessed QODD demonstrated significantly higher quality of dying among patients who did not receive cardiopulmonary resuscitation in the last eight hours of life and for patients who had someone present at their death [65]. Finally, Mularski and colleagues demonstrated moderate inter-rater reliability between family members after a death in the ICU [72]. Although these studies suggest the QODD may be a useful tool for assessing the quality of end-of-life care in the ICU, it is not been demonstrated to be responsive to an intervention. The study of a standardized order form for withdrawal of life-sustaining therapies did not show improvement in the QODD score, either because the intervention was not effective for this outcome or the outcome tool may not be sensitive to a small but clinically important difference [63]. Further studies are needed to determine whether the QODD will be a useful outcome measure for such interventions. There are additional measures of family satisfaction with intensive care that may also be useful outcome measures for studies of interventions to improve the quality of end-of-life care in the ICU, but these measures, while reliable and valid, have also not been assessed for responsive to change [73–75].

Conclusion

End-of-life care is a common occurrence in the ICU setting and is commonly preceded by withholding or withdrawing life-sustaining treatments. Many studies have documented dramatic geographic variations in the prevalence of withdrawal of life-sustaining therapies and some evidence suggests this variation may be driven more by physician attitudes and biases than by factors such as patient preferences or cultural differences. A number of studies of interventions in the ICU setting have provided some evidence that end-of-life care in the ICU is a process that can be improved. However, many of these interventions use surrogate outcomes for quality, such as ICU length of stay. For some of the interventions, for example, ethics consultations or palliative care consultations, the precise mechanisms by which the process of care is improved are not clear. Nonetheless, there is convincing evidence that end-of-life care in the ICU is a process of care that presents opportunities for quality improvement and that interventions are successful at improving this care. Implementation of existing interventions and testing of additional interventions will likely bring about important improvements in the ethics and end-of-life care in the ICU over the next 10 years. The following are a list of action items toward the goal of making this improvement.

- Develop an international consensus on those ethical principles that should guide end-of-life care in the ICU and identify those that are universal and global and those that are region- or culture-specific that should appropriately vary with varying culture, religion, or attitudes.
- Identify the components of high quality communication with patients and families that can be taught to ICU clinicians to improve the quality of care delivered to patients and families.
- Develop methods for improving the interdisciplinary nature of end-of-life care in the ICU to improve the quality of care delivered to patients and their families.
- Identify the components of high quality care in the setting of withholding or withdrawing life-sustaining therapies and develop methods for assessing these processes of care.
- Identify interventions that can improve the quality of end-of-life care delivered in ICUs and identify the aspects of these interventions that are feasible to implement in different types of hospitals and generalizable to many settings and countries.
- Identify reliable, reproducible, and valid measures of quality of end-of-life care that are applicable to the ICU, generalizable to many types of hospitals and countries, and responsive to change with an intervention that improves quality of this care.

Acknowledgement. This manuscript was supported by an RO1 grant from the National Institute of Nursing Research (5 RO1 NR-05226).

References

1. Angus DC, Barnato AE, Linde-Zwirble WT, et al (2004) Use of intensive care at the end of life in the United States: An epidemiologic study. Crit Care Med 32:638–643
2. Danis M, Patrick DL, Southerland LI, Green ML (1988) Patients' and families' preferences for medical intensive care. JAMA 260:797–802
3. The SUPPORT Principal Investigators (1996) A controlled trial to improve care for seriously ill hospitalized patients: The study to understand prognoses and preferences for outcomes and risks of treatments (SUPPORT). JAMA 274:1591–1598

4. Hofmann JC, Wenger NS, Davis RB, et al (1997) Patients' preferences for communication with physicians about end-of-life decisions. Ann Intern Med 127:1–12
5. Nelson JE, Meier D, Oei EJ, et al (2001) Self-reported symptom experience of critically ill cancer patients receiving intensive care. Crit Care Med 29:277–282
6. Azoulay E, Chevret S, Leleu G, et al (2000) Half the families of intensive care unit patients experience inadequate communication with physicians. Crit Care Med 28:3044–3049
7. Kirchhoff KT, Walker L, Hutton A, Spuhler V, Cole BV, Clemmer T (2002) The vortex: families' experiences with death in the intensive care unit. Am J Crit Care 11:200–209
8. Azoulay E, Pochard F, Chevret S, et al (2001) Meeting the needs of intensive care unit patient families: a multicenter study. Am J Respir Crit Care Med 163:135–139
9. Singer PA, Siegler M (1992). Advancing the cause of advance directives. Arch Intern Med 152:22-24
10. Emanuel LL, Barry MJ, Stoeckle JD, Ettelson LM, Emanuel EJ (1991) Advance directives for medical care–a case for greater use. N Engl J Med 324:889–895
11. Schneiderman LJ, Kronick R, Kaplan RM, Anderson JP, Langer RD (1992) Effects of offering advance directives on medical treatment and costs. Ann Intern Med 117:599–606
12. Danis M, Southerland LI, Garrett JM, et al (1991) A prospective study of advance directives for life-sustaining care. N Engl J Med 324:882–888
13. Teno JM, Lynn J, Connors AFJ, et al (1997) The illusion of end-of-life savings with advance directives. J Am Geriatr Soc 45:513–518
14. Teno JM, Lynn J, Wegner N, et al (1997) Advance directives for seriously ill hospitalized patients: Effectiveness with the Patient Self-Determination Act and the SUPPORT Intervention. J Am Geriatr Soc 45:500–507
15. Teno JM (2001) Advance care planning in the outpatient and ICU setting. In: Curtis JR, Rubenfeld GD (eds) Managing Death in the Intensive Care Unit: The Transition from Cure to Comfort. Oxford University Press, New York
16. Grenvik A (1983) "Terminal weaning"; discontinuance of life-support therapy in the terminally ill patient. Crit Care Med 11:394–395
17. Cassem NH (1974) Confronting the decision to let death come. Crit Care Med 2:113–117
18. Lo B (1995) Resolving Ethical Dilemmas: A Guide For Clinicians. Williams & Wilkins, Baltimore
19. Curtis JR, Park DR, Krone MR, Pearlman RA (1995) Use of the medical futility rationale in do-not-attempt-resuscitation orders. JAMA 273:124–128
20. Schneiderman LJ, Jecker NS (1993) Futility in practice. Arch Intern Med 153:437–441
21. Helft PR, Siegler M, Lantos J (2000) The rise and fall of the futility movement. N Engl J Med 343:293–296
22. Truog RD, Brett AS, Frader J (1992) The problem with futility. N Engl J Med 326:1560–1564
23. Sulmasy DP, Pellegrino ED (1999) The rule of double effect: Clearing up the double talk. Arch Intern Med 159:545–550
24. Luce JM, Lemaire F (2001) Two transatlantic viewpoints on an ethical quandary. Am J Respir Crit Care Med 163:818–821
25. Beauchamp TL (1989) Principles Of Biomedical Ethics. Oxford University Press, NewYork, pp 147–150
26. The Hastings Center (1987) Guidelines on the termination of life-sustaining treatment and the care of the dying. The Hastings Center, Briarcliff Manor
27. American Thoracic Society (1991) Withholding and withdrawing life-sustaining therapy. Ann Intern Med 115:478–485
28. American College of Chest Physicians/ Society of Critical Care Medicine Consensus Panel (1990) Ethical and moral guidelines for the initiation, continuation, and withdrawal of intensive care. Chest 97:949–958
29. Sulmasy DP, Sugarman J (1994) Are withholding and withdrawing therapy always morally equivalent? J Med Ethics 20:218–222

30. Melltorp G, Nilstun T (1997) The difference between withholding and withdrawing life-sustaining treatment. Intensive Care Med 23:1264–1267
31. Bleich JD (1979) The Quinlan Case: A Jewish Perspective. In: Rosner F, Bleich JD (eds) Jewish Bioethics. Sanhedrin Press, New York pp 266–276
32. Solomon M, O'Donnell L, Jennings B, et al (1993) Decisions near the end of life: Professionals views on life-sustaining treatments. Am J Public Health 83:14–23
33. Cook DJ, Guyatt GH, Jaeschke R, et al (1995) Determinants in Canadian health care workers of the decision to withdraw life support from the critically ill. JAMA 273:703–708
34. Prendergast TJ, Claessens MT, Luce JM (1998) A national survey of end-of-life care for critically ill patients. Am J Respir Crit Care Med 158:1163–1167
35. Vincent JL (1999) Forgoing life support in western European intensive care units: results of an ethical questionnaire. Crit Care Med 16:1626–1633
36. Sprung CL, Cohen SL, Sjokvist P, et al (2003) End-of-life practices in European intensive care units: the Ethicus Study. JAMA 290:790–797
37. Curtis JR, Bennett CL, Horner RD, Rubenfeld GD, DeHovitz JA, Weinstein RA (1998) Variations in ICU utilization for patients with HIV-related Pneumocystis carinii pneumonia: Importance of hospital characteristics and geographic location. Crit Care Med 26:668–675
38. Engelhardt HT Jr (1998) Critical care: why there is no global bioethics. J Med Philos 23:643–651
39. Thompson BT, Cox PN, Antonelli M, et al (2004) Challenges in end-of-life care in the ICU: Statement of the 5th International Consensus Conference in Critical Care: Brussels, Belgium, April 2003: executive summary. Crit Care Med 32:1781–1784
40. Hickey M (1990) What are the needs of families of critically ill patients? A review of the literature since 1976. Heart Lung 19:401–415
41. Prochard F, Azoulay E, Chevret S, et al (2001) Symptoms of anxiety and depression in family members of intensive care unit patients: Ethical hypothesis regarding decision-making capacity. Crit Care Med 29:1893–1897
42. Swigart V, Lidz C, Butterworth V, Arnold R (1996) Letting go: family willingness to forgo life support. Heart Lung 25:483–494
43. Curtis JR, Engelberg RA, Wenrich MD, et al (2002) Studying communication about end-of-life care during the ICU family conference: Development of a framework. J Crit Care 17:147–160
44. McDonagh JR, Elliott TB, Engelberg RA, et al (2004) Family satisfaction with family conferences about end-of-life care in the ICU: Increased proportion of family speech is associated with increased satisfaction. Crit Care Med 32:1484–1488
45. Curtis JR, Engelberg RA, Wenrich MD, Shannon SE, Treece PD, Rubenfeld GD (2005) Missed opportunities during family conferences about end-of-life care in the intensive care unit. Am J Respir Crit Care Med 171:844–849
46. Abbott KH, Sago JG, Breen CM, Abernethy AP, Tulsky JA (2001) Families looking back: one year after discussion of withdrawal or withholding of life-sustaining support. Crit Care Med 29:197–201
47. Breen CM, Abernethy AP, Abbott KH, Tulsky JA (2001) Conflict associated with decisions to limit life-sustaining treatment in intensive care units. J Gen Intern Med 16:283–289
48. Tilden VP, Tolle SW, Garland MJ, Nelson CA (1995) Decisions about life-sustaining treatment: Impact of physicians' behaviors on the family. Arch Intern Med 155:633–638
49. Asch DA, Shea JA, Jedrziewski MK, Bosk CL (1997) The limits of suffering: critical care nurses' views of hospital care at the end of life. Soc Sci Med 45:1661–1668
50. Meltzer LS, Huckabay LM (2004) Critical care nurses' perceptions of futile care and its effect on burnout. Am J Crit Care 13:202–208
51. Prendergast TJ, Luce JM (1997) Increasing incidence of withholding and withdrawal of life support from the critically ill. Am J Respir Crit Care Med 155:15–20

52. Smedira NG, Evans BH, Grais LS, et al (1990) Withholding and withdrawal of life support from the critically ill. N Engl J Med 322:309–315
53. Vincent JL, Parquier JN, Preiser JC, Brimioulle S, Kahn RJ (1989) Terminal events in the intensive care unit: Review of 258 fatal cases in one year. Crit Care Med 17:530–533
54. Eidelman LA, Jakobson DJ, Pizov R, Geber D, Leibovitz L, Sprung CL(1998) Foregoing life-sustaining treatment in an Israeli ICU. Intensive Care Med 24:162–166
55. Keenan SP, Busche KD, Chen LM, McCarthy L, Inman KJ, Sibbald WJ (1997) A retrospective review of a large cohort of patients undergoing the process of withholding or withdrawal of life support. Crit Care Med 22:1020–1025
56. Cook D, Rocker G, Marshall J, et al (2003) Withdrawal of mechanical ventilation in anticipation of death in the intensive care unit. N Engl J Med 349:1123–1132
57. Christakis NA Asch DA(1995) Physician characteristics associated with decisions to withdraw life support. Am J Public Health 85:367–372
58. Lo B (1995) Improving care near the end of life: Why is it so hard? JAMA 274:1634–1636
59. Schneiderman LJ, Gilmer T, Teetzel HD (2000) Impact of ethics consultations in the intensive care setting: a randomized, controlled trial. Crit Care Med 28:3920–3924
60. Schneiderman LJ, Gilmer T, Teetzel HD, et al (2003) Effect of ethics consultations on nonbeneficial life-sustaining treatments in the intensive care setting: a randomized controlled trial. JAMA 290:1166–1172
61. Campbell ML, Guzman JA (2003) Impact of a proactive approach to improve end-of-life care in a medical ICU. Chest 123:266–271
62. Campbell ML, Guzman JA (2004) A proactive approach to improve end-of-life care in a medical intensive care unit for patients with terminal dementia. Crit Care Med 32:1839–1843
63. Treece PD, Engelberg RA, Crowley L, et al (2004) Evaluation of a standardized order form for the withdrawal of life support in the intensive care unit. Crit Care Med 32:1141–1148
64. Levy CR, Ely EW, Bowman C, Engelberg RA, Patrick DL, Curtis JR (2005) Quality of dying and death in the ICU: perceptions of family and clinicians. Chest 127:1775–1783
65. Hodde NM, Engelberg RA, Treece PD, Steinberg KP, Curtis JR (2004) Factors associated with nurse assessment of the quality of dying and death in the intensive care unit. Crit Care Med 32:1648–1653
66. Lilly CM, De Meo DL, Sonna LA, et al (2000) An intensive communication intervention for the critically ill. Am J Med 109:469–475
67. Lilly CM, Sonna LA, Haley KJ, Massaro AF (2003) Intensive communication: four-year follow-up from a clinical practice study. Crit Care Med 31:S394–399
68. Hall RI, Rocker GM, Murray D (2004) Simple changes can improve conduct of end-of-life care in the intensive care unit. Can J Anaesth 51:631–636
69. Aulisio MP, Chaitin E, Arnold RM (2004) Ethics and palliative care consultation in the intensive care unit. Crit Care Clin 20:505–523
70. Curtis JR, Patrick DL, Engelberg RA, Norris KE, Asp CH, Byock IR (2002) A measure of the quality of dying and death: Initial validation using after-death interviews with family members. J Pain Symptom Manage 24:17–31
71. Patrick DL, Curtis JR, Engelberg RA, Neilsen E, McCown E (2003) Measuring and improving the quality of dying and death. Ann Intern Med 139:410–415
72. Mularski RA, Curtis JR, Osborne ML, Engelberg RA, Ganzini L (2004) Agreement among family members in their assessment of the quality of dying and death. J Pain Symptom Manage 28:306–315
73. Heyland DK, Rocker GM, Dodek PM, et al (2002) Family satisfaction with care in the intensive care unit: results of a multiple center study. Crit Care Med 30:1413–1418
74. Baker R, Wu AW, Teno JM, et al (2000) Family Satisfaction with End-of-Life Care in Seriously Ill Hospitalized Adults. J Am Geriatr Soc 48:S61–S69
75. Johnson D, Wilson M, Cavanaugh B, Bryden C, Gudmundson D, Moodley O (1998) Measuring the ability to meet family needs in an intensive care unit. Crit Care Med 26:266–27

Rationing in the ICU: Fear, Fiction and Fact

M. M. Levy

Introduction

The 'R' word, or rationing brings fear to the hearts of clinicians, politicians, administrators and patients. Politicians fear for their political life, administrators fear for the life and reputation of their institution, clinicians fear for their clinical practice and ethical beliefs, and patients simply fear for their lives. Accordingly, the hospital administrators, physicians, nurses, and, indeed, the public, in general, have been successful at avoiding discussions about rationing [1]. If ignoring the problem were all that was required to make this thorny issue disappear, then patients, clinicians, politicians and administrators would have nothing to fear. Unfortunately, this reflexive avoidance behavior does not lead to the abandonment of the practice of rationing. Only public discussion and debate about rationing is abandoned. And, rationing is driven underground, into whispered hallway conversations, and out to the bedside in a subjective, uncontrolled fashion. As intensive care unit (ICU) costs continue to explode, the need to bring this discussion out into a public forum, where the practice can be examined and evaluated becomes very clear.

This discussion will start first with a definition of rationing, and then evaluate whether rationing is necessary, if it is happening, how it is currently happening and, finally, offer a proposal how guidelines for rationing might be developed.

The Definition of Rationing

Any discussion of rationing must begin with a definition, in order to be sure that the concept is clearly understood. In the attempt to avoid the discussion, many definitions have appeared in the literature that have served to downplay the 'pain' of rationing, and imply that resource allocation may be achieved without any risk to patients. While this may be true in many instances of rationing, by definition, some risk to patients is inherent in all forms of true rationing. Whether that risk is to life or well-being or comfort, depends on the resource being withheld.

By way of background, the Values Ethics and Rationing in Critical Care (VERICC) Task Force was established in 2003. This task force is an interdisciplinary group that includes representatives from bioethics, critical care, hospital administration, and the public [2]. By combining several definitions found in the

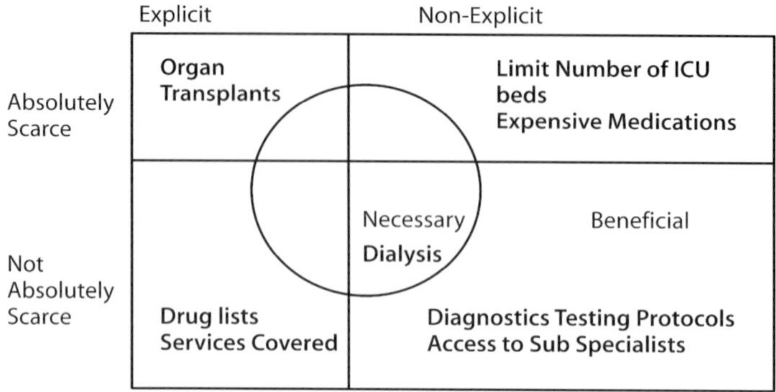

Fig. 1. Examples of rationing from the perspective of explicit vs. non-explicit and absolutely scarce vs. not absolutely scarce (from [3] with permission)

literature, this task force established a definition of rationing: "the allocation of healthcare resources in the face of limited availability, which necessarily means that beneficial interventions are withheld from some individuals".

Rationing can occur in different ways. Rationing may be explicit or non-explicit. Furthermore, rationing can occur with absolutely scare resources or with resources that are not absolutely scarce [3]. Some examples are depicted in Figure 1. For instance, the use of drug lists that limit available drugs to patients enrolled in public assistance programs is a form of explicit rationing of a not absolutely scarce resource. On the other hand, the use of age or medical co-morbidities to limit access to dialysis, prevalent in some countries, is an example of non-explicit rationing of a not absolutely scarce resource.

ICU Costs

Let us look at the costs of health care, in general, and critical care, specifically, using the United States as an example. Much of this discussion will be focused on costs and rationing in the US, but also will include comparison to other cultures. In the US, there are 5.7 million adult ICU admissions per year. There has been a 30% increase in the use of ICU resources for the population over 65 years of age since 1990. In the US, there is a 13% mortality rate across our ICUs. Each year, this statistic translates into 600,000 hospital deaths and 5.1 million survivors or approximately 2% of the population of the United States. Over a 15-year period, from 1985 through 2000, there was a 26% increase in ICU beds and a 70% increase in ICU costs [4]. Thus, about $67 billion or approximately 0.6-1% of the gross domestic product (GDP) is expended every year in the US for the provision of ICU services. Healthcare costs rose dramatically until about 1990, when, for a period of about ten years because of managed care and other factors, healthcare costs stabilized. Over the last several years, however, healthcare spending has been increasing [5] (Fig. 2). The reasons for this increase are multi-factorial

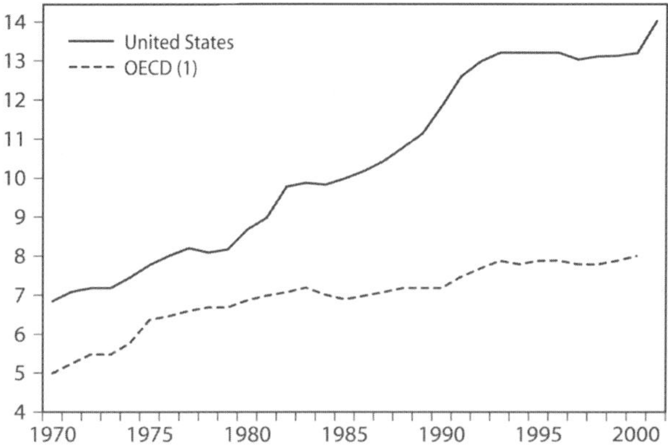

Fig. 2. Rising health costs in the US as a percentage of gross domestic product (GDP). Source: Office of Economic Cooperation and Development (OECD). www.oecd.com

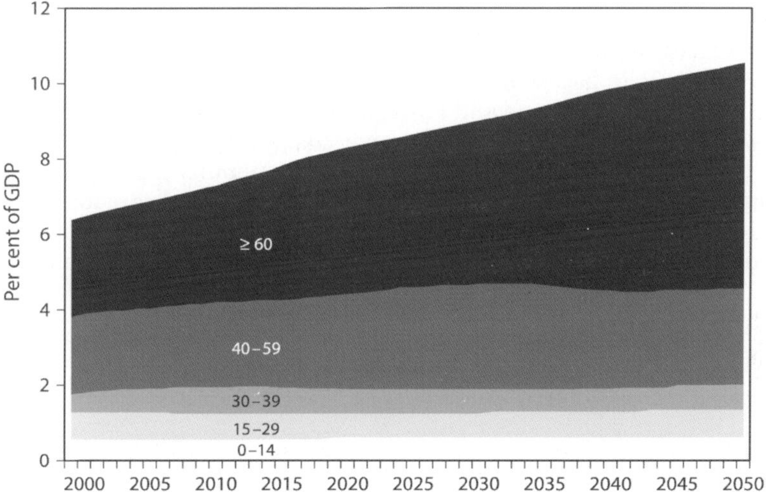

Fig. 3. Predicted rise in health care costs by the year 2050, according to age group. Source: Organization of Economic Development (http//:www.oecd.org)

and, include the introduction of new expensive technologies used in critical care medicine [6, 7]. This trend is expected to continue, in part, because of the aging of populations. In the US alone, the demand for healthcare services among people over 60 is projected to increase by almost 75% by the year 2050 [8] (Fig. 3).

Is Rationing Necessary?

Americans like to believe that rationing must be avoided in order to preserve the health care system, maintain access to excellent health care, and preserve the right to choose physicians as well as all health care options. Without question, the US spends a significantly higher proportion of its GDP on health care than any other nation [8] (Fig. 4). However, a higher level of expenditure does not necessarily correspond to higher quality. The US ranks 26th among countries in the world with regard to infant mortality, 24th in disability-adjusted life expectancy, and the overall quality of the health care system in the United States is ranked 37th by the World Health Organization ranking system [9]. Given the spiraling costs of health care and the rapidly growing national debt in the US, one could argue that failure to ration resources could be catastrophic, quickly paralyzing the ability of clinicians to deliver healthcare of any sort. There are 43 million uninsured Americans; these people have limited access to health care resources, and, in particular, are not receiving good preventative medicine. People without insurance are less likely to see doctors, more likely to be diagnosed with illnesses late, and more likely to report being in fair or poor health [9]. These facts emphasize the importance of a common definition of rationing. The current inequity in access to health care in the United States already reflects a form of rationing. Inequities in access to health care are not unique to the US, and have been well described in Europe and other parts of the world [10, 11]. Simply because the word 'rationing' is avoided does not change the reality of limited access to health care resources for a large segment of the population. Because of the already enormous costs of healthcare, providing all beneficial care for some patients regardless of costs would inevitably prevent us from treating other patients who would benefit more. From this perspective, the ethical peril may lie

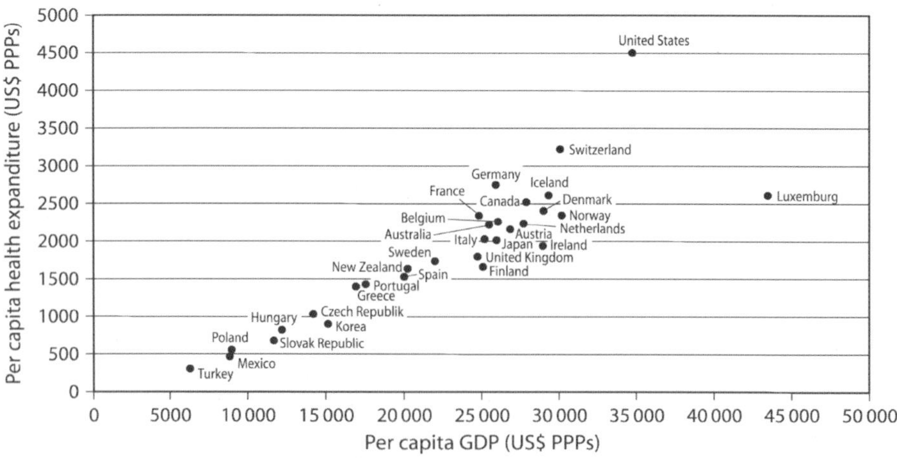

Fig. 4. Per capita gross domestic product (GDP) and per capita health expenditure, 2000. Source: Office of Economic Cooperation and Development (OECD). www.oecd.com

in the persistent view that rationing can be avoided, rather than developing a strategy for allocating resources in ways that optimize medical care, while treating all patients fairly.

Is Rationing Happening?

According to several studies, rationing is already occurring in ICUs [12]. In a study by Hanson and Danis, age-based rationing was found to be a relatively frequent occurrence [13]. Ethnicity-based rationing is also seen in ICUs. In 1993, Whittle et al. reported that racial differences can affect the use of invasive cardiovascular procedures [14]. In a study by Guyatt et al. 78% of patients admitted to the ICU had no explicit resuscitation directive [15]. Severe functional status impairment was associated strongly with an explicit Do Not Resuscitate (DNR) plan. In fact, patients with functional impairment were six times more likely to get a DNR order written in the chart. This study was a multi-cultural study and included centers from France, Australia, the US, and Canada. Thus, the findings could be generalized and were not limited to the US or North America. Furthermore, in this study, patients who were unemployed were 5.5 times more likely to have a DNR order written than those who had a clearly-defined employment status, suggesting that employment may serve as a factor in withholding of resources for patients in an ICU. In a sense, this could be viewed as employment-based rationing at work, influencing the willingness of clinicians to write DNR orders for ICU patients. A recent study by Sinuff et al. from the VERICC Task Force examined the impact of rationing of acute care beds on the process and outcomes of care [16]. Eleven observational studies were included in this systematic review. The conclusions from this study were that patients who are older and sicker are more likely to be refused ICU admission than other patients and that refusal is associated with an increase in mortality. However, during bed shortages, patients refused admission do not have increased mortality. This observation suggests that when faced with bed shortages, critical care clinicians are able to ration resources effectively. Apparently, restricting ICU admission to high-risk patients improves the efficacy of use of critical care resources, while not leading to increased mortality. In 2002, Ward and Levy conducted an anonymous online survey through the Society of Critical Care website [17]. Five hundred members responded. The goal of the survey was to better understand the attitudes of clinicians towards the practice of healthcare rationing. Eighty-four percent of respondents reported that their hospitals did ration procedures, medications, tests, or resources, such as ICU beds. In addition, 54% of the respondents answered that they had withheld a medication, test, or service because they believed that the cost outweighed the potential benefit to a patient. Interestingly, however, 88% of respondents believed that if a fellow healthcare provider withholds a therapy that would be a clear benefit to a patient in order to ration healthcare dollars, this would be unethical. Finally, in this same study, 75% of respondents noted that if a fellow healthcare provider withholds a therapy that would be of limited benefit to a patient in order to ration healthcare, this practice would not be viewed as unethical. These results underscore the ambivalent attitudes of clinicians towards withholding healthcare resources. This ambivalence, while completely understandable, has led to the absence of open dialog and debate about health care rationing and decision-making in resource allocation.

How is Care Rationed?

A recent manuscript by Truog et al. for the VERICC Task Force [18] describes three mechanisms that guide rationing in use in critical care units. They are: 1) external constraints; 2) clinical guidelines; and 3) clinical judgment. *External constraints* consist of hospital and government restrictions on resources, such as medications, diagnostic testing, or admission policies. These constraints are fixed at a level above the critical care unit and do not involve choices made by individual clinicians at the bedside in the ICU but instead reflect constraints placed on ICUs by external sources. *Clinical guidelines* occur at either a societal or a local level. These guidelines may be evidence- or opinion-based and are established either by critical care societies or local societies to guide ICU practices. There are many such examples, including guidelines for the management of sepsis, ventilator-associated pneumonia, or deep venous thrombosis, to cite just a few examples. These guidelines are often not widely adopted, but may also serve as a way in which care in the ICU is rationed. Clinicians may cite these guidelines for choosing a less expensive diagnostic test or denying admission to the ICU for a given patient. *Clinical judgment* represents the so-called 'bedside rationing' approach that occurs when, after operating under external constraints and consistent with clinical guidelines, clinicians at the bedside still withhold potentially beneficial therapy based on their clinical judgment. This practice can occur for illnesses or management for which there are no guidelines written or when there is uncertainty about how to apply guidelines at the bedside. This form of rationing is perhaps the most common and the one that may be of most concern, as it is governed by the subjective attitudes of bedside clinicians [19].

Bedside Rationing

There are many ways clinicians ration care 'at the bedside', some of which may not even be recognized by bedside clinicians as rationing [20, 21]. Certainly, time-based rationing is one of the most common ways that clinicians ration. When a patient in an ICU receives much more of a clinician's attention and time during the rounding process than another patient, this is a form of rationing. There are several factors that bedside clinicians - both nurses and physicians - utilize to prioritize their time with patients. These factors include severity of illness, age, level of pre-admission functional status, and assessment of likelihood of survival. A study by Cook et al. found several clinician- and unit-specific factors that influenced decision-making for withholding and withdrawal of care in the ICU [22]. These factors included the number of years since the clinician graduated, the region in which the clinician was trained, the number of ICU beds, and the clinician's assessment of the likelihood of the withdrawal of life support. Bed allocation is another form of rationing that is commonly seen in ICUs. This strategy is often described as the 'who gets the last bed' approach to rationing. Decisions about ICU admission are clearly a form of rationing, as triage decisions may lead to the withholding of a potentially beneficial therapy for a patient facing ICU admission [23, 24]. Choice of diagnostic testing, prioritization of care and, finally, the level of aggressive care, are also examples of bedside rationing seen in the ICU.

How should Care be Rationed?

The ethical basis for rationing (Table 1) could be viewed as being founded on beneficence and justice. Beneficence, as applied to rationing, is the moral obligation to act for the benefit of others and includes: The rule of rescue, which means rescuing individuals in danger; utility, which is balancing of benefits and drawbacks to produce the best overall results; and cost-effectiveness analysis. The concept of distributive justice is that benefits should be allocated in a fair, equitable, and appropriate way. The idea is 'the greatest good for the greatest number' and ultimately involves the equitable allocation of resources. Allocation can be based on an egalitarian approach, wherein resources are distributed in equitable shares: a libertarian approach, wherein resources are distributed by the will of the free market; or a welfare approach, wherein resources are distributed according to need.

Table 1. Ethical basis for rationing

Beneficence	• Moral obligation to act for the benefit of others
	• Rule of rescue
	  – Rescuing individuals in danger
	• Utility
	  – Balance benefits and drawbacks to produce best overall result
	• Cost-effectiveness analysis

Distributive Justice	• Fair, equitable, and appropriate distribution of benefits – 'Greatest good for the greatest number'

Table 2. Factors in bedside rationing

- Fidelity vs. stewardship
- Patient's medical need for resource
- Likely reversibility of acute problem
- Anticipated duration and quality of subsequent life
- Patient's wishes (to the extent they are known)
- Physician beliefs

Given the reality of bedside rationing, it is important to consider the factors involved in this process (Table 2), which is a matter of striking a balance between fidelity and stewardship. Fidelity, of course, is the duty a health care practitioner has to his or her patient, while stewardship is the responsibility to protect the natural resources of a culture. In addition, factors for guiding the withholding of potentially beneficial resources will also include the patient's medical need for the resource, the likely reversibility of the acute problem, the anticipated duration and quality of subsequent life, the patient's wishes (to the extent they are known), and, finally, the physician's beliefs. All of these are key factors in a clinician's decision to withhold potentially beneficial therapies from any given patient, although they may not be explicitly stated during the decision-making process. As clinicians come under increasing pressure due to high healthcare costs and shrinking budgets, it now becomes extremely important for clinicians to understand and recognize these factors at the bedside during medical decision-making in the ICU. As mentioned already, physicians long have been averse to having these discussions at all, which unfortunately means that bedside rationing continues at an underground level. Exposure to reasoned, intelligent debate and discussion that might ultimately serve to refine this decision-making process is lacking. Is *bedside* rationing necessary? Many ethicists and clinicians feel that decisions about resource allocation should not happen at the bedside, or based on clinicians' judgment, because it prevents physicians from truly representing the best interests of patients. One could argue that rationing by clinicians at the bedside may be beneficial for patients. While far from perfect, bedside rationing allows rationing to account for a patient's individual characteristics and preferences and leaves clinicians with flexibility in decision making at the bedside. In fact, macro-rationing could prevent physicians from individualizing therapies - a situation that would not benefit patients, since bedside clinicians are in the best position to understand the patient's preferences and therefore, most well-suited to make decisions about which therapies might be of benefit to their patients. There is no question that decisions about resource allocation can put clinicians and patients in direct conflict. However, the belief that physicians should not ration at the bedside will not change the reality that it happens with some frequency. In fact, one could make the case, as stated already, that bedside rationing may well be more beneficial for patients in the long run. For this process to become equitable and transparent, ongoing debate and discussion amongst the public and critical care physicians worldwide is needed.

The Oregon Health Plan

In the US, the Oregon Health Plan is often presented as an attempt to ration in an equitable and reasoned manner. In the Oregon Health Plan, the ranking of interventions was first based only on a cost-effective analysis. Unfortunately, based on the first evaluation with cost-effective analysis, tooth caps, surgery for ectopic pregnancy, splints for temporomandibular joint problems, and appendectomy were all ranked the same. Obviously, a cost-effective analysis alone does not provide an adequate basis for rationing. In Oregon, the initial ranking system was then revised according to public and clinical evaluations. This led to the creation of a prioritized list that was more acceptable to both clinicians and the public, and all services below a pre-established line were not covered for patients receiving public assistance in the state of Oregon. In this way, the incorporation of public values was permitted into the ranking. The concept in Oregon was to use savings from rationing to expand insurance coverage [25].

The reality of the Oregon Health Plan showed, in fact, that there was, ultimately, no widespread rationing. There were few excluded services and, in fact, the health care plan was more generous than the old state package, rather than reducing the use of medical resources in the form of rationing. The limits have been difficult to enforce, and there has been little significant savings. Over the first five years of the Oregon Health Plan, there was only a 2% decrease in expenditures, and the expansion in coverage of about 6% was funded by taxes and managed care, not by rationing itself [26].

Lessons learned from the Oregon Health Plan identified some challenges for the future for those who are ready to address rationing and decision-making about resource allocation. First, in order for rationing to become accepted, a public debate must occur. By the same token, the more public the discussion about rationing, the harder it is to ration services to control costs. This should not be a deterrent but must be taken into account when setting out on a course towards healthcare rationing. Realistically speaking, the public must be involved, but there are enormous obstacles to reasoned, public discussions. Second, most legislators do not have the political will to cut services, especially those legislators who are in a current campaign. It is an unpopular topic and one that no politician is enthusiastic to discuss. Unfortunately, most politicians do just the opposite, often playing to the anxiety of the electorate about rationing. This could be viewed as irresponsible; however, it is a political reality, and, as we move forward in this time of high costs and resource allocation, it is important to understand that we will be unlikely to receive any help from politicians in making these decisions. Finally, and most important, in the absence of political and public will, bedside rationing will continue. As has already been discussed, there is ample evidence that bedside rationing is a widespread occurrence in ICUs around the globe. The fact that the public and politicians are unwilling to discuss it will not alter the reality that rationing is an everyday occurrence. Therefore, clinicians must begin to take control of this agenda and be willing to speak of this publicly and acknowledge the fact that simply being unwilling to talk about rationing does not mean it can be avoided. The only way to evolve a more critical and intelligent approach to rationing is to encourage global discussion among the public, clinicians and politicians about the need to track healthcare resource allocation and help guide decision-making for withholding some of these resources.

Guiding Principles for Rationing

Suggestions for principles that might guide rationing are listed in Table 3. Guidelines for rationing could be based on the following: A systematic review of empirical evidence, cost-effective analyses along with public provider and insurer

Table 3. Guiding principles for rationing

- Support by systematic, empirical evidence
- Evaluate with:
  - Cost-effectiveness analysis
  - Public, provider, insurer, hospital input
- Determine scale of likely health benefit
- Availability of services
- General application to population
- Incorporate severity scoring and mortality prediction
- Understand physician and patient preferences

input, assessment of the scale of likely health benefit along with the availability of services. Furthermore, the general application to an entire population could be assessed, taking into account severity scoring and mortality prediction and, finally, incorporating physician and patient preferences into bedside decisions about resource allocation [27].

Several of these principles may be difficult to operationalize in practice at the bedside. This is because high-quality outcomes research for each individual disease and situation is often not available; patients have different co-morbidities; there are variations among patients with respect to the status of their disease, and, finally, there are variations in local treatment patterns.

Conclusion

Rationing, in some form, is already being practiced in the US and globally, both at the bedside and at an institutional level. Furthermore, rationing is not only inevitable but may well be desirable, given the expanding costs of critical care. There is not a clear line between cost containment (eliminating waste) and rationing (limiting beneficial treatments). For the most part, rationing is largely unregulated and undisclosed. Rationing can, at least in part, be based on cost-effectiveness analyses and evidence-based criteria. Finally, and most important, further studies and public discussion are needed. As long as there continues to be an emotional barrier to fostering public debate amongst politicians, clinicians, and the public about rationing, the field will not move forward, and bedside rationing will continue in a haphazard way. Scientific progress in medicine has already made it too expensive for all therapies to be applied to all patients in the ICU. The need for a clear-headed approach to rationing of resources is already evident and is likely to become a dominant force in the daily practice of critical care. As part of the inherent responsibility to patients and their loved ones, it is imperative that clinicians foster this debate, encourage this debate publicly, and help to develop a set of guiding principles for resource allocation that will allow for fair and equitable rationing on a global level.

References

1. Ubel P (1997) Recognizing bedside rationing. Ann Intern Med 126:74-80
2. Values, Ethics & Rationing In Critical Care (VERICC) Task Force. Available at: www.vericc.org Accessed July 2005
3. Ubel P (2000) Pricing Life: Why It's Time for Health Care Rationing. The MIT Press, Massachusetts Institute of Technology, p 13
4. Halpern N, Pastores S, Greenstein R (2004) Critical Care Medicine in the United States 1985-2000: Analysis of bed numbers, use, and costs. Crit Care Med 32:1254-1259
5. OECD (2003) Health at a Glance 2003 - OECD Countries Struggle with Rising Demand for Health Spending. Available at: http://www.oecd.org/document/38/0,2340,en_2825_499502_16560422_1_1_1_1,00.html Accessed July 2005
6. Bloomfied E (2003) The impact of economics on changing medical technology with reference to critical care medicine in the United States. Anesth Analg 96:418-425
7. Gerdtham U, Jönsson B, MacFarlan M, Oxley H (1994) Health Care Reform: Controlling Spending and Increasing Efficiency. OECD Economics Department Working Papers No 149. Available at: http://www.oecd.org/dataoecd/32/20/1862400.pdf Accessed July 2005
8. OECD Health Data 2004. Available at: http://www.oecd.org/findDocument/0,2350,en_2649_33929_1_1_1_1_1,00.html Accessed July 2005
9. Bureau of Labor Education, University of Maine (2001) The US Health Care System: Best in the World, or Just the Most Expensive? Available at: http://dll.umaine.edu/ble/U.S.%20HCweb.pdf Accessed July 2005
10. Income-Related Inequality in the Use of Medical Care in 21 OECD Countries. http://www.oecd.org/dataoecd/14/0/31743034.pdf. Accessed July 2005
11. Organization of Economic Cooperation and Development—member list: http://www.oecd.org/document/58/0,2340,en_2649_201185_1889402_1_1_1_1,00.html. Accessed July 2005
12. Strauss MJ, LoGerfo JP, Yeltatzie JA, Temkin N, Hudson LD (1986) Rationing of intensive care unit services. An everyday occurrence. JAMA 255:1143-1146
13. Hanson LC, Danis M (1991) Use of life-sustaining care for the elderly. J Am Geriatr Soc 39:772-777
14. Whittle J, Conigliaro J, Good CB, Lofgren RP (1993) Racial differences in the use of invasive cardiovascular procedures in the Department of Veterans Affairs medical system. N Engl J Med 329:621-627
15. Guyatt G, Cook D, Weaver B, et al (2003) Influence of perceived functional and employment status on cardiopulmonary resuscitation directives. J Crit Care 18:133-141
16. Sinuff T, Kahnamoui K, Cook D, et al (2004) Rationing critical care beds: A systematic review. Crit Care Med 32:1588–1597
17. Ward N, Levy M (2002) SCCM Rationing Survey. Critical Connections 1:1
18. Truog R, Brock D, Cook D, Danis M, Luce J, Rubenfeld G, Levy M (2005) Rationing in Critical Care (submitted CCM 2004).
19. Caplan A (1995) Straight talk about rationing. Ann Intern Med 122:795-796
20. Light D (1997) The real ethics of rationing. BMJ 315:112-115
21. Marshall MF, Schwenzer KJ, Orsina M, et al (1992) Influence of political power, medical provincialism, and economic incentives on the rationing of surgical intensive care unit beds. Crit Care Med 20:387–394
22. Strosberg MA, Teres D (2003) Intensive care unit admissions do not pass the reasonableness test. Crit Care Med 31:2809–2811
23. Skowronski G (2001) Bed rationing and allocation in the intensive care unit. Curr Opin Crit Care 7:480-484
24. Cook DJ, Guyatt GH, Jaeschke R, et al (1995) Determinants in Canadian health care workers of the decision to withdraw life support from the critically ill. JAMA 273:703-708

25. Ham C (1998) Retracing the Oregon Trail: the experience of rationing and the Oregon health plan. BMJ 316:1965-1969
26. Oberlander J, Marmor T, Jacobs L (2001) Rationing medical care: rhetoric and reality in the Oregon Health Plan. CMAJ 164:1583-1587
27. Little M (2000) Ethonomics: The ethics of the unaffordable. Arch Surg 135:17-21

Training

Training Pathways – Physician and Non-Physician

J. Bion, H. Barrett, and T. Clutton-Brock

The Problem: Changes in Case Mix, Resources and Staffing in Acute Hospital Care

Case Mix

By 2015 several of the contributors to this book will be approaching, or have entered, retirement, joining the growing population of pensioners worldwide who will in time need assistance from their health services. The health care systems on which they depend will have changed in several respects from those of today, with developments in information technology and decision support for both patients and staff, in availability and utility of monitoring and imaging equipment, and in systems for improving patient safety. There are likely to be two streams for patient care: a small and predictable pathway for elective medical care including surgery and complex medical diseases, and a large, heterogeneous group requiring acute and emergent care. If current trends continue [1, 2], this latter component will constitute an even greater component of hospital activity than it does now. Given the aging world population [3], it therefore seems possible that an increasing proportion of the hospital budget may be spent on the emergency care of elderly patients.

Resources

At the same time that demand is increasing, health systems are trying to constrain rising costs, mainly by reducing hospital in-patient beds and increasing throughput [4, 5], by making greater use of day-case or out-patient settings for low-risk interventions [6], or by overt or covert rationing. This has the effect of further focusing hospital care on emergency work, while working to capacity requires meticulous process control if staff are to improve patient safety. This is a particular problem for acute and emergent care [7] because health systems do not have consistent methods for process control of the acutely ill patient, with the consequence that many such patients appear to follow unpredictable pathways. This is not of course true for all acutely ill patients – those who present with clearly characterized syndromes such as acute chest pain or asthma or diabetic ketoacidosis are now much more likely to be recognized early and treated appropriately using evidence-based guidelines. However, this improvement in process control has taken many years to achieve; the management of acutely ill patients with less obvious diagnostic or specialty 'labels' is still far from perfect.

Staffing

In addition to the impact of changing case mix and resources, there are also problems with health care personnel. Many countries at all levels of development are experiencing difficulties with nursing recruitment and retention, for complex reasons which include an aging workforce, suboptimal working conditions, and alternative employment opportunities [8, 9]. Several major developed countries need to expand their physician workforce, but it is unlikely that physician extenders will be able to substitute effectively for doctors in all aspects of a complex healthcare environment [10]. Legislation to reduce hours of work for doctors have also produced additional challenges [11-13]; the potential benefits to patients from reducing medical staff overwork could be offset by failures in medical communication and continuity [14] caused by the transition to shift working and dismantling traditional medical teams, and by less experienced (even though better trained) doctors.

Potential – but partial - solutions to these problems have included the use of physician assistants and non-physician clinicians [15, 16], and new ways of working in acute care, including nurse-led outreach care [17-19], medical emergency teams (METs) [20, 21], hospital-at-night teams [22], and in the USA, the new specialty of 'hospitalists' [23] practising as general physicians. The efficacy of these new approaches remains to be determined [24], though whether improvements in process have to be mirrored by quantifiable improvements in outcomes is a matter of debate [25].

In addition to changes in workforce utilization, the attitude of the public towards doctors is also becoming less deferential, more demanding, and less tolerant of adverse outcomes [26]. Recent events ('high profile failures') in the United Kingdom may have messages for other countries: the enquiries into pediatric cardiac surgery in Bristol [27, 28], post-mortem organ retention at Alder Hey [29], and the mass murderer who was also tragically a general practitioner, Harold Shipman, [30], have done much to undermine the concept of professional regulation and reduce the authority and self-confidence of the medical profession [31], factors which politicians have almost certainly found helpful in 'modernizing' the public health service towards a more commercial model involving the private sector [32]. The fact that a MORI poll has shown that the medical profession is trusted to tell the truth by 92% of the UK population while only 23% of politicians command a similar level of confidence [33] is not an excuse for complacency.

The Challenge: Different Ways of Working

Healthcare workers will need to respond to the problems outlined above by adopting new ways of working. Hospitalized patients, particularly those requiring emergency care, will be attended by transdisciplinary teams whose members will come from a diversity of backgrounds, who will adopt new evidence-based technologies and interventions rapidly, and use electronic systems for information management and decision support. The comparisons often drawn between aviation and healthcare safety, much to the detriment of the latter, should in the case of acute and emergency care perhaps be based on military, not civilian, aviation; and the error rate contrasted with that of 'friendly fire' incidents. Thus the mind set for the new acute hospital will not be the traditional, leisured, linear and hierarchical approach to diagnosis and treatment of disease; it will be open-architectured, flexible, and focused on physiological safety. We will need to improve our management of the unexpected, of planning for uncertainty, and our understanding of risk [34] and its communication to patients and relatives [35, 36]. The care of the acutely ill patient will need to become a coherent entity, rather than remaining 'boxed up' in vertically orientated silos categorized by diagnosis or medical speciality. These developments will need to be reflected by improvements in hospital design to facilitate communication and teamworking.

If this perspective is accurate, it will make major demands on the interpersonal and communication skills of individuals in the healthcare team, including their capacity for collaboration across geographical and professional boundaries [37, 38], and continuing professional development. We will need to find methods for operationalizing two key elements in professional practice: good management (process control), and leadership (direction and policy). Some medical disciplines have achieved effective process control for specific diseases – for example, acute chest pain, asthma, or diabetic ketoacidosis – by introducing protocol-driven care and adopting a systems approach to management from the point of first contact with the patient. Improvements have taken many years to achieve however, and have been made easier by the specialty-specific nature of the diseases. How can we find ways of improving the generic care of the acutely ill patient in the next five to ten years, and how can we ensure that improvements are sustained in an environment of rapid change? Part of the answer lies in training and education. We will now consider how this may be achieved.

Solutions: New (Path)Ways of Training

It would be naive to suggest that all that is required for effective health care delivery is better training and education. Moreover, there is little evidence for the superiority of one educational method over another [39], partly because of the scarcity of appropriate research methodologies, and because so many other confounding factors influence clinician behavior over the course of many years. Despite this, conventional syllabus-based curricula or problem-based learning are gradually being supplemented or replaced by outcomes-based methods for postgraduate and undergraduate education in the UK, Canada, the USA, Australia and New Zealand, and more recently Spain, with intensive care medicine leading the way at postgraduate level [40]. Given the concurrent emphasis on maintenance of professional standards and continuing medical education after specialist appointment, and the developments outlined above, educational systems will need to find ways to facilitate life-long learning of physicians and integrate this with that of non-physician clinicians.

Outcomes-based (competency-based) Training

Outcomes-based training, which we will refer to as competency-based training, has a number of practical and theoretical advantages. Rooted in vocational training and thus in the tradition of craft apprenticeship and practical experience in the workplace, it requires prior definition of the outcomes of training – not 'this is our knowledge base: you can adapt it to later requirements', but 'this is what you must be able to do in your chosen role'. In essence, it demands a 'product specification' as the first step. The product (person) specification can be stated as a collection of competencies (or 'can dos), each of which is described in terms of knowledge, skills and attitudes. Each competence must include a method of assessment to benchmark the level of proficiency expected. The knowledge component essentially defines the syllabus, and the attitudinal elements can be grouped to form behavioral competencies.

There are several advantages to defining training in terms of competencies. First, it makes it clear to the trainee, the trainer, and the customer – patient or employer – what the practitioner will be expected to be able to do. Second, it clarifies the relationship between skills and the knowledge required to support those skills. Third, it makes it easier to monitor progress, correct deficiencies in training, and identify areas that require attention. Fourth, it permits assessment of competence during clinical practice in the workplace, which is a more natural environment than a formal examination. Fifth, assuming a standardized process for assessment in the workplace, it promotes flexibility of the workforce by facilitating free movement of professionals across borders and sharing of skills across professional groups, the latter being an essential element for transdisciplinary team-based care. Sixth, by defining the competence of a specialist, it can also be used as the template for maintenance of professional standards or continuing professional development [41]. Finally and importantly, it is readily modifiable to permit incorporation of new knowledge, thus ensuring that practitioners are kept up to date with progress through research.

Competency-based training has potential weaknesses as well. By defining 'core' (and therefore the minimum) skill sets, it provides a target that most should attain, rather than an aspirational level of excellence. Some clinicians and educators fear that setting a minimum standard will 'level down' the quality of all practitioners. There is no agreed method for deciding which competencies to include, or for setting reproducible standards for assessment of competence. Finding (or funding) the time and support for trainers to make these assessments is a particular challenge. A wide range of educational resources needs to be provided in an accessible format linked to each competence, with further links to the knowledge base (syllabus).

Solutions to these problems are now being developed. Consensus techniques are being used to develop an international training program for intensive care medicine in Europe (CoBaTrICE) and other world regions [40], and it is possible that this methodology might be adopted by other disciplines as well. Input from a large number of 'stakeholders' (specialists, trainees, nurses and other health care professionals, patients and relatives) is being incorporated using a variety of survey techniques. Once the competencies and the workplace-based assessment methods have been agreed, the knowledge base is identified and linked to the other two elements by an electronic curriculum map [42] which also permits integration with the many other aspects of a comprehensive training program. Web-based systems will make this a very powerful and flexible tool for training and education, with considerable stakeholder involvement and 'buy-in'.

'Lateral' Integration with Training of Non-Physician Clinicians

Non-physician clinicians occupy a variety of roles, from medical assistant (for example in operating theaters) through practitioner grades (anesthetic nurses, physician extenders) to independent substitutes (nurse practitioners or nurse consultants) with prescribing and interventional roles. The training programs for many of these groups, (as for physician hospitalists in the USA at present), are varied and often locally-based [16, 43, 44]. Although this diversity may reflect differing needs between services and health systems, the lack of integration with other groups (particularly with the physicians they are intended to supplement or replace) may indicate a desire for professional autonomy and role protection. This is potentially unfortunate at a time of rapid change in health care delivery and in environments such as acute care which require team-working and flexibility in order to deliver care safely. What we need is not more professional barriers, but clear definitions of roles and skills focused on giving the patient the best care.

Before considering how this might be achieved, we should first ask the question – what is it that specifically distinguishes medical doctors from other health care providers? Disregarding specific task- and context-related activities, the main difference is that doctors are expected to diagnose diseases and plan an overall treatment strategy; this requires skills in data integration supported by a substantial body of knowledge. These skills and the associated knowledge base can of course be acquired by non-physicians undertaking clearly defined roles in elective and out-patient settings, or in treating well-characterized emergency conditions such as acute chest pain; in these settings the clinical problem is often characterized by protocols and bounded by standardized treatment pathways. However, the acutely ill patient presents a more complex set of problems in which the combination of clinical uncertainty, urgency and the need for therapeutic intervention before diagnosis makes considerable demands on the practitioner, including the capacity for team leadership when care is delivered outside routine 'office hours'. Do non-physician clinicians have a contribution to make to whole-hospital acute care?

In the USA, the national panel for acute care nurse practitioners has developed competencies that include skills in diagnosis and treatment [45]. The program does not have direct input from physician intensivists, but it is endorsed by the Society of Critical Care Medicine, and the competencies have a firm basis in critical care practice. Given robust training and assessment processes, the intensive care unit (ICU) is an ideal environment for developing practitioners with cross-specialty roles in whole-hospital acute care. In the UK this has already occurred with the development of 'outreach' care, in which critical care nurses provide staff support and patient care in ordinary acute wards, liaising with the ICU when necessary [17]. Discussions are now taking place in the UK about developing national competencies for non-physician clinicians in acute and emergency care, but so far these have not been integrated with medical training programs. It is essential that all such initiatives are coordinated if patient safety in acute care is to be optimized.

'Vertical' Integration: Life-Long Learning

Undergraduate to Specialist

There is no common curriculum for training in resuscitation and acute care at undergraduate level [46, 47]. In the UK the General Medical Council, which has responsibility for undergraduate training, requires [48] that medical students are taught to recognize and manage acute illness. The Acute Care Undergraduate Teaching initiative [49] has used consensus techniques to develop a curriculum in resuscitation and acute care for undergraduates, and this will integrate well with generic (Foundation Years) training in acute care for junior doctors in the UK. The model is transferable to other countries. These developments will provide a continuum with critical care training programs within the next ten years. The challenge lies in resourcing and valuing training and methods of assessment [50-52].

Maintenance of Competence: Continuing Professional Development

At the other end of the spectrum is the issue of how healthcare professionals will maintain, and demonstrate maintenance of, their competence to practice. At present there is considerable international variation, particularly in methods of assessment [53]. Formal recertification is required in Australia & New Zealand, Canada and the United States, the latter by examination in addition to other measures of continued competence in six domains (Table 1). In the UK, the General Medical Council's proposals for 5-year licensing periods have been suspended at the request of the Chief Medical Officer in order to take into account the recommendations of the Shipman enquiry [30]; at present the only benchmark is the disciplinary instrument involving seven domains of fitness to practice (Ta-

Table 1. American Board of Medical Specialities (ABMS) and Accreditation Council for Graduate Medical Education (ACGME).

Six domains of competence for all doctors in practice and in training:
1. Patient care
2. Medical Knowledge
3. Interpersonal and communication skills
4. Professionalism
5. Practice-based learning and improvement
6. Systems-based practice

ABMS Maintenance of Competence program

Requires specialists to demonstrate:
1. Evidence of professional standing
2. Evidence of commitment to lifelong learning and involvement in a periodic self-assessment process
3. Evidence of cognitive expertise
4. Evidence of evaluation of performance in practice

Table 2. General Medical Council (UK) Fitness To Practice (http://www.gmc-uk.org/revalidation/archive/l_and_r_formal_guidance_for_docs.pdf)

The information doctors collect in their folders should show that they have been practising in accordance with the standards of competence, care and conduct set out in *Good Medical Practice*. These are:

- *Good clinical care* – doctors must provide good clinical care, must practise within the limits of their competence, and must ensure that patients are not put at unnecessary risk.
- *Maintaining good medical practice* – doctors must keep up to date and maintain their skills. Doctors must also work with colleagues to monitor and maintain the quality of the care they provide and maintain a high awareness of patient safety.
- *Relationships with patients* – doctors must develop and maintain appropriate relationships with their patients.
- *Working with colleagues* – doctors must work effectively with their colleagues.
- *Teaching and training* – where doctors have teaching responsibilities they must develop the skills, attitudes and practices of a competent teacher.
- *Probity* – doctors must be honest.
- Health – doctors must not allow their own ill health to endanger patients.

ble 2), assessed using a variety of documentation including appraisals and portfolios. The voluntary Australian system of Maintenance of Professional Standards (MOPS) [54] is based on credits for a variety of professional development activities. It seems likely that with time the CoBaTrICE demonstration project for creating a common international competency-based training program for intensive care medicine could be followed by similar convergence for specialist revalidation, at least in terms of the domains which should be evaluated.

Methods of Assessment of Specialist Competence

How should we assess continuing competence of specialists? Should we test theoretical knowledge or the practitioner's practical ability to deliver care to patients? Could we ease the burden of data collection by linking process of care of specific patients (for example, adherence to treatment guidelines) documented in the patients' electronic records to observational databases benchmarking group outcomes? Should we focus on measures of process or outcome, and should these be individual or group assessments? ICU standardized mortality ratios, and cardiac surgeon-specific mortality rates, are examples of group and individual outcomes based assessments, respectively. However, few would argue that either approach adequately measures competence at the level of the individual. Formal knowledge tests, for example using multiple choice examinations, are easy to apply and have the attraction of numerical endpoints which may demonstrate a relationship with practitioner behavior or quality of practice [55], but it does not follow that such tests are appropriate tools for continuing assessment of specialists.

It is likely that the assessment of continuing competence of specialists will be based on a range of metrics combined with regular appraisal. This will require an assessment 'toolbox' containing different measures that can be applied over time by different assessors to common standards. Some of these tools will be predominantly formative (providing feedback and learning), while others will be summative (used for final assessment and documentation). They include direct observation of clinical practice during routine work, mini-clinical examination exercise (mini-CEX), directly observed procedural skills (DOPS), widely-based assessment of attitudes and behaviors (360° assessment), structured clinical encounters using actors or simulators, objective structured clinical examination (OSCE), and annual appraisal combined with personal portfolios containing evidence of educational activities. These forms of personal assessment will be combined with measures of group performance to provide a global assessment of institutional quality. If we are to retain continued public trust in the medical profession, we need to take the initiative in this important matter of effective and transparent professional self-regulation.

References

1. Trends in Hospital Emergency Department Utilization: United States, 1992-1999. Data from the National Health Care Survey. Vital and Health Statistics 13 (150). Centre for Disease Control, Maryland. DHHS publication number (PHS) 2001-1721. Available at: http://www.cdc.gov/nchs/data/series/sr_13/sr13_150.pdf Accessed July 2005
2. Alberti A. Transforming Emergency Care in England. Department of Health, London 2004. Available at: http://www.dh.gov.uk/PolicyAndGuidance/OrganisationPolicy/EmergencyCare/fs/en Accessed July 2005
3. United States Census Bureau, Population Division, International Programs Center. Available at: http://www.census.gov/ipc/www/idbpyr.html Accessed July 2005
4. OECD Health Data 2000: A Comparative Analysis of 29 OECD Countries. Available at: http://www.oecd.org Accessed July 2005

5. WHO Regional Office for Europe's Health Evidence Network (2003) What are the lessons learned by countries that have had dramatic reductions of their hospital bed capacity? Available at: http://www.euro.who.int/document/E82973.pdf Accessed May 2005
6. Ten High Impact Changes for service improvement and delivery: a guide for NHS leaders. NHS Modernisation Agency, Sept 2004. Available at: http://www.content.modern.nhs.uk/cmsWISE/HIC/HIC+Intro.htm Accessed May 2005
7. Bion JF, Heffner J (2004) Improving hospital safety for acutely ill patients. A Lancet quintet. i: current challenges in the care of the acutely ill patient. Lancet 363: 970-977
8. Baumann A, Blythe J, Kolotylo C, Underwood J (2004) Building the Future: An Integrated Strategy for Nursing Human Resources in Canada. The International Nursing Labour Market Report. Available at: http://www.buildingthefuture.ca/e/study/phasel/reports/11E_Intl_Nursing_Labour_Market.pdf Accessed July 2005
9. Buchan J (2002) Global nursing shortages. BMJ 324: 751-752
10. Cooper RA (2004) Weighing the evidence for expanding physician supply. Ann Intern Med 141:705-714
11. Guidance on Implementing the European Working Time Directive for Doctors in Training. Available at: http://www.doh.gov.uk/workingtime/ewtdguidance.htm Accessed July 2005
12. Philibert I, Friedmann P, Williams WT (2002) New requirements for resident duty hours. JAMA 288:1112-1114
13. Steinbrook R (2002) The debate over residents' work hours. N Engl J Med 347:1296-1302
14. Cook RI, Render M, Woods DD (2000) Gaps in the continuity of care and progress on patient safety. BMJ 320:791-794
15. Druss BG, Marcus SC, Olfson M, Tanielian T, Pincus HA (2003) Trends in care by nonphysician clinicians in the United States. N Engl J Med 348:130-137
16. Royal College of Anaesthetists (2004) The Role of Non-medical Staff in the Delivery of Anaesthesia Services. Available at: http://www.rcoa.ac.uk/docs/role_of_non-medical_staff.pdf Accessed July 2005
17. Bright D, Walker W, Bion JF (2004) Outreach - a strategy for improving the care of the acutely ill hospitalised patient. Crit Care 8:33–40
18. Hillman K, Cuthbertson BH (2003) Outreach critical care. Br J Anaesth 90:808-809
19. The National Outreach Report 2003. Available at: http://www.modern.nhs.uk/criticalcare/5021/7117/78001-DoH-CareOutreach.pdf Accessed July 2005
20. Buist MD, Moore GE, Bernard SA, Waxman BP, Anderson JN, Nguyen TU (2002) Effects of medical emergency team on reduction of incidence of and mortality from unexpected cardiac arrests in hospital: preliminary study. BMJ 324:387-390
21. Bellomo R, Goldsmith D, Uchino S, et al (2003) A prospective before-and-after trial of a medical emergency team. Med J Aust 179:283-287
22. 22 NHS Modernisation Agency (2004) Hospital at Night Project: Findings and Recommendations. Available at: http://www.modern.nhs.uk/workingtime/17048/WhatisHospitalatNight/1.1%20Findings%20and%20recommendations.pdf Accessed July 2005
23. Wachter RM, Goldman L (1996) The Emerging Role of "Hospitalists" in the American Health Care System. N Engl J Med 335:514-517
24. Cuthbertson BH (2003) Editorial II: Outreach critical care—cash for no questions? Br J Anaesth 90:5-6
25. Lilford R, Mohammed MA, Spiegelhalter D, Thomson R (2004) Use and misuse of process and outcome data in managing performance of acute medical care: avoiding institutional stigma. Lancet 363:1147-1154
26. Blendon RJ, DesRoches CM, Brodie M, et al (2002) Views of practicing physicians and the public on medical errors. N Engl J Med 347:1933-1940
27. Department of Health (2001) The Bristol Royal Infirmary Enquiry. Available at: http://www.bristol-Inquiry.org.uk/final_report/index.htm Accessed July 2005

28. The Department of Health's Response to the Report of the Public Inquiry into children's heart surgery at the Bristol Royal Infirmary 1984-1995. Available at: http://www.dh.gov.uk/assetRoot/04/05/94/79/04059479.pdf Accessed July 2005
29. The Royal Liverpool Childrens' Enquiry Report 2001. Available at: http://www.rlcinquiry.org.uk/download/index.htm Accessed July 2005
30. The Shipman Enquiry. Available at: http://www.the-shipman-inquiry.org.uk/reports.asp Accessed July 2005
31. Tallis R (2004) Hippocratic Oaths. Atlantic Books, London
32. Pollock AM (2004) NHS plc: The Privatisation of Our Health Care. Verso Books, London
33. Opinion of Professions MORI poll. Available at: http://www.mori.com/polls/trends/truth.shtml Accessed May 2005
34. Chalmers I (2004) Well informed uncertainties about the effects of treatments. BMJ 328:475-476
35. Djulbegovic B (2004) Lifting the fog of uncertainty from the practice of medicine. BMJ 329:1419-1420
36. Sedgwick P, Hall A (2003) Teaching medical students and doctors how to communicate risk BMJ 327:694-695
37. Richard I Cook RI, Render M, Woods DD (2000) Gaps in the continuity of care and progress on patient safety. BMJ 320:791-794
38. Sexton BJ, Thomas EJ, Helmreich RL (2000) Error, stress and teamwork in medicine and aviation: cross sectional surveys. BMJ 320:745-749
39. Chen FM, Bauchner H, Burstin H (2004) A call for outcomes research in medical education. Acad Med 79:955-960
40. Barrett H, Bion JF (2005) An international survey of training in adult intensive care medicine. Intensive Care Med 31:553-561
41. Whitcomb ME (2004) More on competency-based education. Acad Med 79:493-494
42. Harden RM (2001) AMEE Guide No 21: Curriculum Mapping: a tool for transparent and authentic teaching and learning. Med Teach 23:123-137
43. Wachter RM (2004) Hospitalists in the United States – mission accomplished or work in progress? N Engl J Med 350:1935-1936
44. Wachter RM, Goldman L (2002) The hospitalist movement 5 years later. JAMA 287:487-494
45. National Panel for Acute Care Nurse Practitioner Competencies (2004) Acute Care Nurse Practitioner Competencies. National Organization of Nurse Practitioner Faculties, Washington
46. Phillips PS, Nolan JP (2001) Training in basic and advanced life support in UK medical schools: questionnaire survey. BMJ 323:22-23
47. Shen J, Joynt GM, Critchley LAH, Tan IKS, Lee A (2003) Survey of current status of intensive care teaching in English-speaking medical schools. Crit Care Med 31:293–298
48. General Medical Council (2004) Tomorrow's doctors. Recommendations on undergraduate medical education. Available at: http://www.gmc-uk.org/med_ed/tomdoc.htm Accessed July 2005
49. Perkins G, Bion JF on behalf of the ACUTE collaboration (2005) The Acute Care Undergraduate Teaching (ACUTE) Initiative. Crit Care Med 32:A65 (abst)
50. Smith SR, Dollase RH, Boss JA (2003) Assessing students' performances in a competency-based curriculum. Acad Med 78: 97-107
51. Norcini JJ (2003) ABC of learning and teaching in medicine: Work based assessment. BMJ 326:753-755
52. Smee S (2003) ABC of learning and teaching in medicine: Skill based assessment. BMJ 326:703-706
53. Finucane PM, Bourgeois-Law GA, Ineson SL, Kaigas TM (2003) A Comparison of performance assessment programs for medical practitioners in Canada, Australia, New Zealand, and the United Kingdom. Acad Med 78:837-843

54. ANZCA The Maintenance of Standards Program. Available at: http://www.anzca.edu.au/ceqa/mops/ Accessed July 2005
55. Tamblyn R, Abrahamowicz M, Brailovsky C, et al (1998) Association between licensing examination scores and resource use and quality of care in primary care practice. JAMA 280:989-996

Simulation Training in Critical Care Medicine

P. B. Angood

A Safety Revolution is Underway...

For a variety of reasons there are now growing public concerns for safety in healthcare. For one example, it has been estimated that 100,000 lives are lost annually due to medical error in the United States and that 10-15% of medical errors are due to technical incompetence of providers [1]. Patient safety is now at the forefront of healthcare policy development and is rapidly gaining momentum from initiatives within many medical centers on a global basis. The World Health Organization (WHO) has recently initiated the World Alliance for Patient Safety and several individual countries are in the process of organizing or coordinating initiatives in this area as well. The traditional *culture of healthcare*, however, has historically emphasized the acquisition of individual skills by the providers and the demonstration of a commitment towards high quality care – so called professionalism. The presumption being that this professionalism will fundamentally provide safe patient care. The education and training of healthcare professionals has therefore been focused entirely on the acquisition of knowledge and the proficiencies with technical skills. The different disciplines in healthcare have also constructed their individual training environments with associated accreditation and licensure requirements. There has not been any significant effort towards training and education of providers in terms of teamwork function, the integration of systems coordination, or multidisciplinary organizational change. This educational 'silo' system not unexpectedly has created a similar system of 'silos' that are readily pervasive within most all healthcare institutions and continues to carry a dominance of behavior related to physician-based patient care. The *culture of patient safety* will necessarily provide focus on the need to break down historical education strategies and begin to provide solutions for how to implement improved care through a focus upon teamwork, systems management and precipitation of large-scale organizational change.

It is now well recognized that the future of healthcare will involve an increasing burden for the critical care areas of medical centers, that the acuity of patients in these areas will become higher, and that the ability to maintain skilled professionals for critical care areas will be in a crisis because of staffing shortages in several disciplines. Intensive care units (ICUs) are involved with the most critically ill patients and the stakes for outcomes are essentially life, death, and disability. ICUs manage several types of patient but those who carry the highest stakes are the true emergencies and those requiring active physiologic resuscitation. In general, emergencies and active resuscitations are typically characterized by: *uncertainty* due to the nature of the disease process and the patient's responses; *complexity* because of atypical patient responses or the presence of simultaneous problems; acute *time pressure,* and high levels of *provider stress* due to the need for rapid, accurate responses in providing care. ICUs are clearly an environment that require a smooth integration of team responses and ongoing systems improvement in order that positive organizational change can occur with patient safety.

Other high-risk industries have paid particular attention to the efficient management of emergency interventions but until recently healthcare has been relatively late to adopt the lessons learned from other industries. In healthcare there has historically been no conceptual basis concerning crisis management principles. Many medical emergency situations will occur unpredictably; trainees and junior personnel are often left to manage situations without supervision and only occasionally 'moved aside' during crises. Similarly, there is rarely any detailed recording of the actual events or activities that occur in these situations and there is usually no forum for a systematic debriefing about team or individual performances after the situation has been resolved. Gaba et al. [2], have suggested that the key principles for medical crisis management are to teach generic skills in managing critical events, to use full-scale realism to motivate and instill new behaviors, and for liberal use of debriefing with video-taped sessions. Key concepts that are then further developed need to be:

- Roles – clear delineation for the leaders and the followers of a crisis team
- Communication – learning the importance for "closing the communication loops"
- Support – learning that it is important and acceptable to practice calling for help
- Resources – understanding how to get what is needed in a crisis, and from whom
- Global Assessment - avoiding fixation on the same solution for all situations
- Debrief – implementing early debriefing as a tool for improvement and learning

Consider then that traditional forms of healthcare education do not provide an exceptional process for ensuring completely safe or efficient training prior to practitioners' active engagement with critically ill patients. Also consider that the current forms of monitoring competence for all levels and types of practitioners are markedly inconsistent or lacking. Coupled with the previously mentioned 'silo' environment within healthcare, this should give us all pause as we consider how to evaluate the best initiatives for safety, quality, and outcomes of individual ICU patient care in the future. We should begin to construct improved modalities of healthcare training in order to produce better structured and more closely monitored systems of education - systems that are themselves continuously improving. These new approaches need to not only focus on the junior providers but will also need to focus upon the maintenance of competence for experienced providers and to provide the training environments where team integration of performances is emphasized. This change is essential if success is to be achieved in producing the highest level of quality possible for all current and future healthcare practitioners. Ten years from now (2015) is not a long time and so there needs to be a proactive implementation process initiated today.

As one example for a framework of individual learning, Bloom's *Taxonomy of Learning* [3] provides a simple construct to utilize when considering changes for an individual's learning processes. The three primary areas of consideration for learning are the cognitive domain, the attitudinal approaches, and the variable psychomotor skills of the learner. In the cognitive domain, the learner should be provided an environment to progressively move along the spectrum of learning from the simple memorization of facts, to understanding the meaning of the facts and then being able to utilize the facts in some form of application. As the learner continues to mature, there is the ability to analyze the utilization of the factual materials while a gradual synthesis of the information and its uses will ultimately provide the ability for evaluating and comparing the success of utilizing the learned materials. There is now growing recognition that specific attention is also required for the attitudinal approaches of adult learners and that their acquisition of knowledge is considerably different than when acquiring knowledge as children. In general, adults prefer a more interactive and problem-based learning environment, which provides immediate feedback and suggestions for change or improvements. Individuals vary considerably in their attitudinal approaches and so providing options for learning in a training environment should ideally be considered. Similarly, the acquisition of technical skills is also considerably more complex than originally appreciated because of the need for paying attention to the variable psychomotor skills and aptitudes of individual learners. The innate abilities for developing and refining skills related to hand-eye coordination are highly variable among individuals and the ability to retain these skills, once learned, is variable during the course of any one person's life. Anticipating these differences and providing the environments for acquiring, maintaining and evaluating skills throughout the course of careers is therefore an important consideration. Taken together, an appreciation can be gained for the complexity of the components related to successful individual learning.

Crew Resource Management (CRM) [4] is another important framework to consider but it is different in that it provides insights to the complexity of improving team interactions and systems management. The overall goal in crew resource management is to optimize team performances in challenging conditions. The key elements are planning for the optimal utilization of all resources, anticipating the cognitive components required and promoting efficient team management:

- Utilization of all Resources
  - Leadership is required
  - Anticipation and planning for all scenarios
  - Closed-loop communication is essential
  - Monitoring and cross-checking of individual and team responsibilities
  - Prioritization of tasks or responsibilities for the team
- Cognitive Components
  - Understand the team's work environment

  - Anticipate and plan the knowledge required
  - Use all available information and cross-check the information
  - Prevent fixation errors and consider multiple solutions in advance
  - Realize that memory is unreliable and use cognitive aids
- Team Management Components
  - Delineate leadership and follower roles
  - Distribute the workloads with efficiency as the goal
  - Emphasize open communication
  - Anticipate how to deal with conflict management
  - Calling for help early

At the organizational level, lessons are also available to be learned for healthcare from so-called High Reliability Organizations (HROs) [5]. Some organizations perform intrinsically risky activities with low failure rates and industry has come to recognize that there are several key principles for having success in these environments. Healthcare, and particularly the critical care sector of healthcare, potentially has much to learn from these organizations. The high reliability organization principles are:

- There is a strong organizational commitment to safety from the top down
- There are optimized structures and procedures in place in advance
- There is intensive training during operations and with simulation
- There is the maintenance of an active 'culture of safety'
- *REAL* teamwork is recognized as an essential element of the organization
- There is continual learning from all accidents and incidents

Simulation for Healthcare...

Given the above developed context for suggesting the importance of precipitating a change in educational strategies in healthcare, and that consideration in healthcare education must be reviewed in terms of not only educating individuals but also crisis teams and even entire organizations, then the potential opportunity within critical care medicine is enormous. Remember that the stakes are the highest and the potential for creating remarkable outcomes are the largest in ICUs. Simulation is but one component, but an important component, for facilitating this required change in healthcare behaviors and systems improvements. If considered closely, clinical experience, as a portion of the overall processes of healthcare education, has always required supplementation in some fashion. Typical examples have been morbidity and mortality conferences, patient care conferences, clinical-pathology conferences, journal clubs, self-study, and in-training examinations. The application of simulation to healthcare represents a relatively new set of tools for designing and providing supplementation of education for all types of practitioners. It is a novel training environment but it is also an inherently useful modality for the subsequent evaluation and maintenance of competence for healthcare providers. Simulation technologies have now developed to the extent that it is practical to consider their use in healthcare on many levels. Medical and nursing students, residents, physician and nurse practitioners, plus the spectrum of ancillary healthcare providers now have the opportunity to think outside of the traditional concepts or approaches for both training and patient care. Simulation has particular relevance for critical care because the environment and resources in all ICUs are dynamic, the physiology of the patients is highly variable, and the types of practitioners present in the critical care units are often inconsistent. Thus, the environment is perpetually set for the 'perfect storm' and may, on occasion, actually result in unintended consequences of care. It is clearly incumbent on critical care professionals to ensure that their initial education, as well as the ongoing maintenance of competence, focuses only at the highest levels of expertise and skill. As mentioned, educational processes need to change rapidly and simulation technologies now represent one of the most important opportunities for critical care professionals to achieve this change.

Simulation is not simply a set of technologies that provides alternative forms of presenting information but represents a methodology for facilitating education or training with technology. The opportune times for using simulation methodologies are when the cost of experimentation is too high, when the consequences of experimentation are not acceptable and when the complexity of what is being studied or learned requires multiple trials and approaches. Ideally, simulation methodology should:

- never represent a direct risk to patients
- allow for the presentation of a wide variety of scenarios
- include training for common and uncommon events
- have known underlying causes for each situation
- have the same events presented to different/multiple clinicians or teams
- allow for errors in judgment or technical skill to play out realistically
- be required to interact with actual equipment and personnel
- facilitate the recording, tracking and monitoring of performances over time

An excellent resource for learning about the available simulation devices can be found at (www.hmc.psu.edu/simulation/index.html). The essential categorization utilized by the Penn State group is:

- Model-driven simulators
- Instructor-driven simulators
- Computer program simulations
- Task specific models
- Virtual reality/haptic feedback trainers

Model-driven Simulators

Model-driven simulators, also called high fidelity simulators, are those that use a manikin body, or part of a body, to physically represent a patient. These models have physiologic and pharmacologic information systems that direct real-time autonomous reactions of the trainees' interventions and therapies. These types of simulators can also integrate multiple systems in models to produce a complete realistic patient response. These systems can be used to teach normal and abnormal physiology and pharmacology, equipment usage, patient and provider safety, resource management, crisis management, and in many other healthcare areas - at many different educational levels. While this style of simulator is the top of the line, it is also relatively expensive to set up. The simulator is usually sold by itself, so monitors and ancillary equipment must often be purchased separately to create a realistic setting. However, the more time and money spent to outfit the simulation area, the more realistic the experience.

Instructor-driven Simulators

Instructor-driven simulators, also called intermediate fidelity simulators, use a partial or full body manikin as a physical presence on which to practice interventions. The simulators may interact with the user but the bulk of responses are created by the instructor. They use real interventional equipment (probes, i.v. lines, ventilators, etc), and may or may not use real monitoring equipment. The output signals to their displays are consistent with patient anatomy and the conditions being presented, or changed, by the instructor are designed to reflect real-time changes in patient conditions.

The simulators are often set up to teach more than one topic or area and an instructor/operator will adjust the relevant vital signs to accurately reflect patient responses. The user is presented with a much closer approximation to an actual patient and environment than with static partial task trainers. Because the instructor determines what response the patient should show, it may be easier in some cases to bring out a teaching point, especially if the point is regarding a patient whose parameters are out of the normal range. There is significantly more realism and versatility of training topics than with partial task trainers, but less than with model driven simulators. Commensurate with this, the start-up price is also somewhere between part task trainers and model driven systems. It is up to the trainer to determine how much realism is required for an application. It is also trainer-intensive, because the trainer must teach and, at the same time, create patient responses.

Computer-based Simulators

Computer-based simulators contain an interactive patient vital sign screen that responds to user interventions. Computer-based simulations generally are much less expensive than other types of simulators and are easily portable. However, physical skills and tasks cannot be taught on them. Educational content is mainly focused on learning facts, using the information learned to make treatment decisions, and evaluating the effectiveness of that treatment.

Task Specific Models

Task specific models are designed to teach a specific task, procedure, or anatomic region. They often resemble anatomic sections of the body, but this is not necessary. Some are automated, but there is no adjustment based on the user's actions. One benefit of task specific models is their relatively low startup and maintenance cost. The anatomic models are usually affordable enough to allow a center to have many duplicates of many models. This allows concurrent teaching of a large class, broken down into small groups, to increase the hands-on time for each trainee.

Virtual Reality Simulators

Virtual reality simulators use computer modeling and complex programs to cause the user to believe that they are interacting with a patient. The simulator has some type of physical representation with sensing instruments that inform the computer of the user's movements. The program then computes the changes that should take place within the model and projects the correct response onto the screen. Systems may include some sort of three-dimensional (3D) imaging to make the environment more realistic and intuitive. If the model has haptic (touch) feedback, it will also create the illusion that the user is coming into physical contact with the model, and the user will 'feel' the patient as well as see it. Since a virtual reality training system is necessarily run on a computer, there is always the opportunity to collect information on trainee performance. User data can be used to create critiques and to generate an individual's learning curve as well as to compare an individual to a cohort of peers. Virtual reality models have one distinct drawback, however. It is necessary to have a computer programmer create new modules or make significant adjustments to current modules. These simulators are always limited by the number of programs that have already been written and tested.
Other issues to consider are in the so-called 'Options List' for simulators:

- Physical body - Is the user interaction with a physical object (manikin body or part of a body) representing relevant patient anatomy?
- Automatic responses - Does the simulator autonomously respond (give immediate feedback) to basic interventions performed by the user with no instructor input?
- Performance feedback - Can the simulator itself evaluate performance and give feedback to the user after the session without an instructor present?
- Independent learning - Can a user work through a module without an instructor present?
- Start-up cost - What is the average relative start-up cost for a system?

Curriculum development is still in an infancy state for many aspects of medical education with simulation but curriculums need to integrate the use of simulation into the overall training curriculum when considering how to train providers initially, and also for maintenance of competence. It is not wise, nor does it promote success, when the simulators are simply left for open use and then used without specific methodology or education plans. There is a need for competency-based curricula with permissions required to use and perform on simulators – with and without instructors present. The use of metrics for evaluating the learners, as well as the simulation programs, should be tied closely with curriculum development but are also still in an early stage of development. Focused efforts to standardize multi-level metrics are still required in order for simulation to evolve on a successful platform in the long term. These are necessary priorities for the coming decade. Team training strategies are only just beginning to be explored.

Simulation program development for any medical center is a complicated process that requires the setting of explicit program objectives prior to initiating the program and ensuring that the resources will be available for the program's development on an institutional basis. As a result, there is currently not a predominance of schools that have adopted simulation into their education strategy as yet. Issues of developing a program as a stand-alone event or integrating it as a segment of an institution-wide initiative also need to be seriously considered. Success may involve the development of multiple models of education within an institution and the planned sharing of resources. People resources, financial resources, available physical space and mandated time for the trainees are all important issues to resolve prior to opening any new program. Anticipation of known institutional pitfalls and barriers should be included in any business model as well. Recognizing that the initial start-up of a facility is easier than maintaining the cost of operations on an annual basis is an important issue to address in advance. Knowing where the financial support will come from long-term is important to anticipate. Evaluating the success or failure of any simulation program is still highly reliant on the success of the 'bottom-line'.

Assessing the effectiveness of simulation training is complex because rigorous outcomes studies of educational interventions are not easily done and there is still a relative paucity of outcomes studies for simulation in healthcare. Rarely is there a randomized control trial of complex educational models and outcomes. The most important rationale for simulation-based training is improved safety in clinical care but the impact of safety interventions are also difficult to measure. Validation studies demonstrating reductions in clinical error rates would be ideal but consider that definitive proof of effectiveness may also not be required. No prior industry in which human lives depend on the skilled performance of responsible operators has waited for unequivocal proof of the benefits of simulation before embracing it – perhaps neither should critical care medicine.

As a closing perspective, it must be recognized that adoption rates for new technologies are highly variable in different industry sectors (Fig. 1). Healthcare is now recognized to be one of the slowest adoption industries and this needs to be considered when opening simulation programs or planning for longevity of programs. Learning how to manage the conservative expectations and hesitancy to become involved is important for healthcare initiatives that involve technology. Focus upon managing these expectations and then delivering results that are of pragmatic value in the daily routine of education and clinical care are therefore important goals.

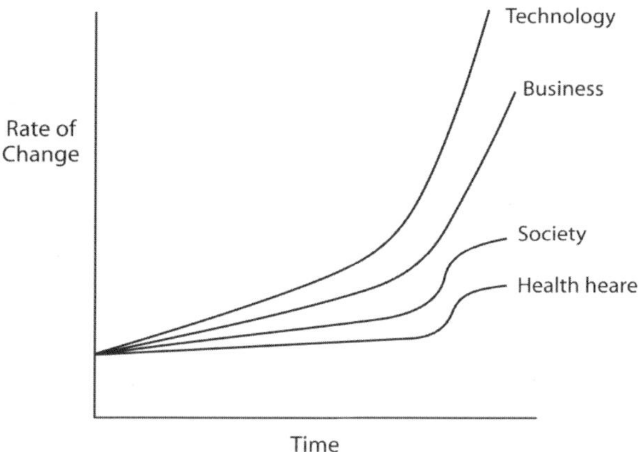

Fig 1. Differing responses to scientific discovery by sector

Conclusion

As a collective term, patient safety has a potentially negative connotation if it is interpreted in such a way that implies that if the patient is left unprotected, harm will occur during interactions with current healthcare systems. Healthcare is a complicated industry, while the processes of providing integrated patient care have become even more complex, and this creates an inherent risk that system failures will occur. The current attention to patient safety is a healthy development for the industry as it has provided the impetus for organizations and individual practitioners to review processes of care and systems management in such a way that patient safety becomes a priority. This can be viewed as a natural evolution of any industry where ongoing change and adaptation to change are necessary components for the ultimate improvement, refinement, and survival of the industry. The root causes of process failures in healthcare are notoriously difficult to identify and the ability to develop tangible solutions for the root causes is equally as difficult to initiate on a long-term basis. Communication failures or losses are the most important component when errors and complications occur in healthcare. Similarly, for improvements and refinements to take place, the element of maintaining an integrated process of communication is essential for high quality care to exist and flourish. Overall, individual institutions have not been efficient as yet in recognizing that employees and healthcare professionals are not trained to function as an integrated team with a culture that has patient care and institutional priorities as the overall goal. Therefore, it is not surprising the net result at times is poor communication and subsequent system failures.

One of the basic future tenets for healthcare system improvement will be the development of improved models of refined communication infrastructures so that all healthcare disciplines become aware of the importance for efficient team communication. With this knowledge, healthcare professionals will be able to contribute to a team-oriented infrastructure in such a way that the patient and institutional needs are placed ahead of individual practitioner preferences. In the interim, professionals from each discipline must make concerted efforts to develop communication practices that reflect efforts to place patient care as the priority and the recognition that interactions as a team will ultimately provide improved outcomes with a lower potential for complications and medical errors. Simulation utilization represents an ideal opportunity to forge these new arenas of improvement in healthcare.

References

1. Institute of Medicine Committee on Quality of Health Care in America (2000) To Err is Human: Building a Safer Health System. National Academies Press, Washington
2. Gaba D, Fish K, Howard SK (1994) Crisis Management in Anesthesia. Churchill Livingstone, New York
3. Merriam SB, Caffarella RS (1999) Learning in Adulthood: A Comprehensive Guide. 2nd ed. John Wiley & Sons, San Francisco
4. Salas E, BurkeC, Bowers C, Wilson K (2001) Team training in the skies: Does crew resource management (CRM) training work? Hum Factors 43:641-674
5. Roberts KH, Rousseau DM, La Porte TR (1991) The culture of high reliability organizations: quantitative and qualitative assessment aboard nuclear powered aircraft carriers. J High Technol Manage Res 5:141-161

Additional Reading

1. Dunn WF (2004) Simulators in Critical Care and Beyond. Society of Critical Care Medicine, Chicago

The Critical Care 'Agenda'

The Agenda for the Intensivist

V. M. Ranieri and G. L. Rosboch

Introduction

We are witnessing an impressive evolution of medicine due to the fast growth rate of bio-technological research; simultaneously, we are facing a substantial reduction in resources and the consequences of the ethical consideration that 'resources are not unlimited'. Cost cutting by governments has sparked an intense debate about its effect on the quality of medical care. Health care rationing is inextricably linked with cost containment. The governments no longer have the financial resources to pay for unlimited medical care for all who need it [1]. These clinical, scientific and sociological changes are exposing intensivists to the new challenges described in the previous chapters. This chapter will focus on what process should select and train the leaders who should guide the discipline through these changes.

The history of critical care medicine as a medical discipline is somewhat similar to army history; the evolution from a non-homogeneous group of clinicians taking care of the critically ill to an independent discipline with a characteristic clinical status and scientific foundation can be considered similar to the evolution from 'mass' (characterized by high numbers of military personnel with limited technology and no or limited training) to 'technology' army (composed of well equipped/trained/armed soldiers). The 'mass army' is the hallmark of ancient Greek and Roman history. Only later, in the first century before Christ, do we have clear testimony of a 'professional army'; Julius Cesar wrote that with only 80-100,000 soldiers he defeated the Vercingetorige's fortress in Alesia; against Cesar were about 3,000,000 barbarians. After that, in the De Bello Gallico, Cesar noted the lack of technology available to his enemies, amazed that that "they weren't able to write!" [2]. Consistently, centuries after, Romolo Augusto defended the 10,000 kilometer borders of the Roman Empire with only 600,000 Roman soldiers. In subsequent centuries, armies again became "mass armies"; during the French Revolution and until World War II large numbers of soldiers were employed in every battle with high human and economic costs. The Korean (1950-1953) and the Vietnam wars (1960-1975) were probably the last fights with 'mass armies'. Nowadays, 'winning' battles are fought using small 'professional armies' characterized by the use of high technological forces (navy and air force). However, no war can be won without having 'boots on the ground'; the use of large armies would be expensive economically but, most important, politically. The consequence of this scenario is the use of 'special forces', small but efficient groups that gain some degree of territorial control with minimal casualties associated with political action in trying to isolate the enemy political structure and enforce local and internal opposition to lead to a change towards a 'friendly' new government.

In this chapter the 'enemy' is the schizophrenic scenario of the request to deal with complex diseases, the reduction of technological and human resources, and the ethical implications of caring at the edge of human biology; the 'mass army' is the current body of the discipline with a non-homogeneous standard of clinical training and practice, a scatter growth of scientific knowledge (from genetics to classic physiology to clinical trials); the 'political framework' is the evolving scenario with new institutions (European Community) and a changing sociology (multi-ethnical, multi-cultural societies); and the 'special forces' are the new leading class we should select and train.

The "Enemy": The Utopia of Higher Results With Lower Resources

It is becoming harder and harder to make choices about health care. On the one hand we have more and newer drugs (often very expensive), higher expectations from the patients and their families, a growing number of people who need to be treated while they suffer from advanced illness (that we were not accustomed to treating in the past). On the other hand we have even lower resources in terms of personnel and funds; as we said before 'resources are not unlimited'.

Intensive care costs per day are often in excess of $1500, with the average admission costing over $10,000 [3]. Though costly, results are often heroic. Lives are saved and there can be little discussion about the value of intensive care unit (ICU) treatment. In Western societies, no one is likely to dispute that $10,000 for a life saved is not offering value for money. But what if a new therapy becomes available that increases the cost by a further $10,000 and for which the number needed to treat is around 100? In that case the costs of saving one additional life are $1,000,000 [4].

Burchardi and Schneider have recently shown that a new biotechnology product with very high costs, drotrecogin-alfa (activated protein C), if targeted to those patients most likely to achieve the greatest benefit, is cost effective by the standards of other well accepted life-saving interventions in sepsis [3]. There is an evident and growing interest in cost-effectiveness in medicine and in intensive care medicine. The cost-effectiveness plane is becoming a travel-mate for physicians (Fig. 1).

The 'Mass Army': The Current Status of Intensive Care Medicine

There are currently few data on the status of critical care medicine training and organization. The American College of Chest Physicians (ACCP) [5] and the European Society of Intensive Care Medicine (ESICM) [6] have recently published guidelines on the content of ICU training. But non-homogeneous formal action has been taken to introduce these standards into practice among the training

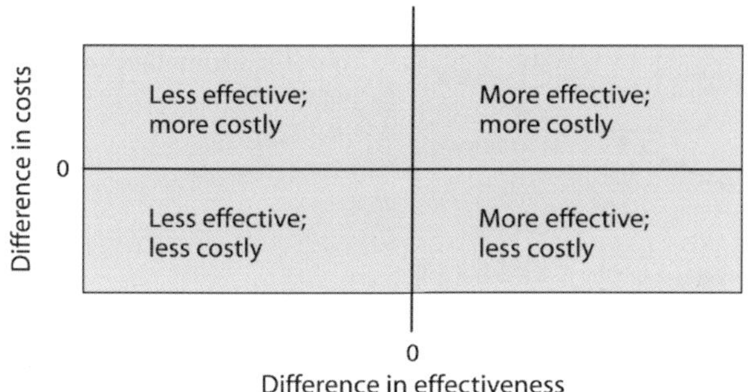

Fig. 1. Cost-effectiveness plan

programs in critical care medicine and the training process has a huge variability worldwide depending overall on the quality and availability of mentors and students.

However, we know that ICUs with dedicated intensivists show considerable cost control with a money saving process of up to 13 million US dollars/year (for a 6 to 18 bed ICU) [7], a lower length of ICU stay [8-9], and, overall, a lower hospital and ICU mortality rate [9]. It is estimated that if intensive care unit physician staffing were implemented in non-rural United States hospitals, 53,000 lives and $5.4 billion would be saved annually [10-11]. Despite the benefits of hiring physicians specialized in the treatment of critically ill patients, many hospitals worry about their ability to hire critical care physicians to staff their ICUs. There are currently too few board-certified intensivists to meet the ICU physician staffing standard at all hospitals [12]. Angus and coworkers [13] determined that only 10% of ICUs had high intensity ICU physician staffing defined as either a closed ICU or mandatory intensivist consultation. Intensivists provide care for at least one patient in 59% of the ICUs and are more likely to provide care in medical ICUs, in hospitals with over 300 beds, and in hospitals with a large percentage of managed care patients. While the supply of intensivists is predicted to remain stable up to year 2030, the COMPACCS study [13] estimates that demand will increase significantly driven largely by the demographics of aging 'baby boomers'. As a result, supply is expected to fall 22% short of demand by year 2020 and 46% by 2030 if nothing changes.

The Political Framework: The 'Bologna Process' and the 'European Higher Education Area'

There are some steps being made in the training of fresh ICU physicians in European countries and worldwide. The first step is the bachelor's degree achieved usually after a six-year course. The second step is the residency program which takes on average 4 to 6 years. The third, facultative, step is the PhD program; to achieve the PhD degree a graduate student usually needs 4 years. Finally there is the postdoc course; in the US an eight-year course is not unusual (the mean is

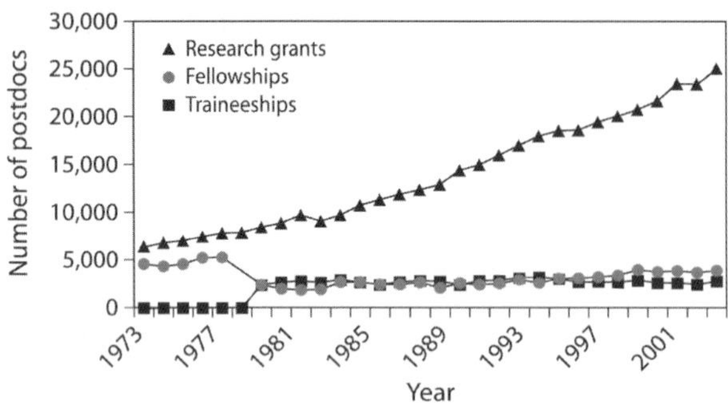

Fig. 2. PhD funding origin (modified from [20] with permission)

approximately 6-7 years) [14] whereas in Europe, the application of the 'Bologna process' is leading to a standardization of the post-bachelor's degree *iter.*

The Bologna Process may be regarded both as the product and continuation of a series of European conferences and a certain number of policy decisions aimed at establishing a European Higher Education Area by 2010 and, overall, a Europe of knowledge. The four main cycles mapping out the Bologna Process so far are those of Paris-La Sorbonne (1998), Bologna (1999), Prague (2001), Berlin (2003), and Bergen (2005). The premises of the Bologna Process are to be found in the Declaration of Paris-la-Sorbonne on 'Harmonisation of the Architecture of the European Higher Education System' signed in May 1998 by the education ministers of four States: France, Germany, Italy and the United Kingdom [15].

The three principles underlying Paris-La Sorbonne are:
1. Facilitating the mobility of students in the European area and their integration into the European labor market, as well as the mobility of teachers;
2. Improving the international transparency of courses and the recognition of qualifications by means of gradual convergence towards a common framework of qualifications and cycles of study;
3. Encouraging a return to studies or their continuation in the same or another institution, in a school or within arrangements for European mobility.

A year later, the Bologna Declaration on the European Higher Education Area, which was largely inspired by the Sorbonne Declaration, was signed. Besides aspects of its content, one of its novel features lay in broadening the debate, increasing to include 29 State signatories (the 15 EU Member States, 3 EFTA countries – Iceland, Norway and Switzerland – and 11 candidate countries) and includes institutions such as the European Commission, the Council of Europe, and associations of universities, rectors or European students.

The six principles of the Bologna Declaration [16] are:
1. Facilitating the readability and comparability of qualifications;
2. Implementing a system based essentially on two main cycles (undergraduate and graduate cycles);
3. Establishing a system of credits;

4. Developing arrangements to support the mobility of students, teachers and researchers;
5. Promoting European cooperation in quality assurance;
6. Promoting the European dimension in higher education (in terms of curricular development and inter-institutional cooperation).

In May 2001, a conference was held in Prague, which included the same categories of participants, now with 33 State signatories (the newcomers were Liechtenstein, Cyprus, Croatia and Turkey). The purpose of this conference was to assess the progress already accomplished (particularly on the basis of national reports) and identify the main principles that should drive the Bologna Process in the years ahead. While the Prague conference confirmed the need to pursue the aims set out in the Bologna Declaration, it nevertheless attached importance to three points in particular [17]:

1. Lifelong learning;
2. The involvement of higher education institutions and students as active partners;
3. The need to enhance the attractiveness of the European Higher Education Area.

When European ministers met again in Berlin (2003) they defined four intermediate priorities for the next two years [18]:

1. Quality assurance including definitions of the responsibilities of the bodies and the institutions involved, evaluation of program or institutions and a system of accreditation and certification;
2. Three cycle system (undergraduate, graduate and doctoral cycle);
3. Recognition of degrees and periods of studies;
4. Synergy between European Higher Education Area and European Research Area.

The last priority of the Berlin congress was a milestone in the Bologna process; European ministers emphasized the importance of research and research training and the promotion of interdisciplinarity in maintaining and improving the quality of higher education and in enhancing the competitiveness of European higher education more generally. Research and education became 'two pillars of the knowledge based society'.

The 'Special Forces': The Leading Class for the New Millennium of Intensive Care Medicine

Several factors are needed to ride and to embrace the new wave of modernization and to create a novel ICU physician: money, mobility, flexibility, time, mentorship and partnership between science and clinic. First, funding for education. In the US, where research funding are proportionally higher than in Europe, money is concentrated in relatively fewer institutions. In addition, US science and education are based on a diversity of independent public and private funding sources grater than in Europe that allows a great ease of hiring foreign researchers and PhD students [19]. Moreover, 80% of postdoctorate positions are paid from a principal investigator grant [20]. Second, mobility is a key feature of the new educational profile; as outlined by the Bologna process, which suggest a 6-month outdoor period; external experiences should be strongly encouraged. Moreover, flexibility is another hallmark of the learning process; money, mobility and flexibility prevent the ossification of research institutions and fuel productivity and innovation [19].

Tobin recently defined the ideal mentor profile as someone who should be at the same time a teacher, an advisor, an agent, a role model, a coach, and a confidante customizing each role to match the characteristics of the fellow [21]. The importance of mentoring has been acknowledged for decades. Many successful senior investigators identify early positive role models and mentors as critical to their success [22-26]. More recently, in a survey of over 1100 junior faculty from 24 nationally representative US medical schools, faculty with mentors reported more professional support from their institutions for teaching, research, and administrative activities [27]. Faculty who were mentored also had a higher perception of their research skills and an increased likelihood of being awarded research grants. Mentoring is often divided into two categories: *research* and *career* [26]. It is important to distinguish between research and career mentoring because they differ in:
1. goals;
2. skills;
3. the fundamental relationship between mentor and mentee.

The goal of the *research mentor* is to develop the research career of the mentee. This involves the acquisition of research skills, selecting and conducting research projects, presenting research findings at national meetings, ensuring the completion and submission of manuscripts, assisting in networking and finally, teaching the mentee how to obtain extramural funding. This contrasts with the *career mentor* who focuses on more global aspects of an academic career, including balancing family demands and work, career promotion, juggling the different aspects of academic life (teaching, administration, clinical care, and research) and major career decisions, such as changing institutions or research direction. Different skills are needed for each type of mentor. Commonly, career mentors have accumulated years of experience and wisdom in academia. This may not be true for research mentors, who may be well versed in epidemiology, biostatistics and other research methods, but lack comparable years of experience in academic medicine. Although, many mentors are often involved in both aspects of providing support and guidance, fellows and junior faculty should understand the difference between these two types of mentors. The research mentor-mentee relationship can also be divided into two categories - informal and formal. Informal mentors are important, but for various reasons, the relationship lacks the intensity and commitment that is necessary to ensure that the mentee has a successful research career.

Finally, as outlined by the Bologna process where research and education are considered as 'two pillars of the knowledge based society', partnership between science and clinic should represent the milestone of young physicians' training. As Leonardo da Vinci noted a long time ago: "quelli che si innamoran di pratica senza scienza son come il nocchier ch'entra in naviglio senza timone o bussola, che mai ha certezza dove si vada".

In the US over the past decade, there has been increasing recognition of the importance of clinical research as evidenced by the birth of a new federal agency (The Agency for Healthcare Research and Quality (AHRQ) (http://www.ahcpr.gov/), which provides an array of intramural and extramural predoctoral and postdoctoral educational and career development grants and opportunities in health services research and supports the development of health services research infrastructure in emerging centers of excellence and works with Federal and academic partners to develop innovative curricula and educational models) and commitment of funds from the National Institutes of Health (NIH) (http://www.nih.gov/grants/) and private foundations (such as The Robert Wood Johnson Foundation, Princeton, New Jersey).

Clinical research is the linchpin of the nation's biomedical research enterprise. Before a therapy is approved for general use, it must be studied carefully in the laboratory to understand how the treatment works, how effective it is, and what potential risks may exist. The safety and benefits of the therapy for humans must then be proven through an orderly series of tests in people. Over the years, medical research has succeeded in converting many diseases once considered uniformly lethal into more chronic, treatable conditions. As noted by the NIH committee, clinical research has become increasingly difficult to do and it has become clear to the scientific community that the US must recast its entire system of clinical research if such efforts are to remain as successful as they have been in the past.

To accelerate and strengthen the clinical research process, a set of NIH Roadmap (http://nihroadmap.nih.gov/) initiatives will work toward improving the clinical research enterprise by adopting a systematic infrastructure that will better serve the evolving field of scientific discovery. This effort, which complements the other initiatives that comprise the NIH Roadmap, will provide the necessary foundation for advancing basic and clinical research. With the NIH Roadmap in action, investigators will be better poised to translate basic discoveries into the reality of better health. The two main pillars of NIH roadmap are: clinical research workforce training and translational research.

Clinical research workforce training:

According to the NIH roadmap, the ability of the US to fully explore the ever-expanding opportunities for medical advances are limited only by resources, the most important of which is the scientific workforce. To fulfill the promise of 21st century medicine and to make further progress in controlling major human diseases, we must cultivate and train a cadre of clinical researchers with skills that match the increasing complexity and needs of the research enterprise. The clinical research workforce must be large enough to facilitate bench-to-bedside research, the phased testing of approaches from small to large studies, and the translation of proven concepts into medical practice at the community level. Clinicians must be trained to work in the interdisciplinary, team-oriented environments that characterize today's emerging research efforts. Clinical researchers need to be trained in an array of disciplines important to the conduct of clinical studies, including epidemiology, behavioral medicine, and patient-oriented research. This NIH Roadmap effort envisions several major programs to expand, enhance and empower the clinical research workforce: the establishment of an agency-wide Multidisciplinary Clinical Research Career Development Program, a cadre of National Clinical Research Associates, and a clinical research training program for medical students.

- Multidisciplinary Research Career Development Program. The purpose of this program is to support the early career development of clinical researchers from a variety of disciplines, including patient oriented research, translational research, small and large scale clinical investigation and trials, and epidemiologic and natural history studies. The program will fund doctoral level professionals to learn how best to design and oversee research in multidisciplinary, collaborative team settings. As such, these researchers will have a high potential for becoming leaders of various fields of clinical research critical to the NIH mission. Each of the research career development grants will include a broad representation of clinical disciplines and professions (e.g., internal medicine, surgery, pediatrics, obstetrics/gynecology, dentistry, pharmacy, statistics, nursing, psychology) and the various specialties and sub specialties within each of these areas. The programs will include a structured, core didactic component and a practical, training component suited to various aspects of the design, conduct, and analysis of clinical research.
- National Clinical Research Associates. The clinical research workforce also must be broad enough to support the testing of ideas in large-scale studies and the translation of proven concepts into medical practice, both at the community level. The National Clinical Research Associates (NCRA) Program will help increase the number of clinical investigators and diversify the settings in which clinical research is conducted. Community practitioners (physicians, dentists, and nurse practitioners) will be recruited to refer and follow their patients in clinical research.
- Clinical Research Training in Medical Schools. To encourage and support clinical research workforce development among physicians, dentists, and nurses, a national meeting was held on May 11–12, 2004 to consult with the extramural community on ways to expand the pipeline of students entering clinical research, train future leaders and other team members, and create a viable career pathway for clinical researchers. Meeting participants discussed specific uses, strengths, and weaknesses of existing clinical research training programs and general medical scientist training programs. NIH staff are now examining how to balance the various options for enhancing the teaching of clinical research. These include short courses, one-year pull-out programs, master's level programs, and modifications of the existing Medical Scientist Training Program.

Translational research:

To improve human health, scientific discoveries must be translated into practical applications. Such discoveries typically begin at 'the bench' with basic research - in which scientists study disease at a molecular or cellular level - then progress to the clinical level, or the patient's 'bedside'. Scientists are increasingly aware that this bench-to-bedside approach to translational research is really a two-way street. Basic scientists provide clinicians with new tools for use in patients and for assessment of their impact, and clinical researchers make novel observations about the nature and progression of disease that often stimulate basic investigations. Translational research has proven to be a powerful process that drives the clinical research engine. However, a stronger research infrastructure could strengthen and accelerate this critical part of the clinical research enterprise. The NIH Roadmap attempts to catalyze translational research in various ways, including the following two projects:

- Regional Translational Research Centers. Key to building a strong infrastructure is increasing interactions between basic and clinical scientists and easing the movement of powerful new tools from the laboratory to the clinic. One strategy to achieve this involves NIH facilitating the development of Regional Translational Research Centers, or RTRCs. These centers will provide sophisticated advice and resources to help scientists master the many steps involved in bringing a new product from the bench to medical practice. Such steps involve laboratory studies to understand how a therapy works and animal studies to determine how well a therapeutic agent is absorbed into the body, how it is distributed to target tissues, how effective it is, and how likely it may be to cause unanticipated side effects.
- Translational Research Core Services - The NIH-RAID Pilot Program. Promising ideas for novel therapeutic interventions may encounter roadblocks in bench-to-bedside testing. While translation is sometimes facilitated by public-private partnerships, high-risk ideas or therapies for uncommon disorders frequently do not attract private sector investment. Where private sector capacity is limited or not available, public resources can bridge the gap between discovery and clinical testing so that more efficient translation of promising discoveries may take place. To help address this need, the NIH is establishing a pilot program to make available, on a competitive basis, certain critical resources needed for the development of new small molecule therapeutic agents. The NIH Rapid Access to Interventional Development (RAID) Pilot Program is intended to reduce some of the common barriers between laboratory discoveries and clinical trials for new therapies. Projects in both the early and late stages of pre-clinical development are suitable for NIH-RAID applications.

Conclusion

The successful leader has to plan the evolution of his/her leadership to the new challenges and set up a training/selection process that will guarantee its evolution. Critical care medicine has finally and through an essentially non-planned process reached the status of an independent discipline. Markers of this maturity are the impact of critical care medicine in health management, the numbers of papers on critical care related issues published in general medical journals, and the growing interest for basic research to investigate the pathological processes 'cured' in ICUs. Within the sociological and cultural evolution of modern societies, critical care medicine must plan the training/selection process of the new leading class. Critical care societies and intensivists of the highest academic rank must define and formalize the optimal curricula of the future leaders of the discipline.

References

1. Rosner F (1994) The rationing of medical care in United States. Chest 105:984-985
2. Caio Giulio Cesare: De Bello Gallico, Liber VII
3. Burchardi H, Schneider H (2004) Economic aspects of severe sepsis: a review of intensive care unit costs, cost of illness and cost effectiveness of therapy. Pharmacoeconomics 22:793-813
4. Van Hout BA (2003) Whom and how to treat: Weighing the costs and the effects. Scand J Gastroenterol 38:3-10
5. Dorman T, Angood PB, Angus DC, et al (2004) Guidelines for critical care medicine training and continuing medical education. Crit Care Med 32: 263-272
6. European Society of Intensive Care Medicine (1996) Guidelines for a training programme in intensive care medicine. Intensive Care Med 22:166-172
7. Pronovost PJ, Needham DM, Waters H, et al (2004) Intensive care unit physician staffing: financial modelling of the Leapfrog standard. Crit Care Med 32:1247-1253
8. Higgins TL, McGee WT, Steingrub JS, Rapoport J, Lemeshow S, Teres D (2005) Early indicators of prolonged intensive care unit stay: impact of illness severity, physician staffing, and pre-intensive care unit length of stay. Crit Care Med 31:45-51
9. Pronovost PJ, Angus DC, Dorman T, Robinson KA, Dremsizov TT, Young TL (2002) Physician staffing patterns and clinical outcomes in critically ill patients: a systematic review. JAMA 288:2151-2162
10. Birkmeyer JD, Birkmeyer CM, Wennberg DE, Young M (2000) Leapfrog patient safety standards. The potential benefits of universal adoption. The Leapfrog Group, Washington
11. Pronovost PJ, Waters H, Dorman T (2001) Economic implications of the Leapfrog standard for ICU physician staffing. In. Birkmeyer JD, Birkmeyer CM, Skinner J (eds) Economic Implications of the Leapfrog Safety Standards. The Leapfrog Group. Washington
12. Pronovost PJ, Waters H, Dorman T (2001) Impact of critical care physician workforce for intensive care unit physician staffing. Curr Opin Crit Care 7:456-459
13. Angus DC, Kelly MA, Schmitz RJ, White A, Popovich J, for the Committee on Manpower for Pulmonary and Critical Care Societies (COMPACCS) (2000) Current and projected workforce requirements for care of the critically ill and patients with pulmonary disease: can we meet the requirements of an aging population? JAMA 284:2762–2770
14. Russo E (2004) Fast Track PhDs. Nature 431:382-383
15. Sorbonne Joint Declaration; joint declaration on harmonisation of the architecture of European higher education system. Paris, May 25 1998. Available at: http://www.bologna-berlin2003.de/pdf/Sorbonne_declaration.pdf Accessed May 2005
16. European ministers of education: Bologna declaration. Bologna, June 19 1999 Available at: http://www.bologna-berlin2003.de/pdf/bologna_declaration.pdf Accessed July 2005

17. European ministers of education: Towards the European higher education area. Prague May 19 2001. Available at: http://www.bologna-berlin2003.de/pdf/Prague_communiquTheta.pdf Accessed July 2005
18. European ministers of education: Realising the European higher education area. Berlin September 19 2003. Available at: http://www.bologna-berlin2003.de/pdf/Communique1.pdf Accessed July 2005
19. Andras P, Charlton BG (2004) European science must embrace modernization. Nature 429: 699
20. Singer M (2004) The evolution of postdocs. Science 306:232
21. Tobin M (2004) Mentoring. Seven roles and some specifics. Am J Crit Care Med 170:114-117
22. Barondess JA (1997) Mentoring in biomedicine. J Lab Clin Med 129:487–491
23. Bland CJ, Schmitz CC (1986) Characteristics of the successful researcher and implications for faculty development. J Med Educ 61:22–31
24. Rogers JC, Holloway RL, Miller SM (1990) Academic mentoring and family medicine's research productivity. Fam Med 22:186–190
25. Barondess JA (1997) On mentoring. J R Soc Med 90: 347–349
26. Applegate WB (1990) Career development in academic medicine. Am J Med 88:263–267
27. Palepu A, Friedman RH, Barnett RC, et al (1998) Junior faculty members mentoring relationships and their professional development in U.S. medical schools. Acad Med 73: 318–323

Transforming Adult Critical Care Service Delivery in Ontario

H. MacLeod

Introduction

This chapter is about how we are going to achieve our dreams of the 'ICU of the future'. By writing in the first person, I hope that it will spark some 'first person' reflections in you. As a jumping off point, I want to pose a somewhat rhetorical question: in order to realize the 'ICU of the future', what will be more difficult: the challenge of scientific discovery or the challenge of changing human behavior? That may seem like an odd question. Obviously, scientific progress is essential but so is change. I believe that health professionals and health system managers need to take change as seriously as we do scientific discovery. To achieve the promise of the 'ICU of the future', change will be required at several levels. I will touch on changes in our personal behavior, changes in our institutional cultures, and changes at the level of our health care systems. In particular, I want to talk about leadership in creating the conditions for positive change in health care settings. Throughout, I will refer to the work we are leading in Ontario as we try to put in place the foundations of our ICU of the future.

In Ontario, we recently had an experience that exposed the extent to which we do not really have a health care *system*. Our battle with severe acute respiratory syndrome (SARS) tore up some of our illusions in this regard. Nowhere was this more evident than in our critical care services. SARS also revealed our strengths, primarily in terms of the dedication, resourcefulness and bravery of our people. Perhaps most importantly, it brought us together and got us talking in a new way. Our crisis has become an opportunity for transformation. In terms of the provision of adult critical care services, we are experimenting with innovative service delivery options and have developed a blueprint for system-level transformations. At the core of this initiative, we are explicitly recognizing the need to cultivate the leadership potential in our clinicians and administrators.

Health Care in Ontario

A Sketch of the Health Care Delivery System in Ontario

Before describing Ontario's critical care transformation initiative, I want to provide you with some sense of the context that we are working in and sketch out some of our key challenges. In particular, I want to focus on one aspect of our health human resources challenge, which underscores the many linkages between leadership and critical care.

Canada's health care system is governed by the five principles of the Canada Health Act (CHA). This Act is enforced by the federal government and is designed to ensure that we have a universal, comprehensive, accessible, portable, and publicly-administered system. The federal government provides some funds, but it is the individual provinces that are responsible for the administration and delivery of health care services. Each provincial government sets policy, establishes legislative and regulatory frameworks for health professions and other services (e.g., public hospitals) and transfers funding to the organizations that actually deliver most services. Ninety seven percent of health care programs in Ontario are provided by transfer payment organizations, not by the government. The provision of services is by both 'for-profit' organizations (e.g., independent health facilities, pharmacies) and 'not-for-profit' entities (e.g., hospitals). Private sector financing (approximately 32%) includes third-party insurers (e.g., insurance companies), out-of-pocket expenses, concentrated on drugs, vision care, dental services and homecare.

The Ontario health care system is complex. It serves the needs of approximately 12 million people and can be understood as the largest and most comprehensive Health Management Organization (HMO) in North America. Our system is analogous to an HMO in that it has a similar financial structure in which a single funding body manages the provision of a range of health care services for plan subscribers. In our case, the funding body is the provincial government and the plan subscribers are the taxpayers of Ontario. However, unlike many HMOs, our plan covers everyone, ensuring all members of our communities have equal access to health care services.

Ontario has over 230,000 regulated health care providers including 23,000 physicians and over 135,000 nurses. There are currently 152 hospital corporations across the province operating 228 sites. We fund approximately 32,714 beds in all hospitals of which 20,522 are considered 'acute care beds' and of which about 1100 are intensive care beds capable of supporting mechanical ventilation. Government transfers to hospitals are the largest single transfer payment in Ontario, amounting to approximately \$11.3 billion in 2004/05. These funds, representing 85% of the total hospital sector spending, cover all core health services. Hospitals also generate revenue from other sources, including private and semi-private accommodation, chronic care co-payment, workers' compensation and fundraising. This additional funding is used for ancillary costs such as research projects.

System-Level Challenges – Health Human Resources

The Ontario health care system faces a variety of key systems-level challenges leading to widespread concerns that our publicly funded system is not sustainable. Funding increases of between 8 to 9.5% per year have been required to maintain services. Cost drivers include population growth and aging, emergence of new diseases, increasing pharmaceutical costs, accelerated use of new and existing technologies and the need for infrastructure investments. Additional challenges include a shortage of health care workers, an aging workforce, silo-based delivery and funding, ethnic diversity and changing public expectations. I cannot explore all these issues in this chapter, but I draw attention to one issue that is of vital importance to critical care and emphasizes the many interesting linkages between leadership and our critical care transformation agenda.

We must remind ourselves that 65 to 70% of the asset value of our healthcare delivery system is human capital. Only 30 to 35% of the value we offer are our capital assets of building and equipment plus supplies and drugs. As leaders, we need to be responsible for creating healthy workplace environments for our human capital assets, the people who self-selected to work in healthcare. Healthier work environments increase the resiliency, adaptability, creativity, satisfaction, morale and productivity of individual workers. At the organizational level, this translates into improved performance, decreased costs and increased quality. In other words, employee and workplace health is inextricably linked to productivity, high performance and success. All of this is especially relevant for adult critical care services where there are high staff/patient ratios, inherently stressful working conditions and potential exposure to infections. As we look forward to meeting increased demands for critical care services in the future, we will need to demonstrate improved employee and workplace health in order to recruit and retain the required personnel.

SARS – Ontario's "Burning Platform"

The Concept of the Burning Platform

The concept of the "burning platform" as an impetus for change was introduced by Darryl Conner [1] and is based on an incident involving an oilfield driller who jumped 50 meters into the freezing North Sea from a burning oil drilling platform. When asked how he found the courage to leap, the worker replied: "I could go into the water and have a minimal chance of survival, or I could stay on the platform and face certain death as my coworkers did. It took no courage at all."

The image has captured people's imaginations for what it highlights about human nature, change and crisis. Change is inherently difficult. To achieve major innovation, we need something akin to a 'visible crisis'. This focuses our resolve and enables us to 'take the leap' that we now see as vital. For Ontario's health care system, SARS was our burning platform.

SARS and Critical Care

SARS was my introduction to public service in the Ontario healthcare system. I was given a front row seat at an incredible learning experience that was filled with genuine heroism, courage and love at the front line and genuine stewardship within the governance, managerial and public service leadership at the top of our system hierarchy.

In many ways, SARS unmasked some painful truths about our existing system. Throughout the crisis, we had to face head-on the unintended outcomes that flow from how we have historically designed the health care delivery system as a series of unconnected and relatively autonomous silos. Prior to SARS we had been discussing this and using language like ‘service fragmentation’, ‘lack of coordination’, and ‘silo orientation’ for years. SARS made us face the consequences of these system design choices.

Hospitals, community care access centers, community service providers and public health units all discovered that their individual silos could be dramatically impacted by other silos. In our vulnerability, we could see how interconnected we are, how like an organic system we are. Our ‘relative autonomy’ had given us the illusion of being independent but we are very connected, even if these connections are poorly designed.

While the current component parts of the system were never intentionally designed to create synergy, coordination and cooperation, individual leaders across the system pulled together, despite the disincentives and the barriers to fight and ultimately, it was as a system, that we defeated SARS. I think we succeeded because on a very human level, we were able to combine our collective intelligence to solve real problems. Many people and several organizations achieved remarkable results through actions that were executed within accelerated timeframes.

While it was a major crisis, SARS involved a relatively small number of actual patients. The outbreak – really one outbreak with two peaks – occurred from March 5 to June 12, 2003. We had about 400 probable and suspect cases and in total 44 people died. Hospital based transmission of SARS led to a majority of our cases, including patients, visitors and healthcare workers. Issues such as loss of healthcare workers to quarantine or illness resulted in enormous challenges delivering care to patients with and without SARS. Our health system was pushed to the limit. We were faced with closures of hospitals and critical care units, and cancellation of elective surgeries.

A useful article co-written by C. Booth and Dr. T. Stewart highlights the issues that SARS revealed about our critical care service delivery [2]. They suggest that the lack of a coordinated leadership and communication infrastructure was the most important limitation to Ontario’s response to SARS from a critical care perspective. For example, they noted how the critical care community had not carefully thought through nor communicated our approach to a crisis that impacted critical care beds. Hospitals, clinicians, public health, researchers and government officials were left unsure of what each other was doing.

The silo-oriented management of the critical care system meant that we did not have a clear picture of the availability of critical care beds across the province. I was the Assistant Deputy Minister of the Acute Services Division and I could not get a timely accurate number and location of critical care beds across the province. As the number of unavailable intensive care beds grew – a total of 73 intensive care unit (ICU) beds were closed at different points during the SARS outbreak [2], this gap in our critical care information system limited our ability to relocate patients with low-acuity complaints.

In the midst of all this, I discovered many people who were going through this experience with a 'third' eye – an eye focused on the underlying systemic issues that were being exposed on a daily basis as we moved through this crisis. Healthcare leaders I spoke with throughout the SARS crisis were asking some very probing questions about system design: about roles and responsibility; about accountability and empowerment and about the need for fundamental strategic changes that would enable us to move forward. SARS became the burning platform for our health system change, in particular for critical care.

Post-SARS Assessments and Critical Care

Democratic traditions are strong in Canada and in Ontario and following SARS, we engaged in some very honest and open discussions at a very public level. In particular, two processes helped us articulate and formulate what we had learned:

a) The federal process led by the National Advisory Committee on SARS (the Naylor Committee) which generated the October 2003 report entitled *Learning from SARS* [3]
b) The provincial process led by the Expert Panel on SARS and Infectious Diseases (the Walker Panel) which generated the December 2003 report entitled *For the Public's Health* [4]

The public nature of these reports helped to give those whose 'third eye' had opened a chance to make their insights public. Many useful insights into how we might improve our system were recorded in these documents. Ontario's lack of planned surge capacity in critical care was repeatedly mentioned. The key ideas from these reports were picked up in subsequent discussions and have been woven into the blueprint for transforming critical care that I will describe below.

In addition to these public discussions, I have engaged in hundreds of dialogs with hospital board members, front line staff and senior managers. The consensus view of the leadership of Ontario's healthcare system was clear – after SARS, the system will never be the same again. The leaders were ready to jump. With respect to critical care, I gathered a group of leaders to discuss how to move forward. There was a remarkable readiness amongst the critical care leadership. There was consensus diagnosis regarding:

- Our lack of surge capacity – 90% to 95% critical care bed occupancy combined with no 'surge' plans left us vulnerable. We had no way to leverage the aggregate of our resources.
- Our lack of standardization – Specific concerns regarding infection control opened up into broader discussions regarding patient safety and variability in best practices in critical care units across the province.
- Our lack of data – We had not collected even a minimum dataset that would allow us to engage in accountability/knowledge transfer and quality improvement initiatives. We could not manage what we could not measure.

Leverage Actions vs. Strategic Directions

Leveraged actions are those actions we can take that:

- Create maximum impact for minimum effort;
- Provide the highest return-on-investment (ROI); and,
- Produce the 'biggest bang-for-the-buck' – with the least number of unintended consequences.

Senge's *The Fifth Discipline, The Art & Practice of The Learning Organization* [5] describes leveraged actions as small, well-focused actions that can sometimes produce significant, enduring improvements if they're in the right place. For example, the 'trim tab', or small 'rudder on the rudder' of a ship is an excellent metaphor for leverage. This tiny tab is what makes it easier to turn the rudder, which in turn makes it easier to turn the ship.

Just like the trim tab, high-leverage changes are usually highly non-obvious to most people in the system. Unless you understood the force of hydrodynamics, it is unlikely that you would think of pushing a tiny trim tab at the back of a huge ocean tanker in order to make it move in the direction you wanted. The more obvious course of action might be to push the bow of the tanker to the left if that was the direction you wanted it to go. Yet, the amount of force required to move the tanker would be tremendous. Instead, the leverage lies in going to the stern and pushing the trim tab and the rudder to the right in order for the bow to point to the left.

Like the trim tab, leveraged actions are usually not 'close in time and space' to obvious problem symptoms. There are no simple rules for finding high-leverage changes. However, learning to see underlying structures rather than events -- and thinking in terms of processes of change rather than snapshots -- is a way of thinking that makes identifying leveraged actions more likely. Another helpful tip is that leverage most often exists at the point of intersection between things. Therefore, an understanding of the different variables in the system and their inter-relationships is crucial in identifying areas for organizational leverage.

What I am advocating is that we focus our attention on a smaller number of highly leveraged actions that will have the highest impact on the way the system is governed and managed, and on the customer outcomes. I am saying that by making small changes to the basic DNA of the Ontario healthcare system, we can achieve dramatic changes within a four-year timeframe.

Before describing the transformation process, I want to share some comments on 'structure'. Structure is like the DNA of the system: whatever you design into it, it will produce the outcome or results. If you design mechanisms and different silos, holding different assumptions, you will create a fragmented silo-oriented system that is out of alignment, dysfunctional, or at least sub-optimal in performance. Structure, of course, has several components: design, decision-making, information systems and rewards and incentives.

Let's start with 'design'. An organization's design is composed of what it does (its functional design), who does what (its structural design) and how work is done (work process design). In doing functional design work, a determination must be made about what services or capabilities the organization wants to make available as well as what services or capabilities it needs itself to operate effectively.

Turning to 'decision making', this component of structure includes what decisions are made, and who is involved in making them. It is really an expression of how power and authority are distributed in an organization or in a system.

'Information systems' are a very important component of structure. In the knowledge economy, information systems need to evolve to support leveraged managerial decision making that propels the organization towards achievement of outcome. Effective and efficient organizations therefore, must have information systems to track indicators, set targets, monitor their progress and make adjustments to strategy on an ongoing and continuous basis.

And finally, 'rewards and incentives'. The culture of an organization, particularly its behavioral norms, is very much affected by what and how the organization rewards people. Consequently, it is important to insure that the organization's rewards and incentives system is actually encouraging the kind of behavior the organization or the system needs to enable its strategies.

Getting a Transformation Process Rolling

The way Ontario is approaching its Critical Care Transformation Strategy may prove to be a template we can follow in other areas of health care transformation. We are trying something new. If it works, and I am very optimistic that it will, we may be able to expand it to other areas, especially in the acute care system.

If you are aiming for transformation, not incremental change, you often have to change the way you do things in addition to just trying harder. For the ministry, this meant lowering our drawbridge and forging an even closer link with the innovative leaders in the critical care medicine field. We obtained the services of two respected opinion leaders in our deliberations. Dr. William Sibbald and Dr. Thomas Stewart were asked to chair an internal Critical Care Working Group. This is a rare arrangement in government. Drs. Sibbald and Stewart retained their clinical positions in the community while at the same time participating in internal planning initiatives. This hybrid was a risk for the ministry managers as it threatened to blur the line between system funder and system provider. I was strongly supportive as I believed that this was the only way we could start addressing the lack of standardization in Critical Care in Ontario. Let me explain.

It was well know that the various sorts of critical care units have evolved somewhat idiosyncratically in Ontario hospitals over recent decades. This evolution has been driven by a number of factors including hospital size, community need, other hospital priorities, physician interest and hospital funding levels and methods. Ontario ICUs and step-down units exhibit a wide variety of patient type, unit size, technological sophistication, physician management structure, staffing levels and clinical procedures. There is a real concern supported by expert opinion and anecdotal evidence that this level of customization has come at the price of inconsistency in standards of care across the province. As a general principle in health care service delivery, I would argue that useful customization can only be achieved against a backdrop of standardization. It might seem that a 'top down' approach is the natural way to achieve standardization but through discussions with our physician champions, it became quite clear that any top down initiatives would have to be supplemented by 'sideways' support. For the critical care field to work toward standardization, it would help to get them talking together in even more engaged and open ways. Having each institution defending their 'uniqueness' to the ministry would be counterproductive. We needed to find ways of sparking system-level thinking, it had to be engendered from within the 'silos' of care, and we knew that following SARS the field was ready.

In order to facilitate this system level thinking, we embarked on a two-prong approach:

1. We funded service innovation initiatives with a view to promoting inter-hospital integration and cooperation.
2. We organized a group of leaders from the field and supported them in developing a broader 'blue print' for transformation of adult critical care services.

With respect to the service innovation initiatives, we began looking at three projects:

a) ICU Outreach Teams
b) Telemedicine
c) eICU technology.

We have already launched the first two and are actively reviewing how eICU might be useful in Ontario. Our approach to ICU outreach teams (or medical emergency teams as they are sometimes called) has been to emphasize the knowledge transfer and inter-institution learning opportunities. Our Telemedicine initiative directly links institutions and is particularly designed to encourage standardization of best practices between and within hospital critical care units.

With respect to the broader blueprint for transformation, we gathered representatives from institutions across the province and from the key health care professions and asked them to prepare comprehensive recommendations for improving safety, access, efficiency and quality. The ministry provided staff and research support and was a player at the table - but was not directive. The results, as I shall detail below, are impressive. Within a year, the stakeholder group, known as the Ontario Critical Care Steering Committee, produced a very useful report that is currently being reviewed by government prior to formal decisions regarding implementation.

The Quality Improvement Cycle and the Committee Report

The Stages of a Quality Improvement Cycle

The Ontario Critical Care Steering Committee followed a version of the Continuous Quality Improvement (CQI) management philosophy. Originating in industry, CQI has received increasing attention from the health care system involving

management, staff and health professionals in the continuous improvement of work processes to achieve improved patient outcomes. To put the stages of this cycle in a nutshell, you work your way through the following questions:
a) What are we doing now?
b) What are best practices in the given area of endeavor?
c) What is the gap between what we are doing and best practices?
d) How do we bridge the gap?

This then leads to a round of implementation and monitoring which, in due course leads back to the assessment again. The Ontario Critical Care Steering Committee has done an excellent job in taking us up to the point of implementation.

What Have We Learned about Critical Care Delivery in Ontario?

The Steering Committee began by measuring our current capacity and practices. This involved original research, data gathering and analysis. In addition, the Committee completed over 20 papers, which mined the available scientific literature and other health planning documents for ideas that might help us in designing our made-in-Ontario blueprint. We were determined not to reinvent the wheel. Certain aspects of the National Health Service (NHS) Modernisation Agency's Critical Care Programme were especially useful for us. The UK approach helped us explore alternate 'systems-level' thinking in critical care, consider new approaches to standardizing practice across institutions, and reconsider a wider range of accountability measures [6].

a) Critical care capacity audit

The critical care capacity audit collected information on the functioning characteristics, bed capacity, and administrative structure of critical care units across Ontario. The audit focused on critical care bed capacities; the availability of diagnostic, monitoring and therapeutic technologies; and the organizational structure of critical care services. A questionnaire was developed in collaboration with the Critical Care Research Network (http://www.criticalcareresearch.net), an innovative consortium of Ontario hospitals that coordinate on critical care research projects. Hospitals reported on any beds physically aggregated into a discrete unit to provide care to higher acuity patients, including ICUs, intermediate or step-down units, and subspecialty units (e.g., coronary care, trauma, cardiovascular).

The audit suggests that the availability of critical care resources varies across the province. In particular, there appears to be marked variations in per capita bed capacity across the different regions. The data also suggest that the availability of critical care technologies is less than optimal within acute care hospitals. Many hospitals have both general and specialized critical care units (e.g., cardiovascular, neurosurgery, etc.). The majority of these units report to and are managed by different program areas. The audit also demonstrates that a minority of the province's critical care units were 'closed' and employed an intensivist model for care. While it is true that a large number of our ICUs are of insufficient size to justify a 'closed' model of care, many of our larger ICUs were not yet employing a 'closed' model.

b) Critical care HHR audit and gap analysis

A critical care medicine and allied health workforce survey was sent out to hospitals in early January 2005. The survey asks hospitals to provide information on:

- critical care unit staffing (e.g., registered nurses, respiratory therapists, intensivists, pharmacists, dieticians/nutritionists, social workers and physiotherapists)
- patient acuity and the acuity measurement tool used, and
- the impact of work force shortages on the number of staffed beds, diverted emergency department patients and cancelled surgery.

Results of the survey are expected by March 2005 but were not available in time for inclusion in this chapter. These results will help develop a profile of current critical care human resources, project future requirements and identify critical care issues. Human resource projections for Ontario will be based on the assumptions that critical care services in hospitals will be organized by patient acuity. Critical care units will ideally operate at an 85% occupancy which will allow units to maintain surge capacity and core staffing guideline ratios will be used in developing projections.

c) Critical care service demand forecasting

Two separate studies were conducted using different data sources in an attempt to determine the future demand for adult critical care services and in particular, the requirement for beds capable of supporting mechanical ventilation. Ontario's population is growing and aging and we know that both these factors will drive increased service needs and that critical care in particular will be affected by the demographic shift Ontario is experiencing. Projections suggest that to achieve an 80% occupancy rate for our critical care beds capable of supporting mechanical ventilation, Ontario will need to add new critical care beds to our system each year.

While this is an impressive growth requirement, we are very aware that in advance of gathering stronger data demonstrating the appropriateness and efficiency of critical care resource utilization, these projections are at best preliminary.

An Overview of our Blueprint for Transformation

As noted, the Committee's blueprint for transformation emphasized the newly emerging systems approach. The blueprint maps out how critical care can be managed from a systems perspective in which groups of hospitals work together to meet the needs of the critically ill patients in their catchment area. It is linked up with other system-level transformations that are underway, including the creation of 'Local Health Integration Networks' (LHINs) and improved services for the chronically ill.

The goals of the LHINs and what they will be expected to do can be summarized as follows:

1) manage the development of an integrated local health system to deliver coordinated health services at the local level
2) improve the accessibility of health services to allow people to move more easily through the health system
3) bring economic efficiencies to the delivery of health services, promote service innovation and improve the quality of care, and make the health care system more sustainable and accountable;
4) engage the community in local health system planning and setting of priorities, including establishing formal channels for citizen input and community consultation.

What follows are some highlights of the report's Executive Summary of the "Blue Print For Transformation":

- Access To Critical Care Through Greater Efficiency And Effectiveness

  – System-level solutions

System-level recommendations to improve access include establishing critical care networks in Ontario, with hospitals categorized by the level of critical care they provide (Our debt to the U.K. NHS Critical Care Modernisation Programme [6] is explicit here. Our Committee reviewed various alternatives and determined that the British nomenclature for critical care patient acuity best fit with our overall strategic direction). These levels will clearly delineate the capacity of hospitals to care for patients with different acuities of illness. In addition, critically ill patients will be categorized by their level of acuity using a standardized four level system that mirrors the hospital classification.

  – Organization-level solutions

Access to safe, quality care will be improved at the organizational level by the recommendation for Ontario hospitals to manage their critical care resources using an intensivist-led management model, which has been shown to result in better patient outcomes. In addition, hospitals will improve access to critical care services, the flow of patients, and the efficient and effective use of resources by establishing a single point of accountability for their critical care areas, and a unified approach to the utilization of critical care resources. Other recommendations to improve organization-level access include expanding outreach team pilots to include other hospitals in Ontario, funding the 24 month telemedicine demonstration project to disseminate critical care best practices, funding the proposal to conduct a three year evaluation of electronic ICU technology in remote hospitals,[1] and increasing critical care capacity by increasing the number of chronically ventilated beds in Ontario, in a timely fashion, in the area of most need – the central Ontario corridor.

- Surge

A number of recommendations address the need to equip the critical care system to respond to surges in demand. Recognizing minor, moderate and major surges is recommended along with requirements for accountability, human resources, physical plant and process improvements at each level. Hospitals will be expected to develop contractual agreements with their LHIN or critical care networks, as appropriate, that outline each hospital's role and responsibilities in surge situations. To prepare the province to respond in the event of major surge, it is recommended that the Ministry create additional Emergency Medical Assistance Teams (EMATs) and that hospitals encourage and facilitate their staff to become EMAT volunteers.

- Ethical considerations for access

The increasing demand for critical care services in the face of resource limitations highlights serious ethical issues. It is recommended that the critical care community convene an annual conference on ethical issues in accessing critical care services and identify solutions. The need here is to bring the discussion out beyond the medical community to society as a whole. The relevant issues go beyond medical decisions to societal discussion as to how we are going to use our resources. There is a need to create a dialog between funding organizations, patients, clinicians and opinion leaders from all walks of life.

- Quality and Safety Through a Framework to Improve Critical Care Performance

The Committee recommends a framework to improve critical care performance that includes establishing evidence-based benchmarks, best practice guidelines and standards, and identifying indicators to assess critical care performance against these measures. It is also recommended that hospital boards be held accountable for governing their organization's critical care resources including access, appropriate use, quality and ongoing improvements. The Ministry will monitor performance against established goals. In addition, individual critical

[1] While the Ministry is still in the process of reviewing eICU approaches, there are several aspects of our system that make eICU attractive. To begin with, Ontario has several remote areas, notably the north, where our population is sparse. For such areas, eICU may help us provide standardized care to these remote areas, by 'coaching' the physician workforce they have available to them. This technology should also reduce the 'toxicity' of the workplace, for example, in medium-size cities where providing 24/7 coverage is a huge burden. By providing these hospitals with an eICU option, we may be able to provide a better quality of life for the physician workforce in these cities.

care units and LHIN will measure their performance, and institute quality improvement initiatives tailored to their specific local needs.

- Sufficient and Appropriate Human Resources to Meet the Need for Critical Care

The importance of ensuring that sufficient numbers of appropriate human resources are available to work in critical areas resulted in recommendations to explore measuring the workload of critical care professionals, and adopt core staffing ratios as minimum guidelines for critical care. With regard to practice, it is recommended that professional staff working in critical care meet provincially-recognized standards and core competencies.

- Critical Care Technologies

Since a great deal of healthcare-related evaluation activity is already occurring, the Committee recommended that the critical care community should review the evaluations conducted by these groups to inform the adoption, diffusion and withdrawal of critical care technologies. These evaluations should also be used to identify the standard technologies that hospitals should acquire or retire. Suggestions on technologies to evaluate should be forwarded to these groups. In addition, it is recommended that the critical care community offer to participate in the evaluation of current critical care technologies in partnership with existing evaluation bodies. This sharing of information should go beyond provincial borders and indeed beyond national borders.

Leadership

Leadership and Reflection

At the personal level, I believe leadership starts with self-reflection. Moments of self-reflection restore personal balance and make it possible for us to take the next risk. We have to create the conditions for change in ourselves before we can foster them to our colleagues. Join me in a thought experiment. Imagine that you could step out of your day to day role for a moment. Leave the lab or the bedside or the desk or the board table and come with me up a steep flight of stairs. At the top of the stairs, you will see that we have emerged onto a wide balcony. Below us is spread the entire health care system. From here we can see all its components. We can see the degree to which it is a system and the degree to which it is not. We can see the strengths and we can see the problems. We can see the providers, working in their manifold tasks and we can see the patients and their families. On this balcony we are joined by our muse, a challenging voice who lives on the periphery of our consciousness and in the comments of our colleagues. Sometime we cannot wait to hear from our muse. Sometimes we try to ignore our muse. Generally, to hear the muse, it is best to free ourselves of the day to day pressures, if only for a moment. Every conversation with a muse is different. Here is one sample:

Muse: You look terrible.

Self: Gee, thanks. I'm feeling overwhelmed and seem to be out of ideas. I thought coming up here and looking things over would help.

Muse: That's good news. That you are out of ideas, I mean. That's good soil for a new vision to take root.

Self: What are you talking about? We already have a vision. We wrote it all down. I've got it here somewhere. Let me read it to you. "Health care in Ontario is a multi-faceted..."

Muse: Oh, please, not again! That thing sounds like a badly written obituary. It doesn't capture the essence of what drives you.

Self: You think a slogan is going to save us?

Muse: No, but it could make your hopes more visible. It could help free up your colleagues' imaginations. You are all still afraid to try new approaches. Nay-sayers get the most air time with you.

Self: Well, this is no sandbox. We are accountable...

Muse: Yes, yes but what is your accountability really for? Is it primarily about blame or is it primarily about learning? For sure, if you try something new, you have to monitor the results and shut it down if necessary but when accountability chokes out experimentation you are in big trouble.

Self: Well, truth is that I am concerned that I will lose control. I am supposed to be leading this thing.

Muse: When you were in your 30s and you were brimming with answers, I didn't bug you too much but now that you are in your 50s, you really have to get over yourself.

Self: True - heaven help us if I have to come up with all the answers. I could do more to encourage the risk takers. I could help them shape their ideas...

Muse: All right! Welcome to the gray zone! This is where the good stuff comes from...By the way, do you know why you keep coming up here?

Self: Yes. From here I look on to the vista of the system from the perspective of my professional life. I ask myself over and over again... "What do you see?"

The other comment I want to make about leadership at the personal level is the importance of how we treat each other. As leaders, whether bureaucratic, clinical or managerial, we are working in various sorts of hierarchies. It is my experience that as leaders, our behavior is standard setting and is imitated up and down the chain of command. As leaders, we have to think about how the way we treat others feeds strongly into our institutional culture.

Leadership and a Culture of Innovation

Based on moments of personal reflection, as leaders, we can undertake our key responsibility which is to create the systemic conditions within the health care system that provide solutions to today's challenges. Leaders foster conditions in which systems can outgrow constraints in current approaches. So much of society and health care is geared to recognizing the right answer and 'hang your head low' if you do not have it. We must continually ask: How can we as leaders meaningfully tap into and create a culture that encourages the expression of intellect, passion, commitment and experience by all levels of the delivery system to make real change that satisfy healthcare consumer needs and expectations? The change management thought leaders tell us that change requires a literal opening and emptying that creates a space for new vision to emerge, which articulates new shared values. This opening requires discipline and courage: discipline to look at what is not working and to resist knee jerk reactions to new ideas; and courage to separate from old patterns, structures and processes which are no longer useful to a health care system that is being compelled to evolve.

The challenge ahead for the leadership of our healthcare system is about learning how to lead, manage, guide, and coach others through the change process. Leadership and change management have been my passion for a good number of years but the more I learn, the more I truly understand how little I really do know about it. I learn a little bit more each day – particularly from people who tell me what is really going on at the front line, from the hospital board perspective and from the senior management and physician leadership. They provide me with feedback on 'lessons learned' from our own 'best mistakes' of the past.

Instead of thinking and acting as isolated silos under siege, governance and managerial leaders can choose to see themselves through another lens, a lens in which you can see yourself in relationship to a local health service delivery system, your community partners in the delivery of care. If we are going to be successful at managing change over the next four or five years in Ontario, we will need to reflect on and learn from our 'best mistakes' of the past. We also need to be carefully examining the basic assumptions that we are holding about our existing and future healthcare delivery system. Assumptions are not facts. They are the beliefs we hold about our reality and our vision. For system leaders, in Ontario and other jurisdictions, the first assumption that must be tested is 'Do you have all the answers to the challenges and dilemmas that you face?' Of course you don't.

What I know for a certainty is that healthcare people are capable of brilliance. I know that the answers to the questions we need to ask are within the hearts and minds of the people in the healthcare system. The answers to the dilemmas that you face are within your own organization – from your front-line healthcare providers, from your managers, and from your boards.

Leadership and Health Care as a Brand

It is interesting to reflect on the fact that while there is general confidence that science will continue to make progress, there is general concern around whether we can hope for ever improving health care. From a historical perspective, this is puzzling. The last few hundred years of scientific progress has been roughly paralleled by equally dramatic improvements in the delivery of health care. Without in anyway underestimating the tremendous effort required, it is reasonable to assume we will continue to make medical and scientific discoveries. It would seem that in the longer historical view, there is basis for a similar optimism with respect to improvements in the delivery of health care services. Yet, in many jurisdictions, the contemporary assessment of the health care system and its future is not very optimistic. There is a constant expression of concern about the quality of health care, or about the cost of the health care system, or the level of funding for health care, or about equity of access to health resources and so on. Many commentators, including leaders in the health care system, voice these concerns in rather negative tones. There is precious little in the way of optimism that these concerns represent opportunities for new thinking, for creativity and change.

I think it is understandable that people's concern with health care is of the moment, not historical. Whether my loved one is going to get the care he or she needs is my concern. My historical consciousness is not involved. Healthcare must become more consumer quality focused. To quote Roy Romanow, who led Canadians through a deep review of our commitment to a publicly funded system: "The most important work in providing quality healthcare happens in every interaction that our citizens have with healthcare providers and people working on the front lines of service delivery" [7].

Customer service includes cultivating brand satisfaction. Our system leaders need to be constantly emphasizing the excellent work being done by our frontline. This is, ultimately, the product we are bringing to market. Imagine if everyone who worked at General Motors, including the senior engineers and managers, spoke to the public constantly and in negative tones about the many problems GM faces as a company. Imagine the impact that would have on car sales and on company morale. In many jurisdictions, certain institutions and some larger Health Maintenance Organizations (HMOs) have this sense of caring for their brand, but where this pride exists, it remains in silos and blame is shifted to the next level up. The general public needs to see us working together. They need to see evidence of the existence of a real health care system.

Conclusion

In closing, the leaders I talked to throughout the SARS crisis were asking some very probing questions about system design, roles and responsibilities, accountability and empowerment, and about the need for fundamental strategic changes that will enable us to modernize and update our traditional industrial-age approach to healthcare delivery.

When time frames accelerate, leadership emerges at all levels as people ask complete questions to compel everyone to think differently about the challenges. When we stick to the same old mental models, we come up with the same old solutions - which inevitably fail us again and again.

We must remember that anxiety includes undiscovered skills, potentialities, incredible energy and many aspects of a healthy life that long to be lived. It takes great courage for leaders to ask 'wicked' probing questions in search for the truth – and do so without blaming. Leaders must become very vulnerable themselves to enable truth to heal the system from within.

Imagine the system to be a multi-story building. Most of the leaders of the healthcare system have been far more concerned with the dramas taking place in the upper rooms and halls of the building than the flaws in the design of the building. These flaws are the true source of unbalanced patterns of energy flow. Can you describe, in terms of paradox, the fundamental drama on the first floor, where the true owners of the system reside, the tax-payers?

Bottom line, we have a fundamental paradox which is a conflict between independence vs. interdependence. But my argument is, can we not redesign the building to have both principles supporting each other? There are three choices in this metaphor: You may continue to accept the building as it is; you may change the building; or, you may tear it down and re-build. To make the choice that enables you to outgrow this knowledge management paradox, the system needs to learn how to experience unity in diversity.

References

1. Conner DR (1993) Managing at the Speed of Change. Villard Books, New York, p. 92
2. Booth CM, Stewart TE (2005) Severe acute respiratory syndrome and critical care medicine: the Toronto experience. Crit Care Med 33 (suppl 1):S53–60
3. Learning from SARS – Renewal of Public Health in Canada. A report of the National Advisory Committee on SARS and Public Health October 2003. Available at: http://www.phac-aspc.gc.ca/publicat/sars-sras/naylor/index.html Accessed July 2005
4. For the Public's Health – Initial Report of the Ontario Expert Panel on SARS and Infectious Disease Control. Available at: http://www.health.gov.on.ca/english/public/pub/ministry_reports/walker_panel_2003/walker_panel.html Accessed July 2005
5. Senge PM (1994) The Fifth Discipline, The Art & Practice of The Learning Organization. Currency-Doubleday, New York
6. National Health Service (NHS) Modernisation Agency's Critical Care Programme. Available at: http://www.modern.nhs.uk/scripts/default.asp?site_id=20 Accessed July 2005
7. Romanow R (2002) Building on Values. The Future of Health Care in Canada. Available at: http://www.hc-sc.gc.ca/english/pdf/care/romanow_e.pdf Accessed July 2005

Subject Index

A
activated protein C 5, 49, 95, 192, 402
acuity system 147
acute lung injury (ALI) 158, 197
- normovolemic hemodilution (ANH) 170
- respiratory distress syndrome (ARDS) 3, 207, 213, 307
- - failure 4
adaptive support ventilation (ASV) 232
advance directive 345
albumin 14
alveolar stress 218
ambulance 268, 284
aminoglycoside 75
anesthesiology 62
antibiotic 16, 184
- resistance 69, 178
antigen detection 179
antioxidant 208
APACHE II score 192, 283
arterial waveform analysis 8
artificial intelligence 231
asthma 107
asynchrony 228
audit 421

B
bacteria 73
barbiturate 12
beneficence 369
beta-lactamase activity 71
biomarker 250
bioterrorist 258
bronchoalveolar lavage (BAL) fluid 189
budget 282, 330
bundles 47

C
capnography 170
carbenicillinase 72
carbon monoxide 268
cardiopulmonary resuscitation 11
cardiorespiratory performance 153
care delivery 41
cellular energy 157
central nervous system (CNS) 239
- venous oxygen saturation ($ScvO_2$) 7, 155, 169
- - pressure (CVP) 159
cephalosporinase 72
cerebral blood flow (CBF) 243
- perfusion pressure (CPP) 241
- resuscitation 12
circulatory shock 156
clinical decision support (CDS)
- information system (CIS) 139
- trial 291
closed-loop communication 143, 391
- technology 141, 227
comfort 91
communication 25, 34, 63, 65, 126, 390
community acquired infection 76
- expectations 56
compliance 217
computer 65, 125, 136, 299, 394
- simulation 306
confidentiality 148
conflict 36
contiuing medical education 30
core processes 118
coronary care unit 45
corticosteroid 168
cost 90
- effectiveness 141
- minimization analysis 90
- utility analysis 90

C-reactive protein (CRP) 178
cytochrome 157
cytokines 191

D
dead space 214
delirium 50
design 115
diagnosis 91
diagnostic technology 153
dialysis 13, 58
differential gel electrophoresis (DIGE) 197
diffusion-weighted MRI (DWI) 243
directly observed procedural skills (DOPS) 384
disaster medicine 257
disseminated intravascular coagulation (DIC) 202
diuretics 13
DNA gyrase 77
– polymerase 72
dobutamine 159, 205
dopamine 13

E
economic constraint 292
education 129, 136
effectiveness 89
efficiency 89
electronic communication 316
– medical record (EMR) 136
– systems 379
emergency department (ED) 121, 273
– medical system (EMS) 259
– medicine 275
– – physicians 49
– team 43
end-expiratory lung volume (EELV) 218
end-of-life care 345
endotracheal intubation 100
enteral feeding 9
enzyme-linked immunosorbent assay (ELISA) 180, 189
epiglottis 99
epinephrine 11
error 341
esophageal Doppler 8
ethics 318, 345
– consultation 351
etomidate 206
evidence-based medicine (EBM) 95, 138
extracorporeal membrane oxygenation (ECMO) 45, 219

F
factor VIIa 12
family 31, 50, 346, 348
– conference 355
flagellin 190
fluid overload 16
funding 92, 311, 325
– sources 303
fungi 73
future demand 47

G
gas exchange 213, 230
gastric tonometry 156, 168
genomics 189
genotypic variation 247
globalization 300
glucose control 8
guidelines 27, 160

H
Haemophilus influenzae 100
handheld computing 144
head trauma 12
healthcare 116, 366, 412
– insurance 88
– resource 47
– systems 24
health maintenance organization (HMO) 279
– technology assessment 88
hemodynamic monitoring 8
hemofiltration 206
hibernation 204
high frequency jet ventilation 222
mobility group box protein 1 (HMBG1) 194
hospital 42
hospitalist 49, 297
hydroxyethyl starch solution 14
hygiene measures 10
hyperlactatemia 155
hypothermia 12, 244, 251
hypoxemia 157

I
immuno-enhancing diet 9
immunological monitoring 189
immuno-suppression 282
infections 69, 177
information systems 37
– technology 133
informed consent 317
intensive care unit (ICU) admissions 15
– – – core processes 118

– – – design 115
– – – rationing 363
– – – resources 117
intensivist 56, 67, 133, 240, 277, 279, 330, 401
– physician staffing 45
international study 314
internet 135
intracranial hemorrhage 246
– hypertension 241, 251
intrapulmonary shunt 214
ischemia 155
isolation 129
isotype ratio mass spectrometry (IRMS) 197

J
jugular oximetry 242

L
lactic acidosis 202
leadership 23, 31, 32, 425
leukotrienes 191
lipopolysaccharide (LPS) 74, 178, 190
liver failure 11
lobbying 286
lung mechanics 215
– protective strategy 220

M
macrophage 193
magnetic resonance imaging (MRI) 121, 243
management 23, 30
mass spectrometry 196
mechanical ventilation 4, 10, 217, 227
medical education 30
– emergency team (MET) 15, 43, 49, 57, 277, 378
– staff 59
medication error 138
methicillin-resistant *Staphylococcus aureus* (MRSA) 10, 129, 181, 264
microarray analysis 301
microbiology 181
microcirculatory distress 165
microdialysis 249
mistakes 62
mitochondrial dysfunction 166, 203
mixed venous oxygen saturation (SvO2) 154
molecular adsorbent recirculating system (MARS) 11
monitoring 165, 182, 248
morbidity and mortality conferences 392
mortality 3, 14, 91, 117, 148, 241, 281, 318, 335, 339
motivation 36
multi-organ failure 204

N
near infrared spectroscopy (NIRS) 169, 242
neonatal critical care 99
networking 26
neuroprotection 243
nicotinamide adenine dinucleotide (NADH) 169
nimodipine 243
nitric oxide (NO) 167, 204
non-invasive ventilation (NIV) 228, 231
nosocomial infections 10, 46, 207
nuclear factor-kappa B (NF-κB) 191
– magnetic resonance 215
nursing staff 58
– station 125
nutritional support 9

O
obesity 108
open design 127
operating room 121, 273
optical spectroscopy 169
organ function 201
organization 273
orthogonal polarization spectral (OPS) imaging 166
outcome 91, 147, 338
oxygen delivery (DO_2) 7, 154
– toxicity 219
– transport 204

P
palliative care 351
paramedics 268
passwords 146
patient data management system (PDMS) 131
– process 115
– ventilator synchronization 227
pediatric intensive care 99
penicillin-binding protein (PBP) 77
peptidoglycan 77
performance 30, 335
perfusion-weighted MRI (PWI) 243
permissive hypercapnia 220

personal data assistant (PDA) 144
- protective equipment (PPE) 266
phosphorescence 169
photoaptamer 197
physician staffing 279
picture archiving and communication system (PACS) 140
planning 26, 28
plasmid 79
pneumonia 93, 104
polymerase chain reaction (PCR) 180, 193, 299
polytrauma 12
positive end-expiratory pressure (PEEP) 5, 158, 216, 232
positron emission tomography (PET) 193, 215, 243
preload responsiveness 158
pressure volume (PV) curve 229
problem-solving 28
procalcitonin 178
procedure 58, 148
process 306, 338
- of care 14
professional support 94
professionalism 25
prophylaxis 184, 208
proportional-assisted ventilation 233
proteomics 189
protocol 160, 246
protocolized care 154
Pseudomonas 72, 177
publication 316
purpura fulminans 100

Q
quality 24, 33, 61, 141, 252, 335
- improvement 141, 356, 420
- of end-of-life care 357
- of life 335

R
radiation 263
radiofrequency identification (RFID) 146
rationing 363
receptor for advanced glycation endproducts (RAGE) 195
record keeping 139
reductionism 208
reflectance spectrophotometry 169
regional blood flow 156
regionalization 46, 101
renal failure 12
research 291, 311, 332, 407
resource 47, 377, 390
- allocation 117, 370
- utilization 91
respiratory syncytial virus (RSV) 103
resuscitation 57, 155
ribosomal RNA probes 179
rounds 67, 139
Safety 61, 88, 294, 389, 424
sedation 10, 355
sepsis 3, 103
septic shock 5, 6, 156
serum bactericidal assay 183
severe acute respiratory syndrome (SARS) 69, 265, 413
Sidestream Dark Field (SDF) imaging 173
simulation training 145, 389
staffing 28, 378
standardized mortality ratio (SMR) 339
Staphylococcus aureus 71
step-down facility 121
steroids 5
storage room 125
stroke 13, 239, 249
subarachnoid hemorrhage (SAH) 242
sublingual capnography 170
- PCO_2 156

T
tagging 120
teaching 326
team building 36
- management 392
teamwork 389
technology 298, 425
- advancement 292
- assessment 87
telecommunication 301
telemedicine 420
tetracycline resistance 78
Therapeutic Intervention Scoring System (TISS) 357
thrombolysis 246, 251
tidal volume 94, 143, 205, 221, 283
time-to-positivity (TPOS) 183
tissue PCO_2 156
- perfusion 153
training 26, 267, 275, 377, 402
transcranial Doppler 156, 248
transfusions 14, 206
translational research 408
transport 122
transposable genetic elements 80
trauma 153, 264
traumatic brain injury (TBI) 239

treatment algorithm 160
trophic factor 251
tumor necrosis factor (TNF) 185

V
vaccine 264
vancomycin 76
– resistant enterococci (VRE) 10
vasoconstriction 153
vasodilator 168
vasopressin 6
vasopressors 168
ventilator-associated lung injury (VALI) 228
– – pneumonia (VAP) 4, 177
– induced lung injury (VILI) 218
Virtual Center 314
– reality simulator 395
viruses 73
voice recognition 144
volume challenge 158
volumetric capnography 230

W
West Nile Virus 70
wireless technology 148
withdrawing 346